Dietary Fibers: Nutritional Function in Health and Disease

Edited by Albie Copeland

hayle medical

New York

Hayle Medical,
750 Third Avenue, 9th Floor,
New York, NY 10017, USA

Visit us on the World Wide Web at:
www.haylemedical.com

ISBN: 978-1-64647-534-6

Cataloging-in-Publication Data

Dietary fibers : nutritional function in health and disease / edited by Albie Copeland.
p. cm.
Includes bibliographical references and index.
ISBN 978-1-64647-534-6
1. Fiber in human nutrition. 2. Food--Fiber content. 3. Nutritionally induced diseases.
4. Diet therapy. I. Copeland, Albie.
QP144.F52 D543 2023
612.3--dc23

Table of Contents

Preface

In my initial years as a student, I used to run to the library at every possible instance to grab a book and learn something new. Books were my primary source of knowledge and I would not have come such a long way without all that I learnt from them. Thus, when I was approached to edit this book; I became understandably nostalgic. It was an absolute honor to be considered worthy of guiding the current generation as well as those to come. I put all my knowledge and hard work into making this book most beneficial for its readers.

Dietary fiber, also called roughage, includes the parts of plant-based foods that the body cannot digest or absorb. It can be broadly categorized into soluble fiber and insoluble fiber. Soluble fiber dissolves in water to form a gel-like material in the digestive system. Oats, peas, beans, apples, citrus fruits, carrots, barley, and psyllium are good sources of soluble fiber. It helps lower blood cholesterol and regulates the blood sugar levels. Insoluble fiber is a type of fiber that does not dissolve in water and promotes the movement of stool through the digestive system. It is found in whole-wheat flour, wheat bran, nuts, beans, and in vegetables such as cauliflower, green beans, and potatoes. Insoluble fiber adds bulk to the stool and prevents constipation. The book aims to shed light on the nutritional function of dietary fibers in promoting human health. Its extensive content provides the readers with a thorough understanding of the subject.

I wish to thank my publisher for supporting me at every step. I would also like to thank all the authors who have contributed their researches in this book. I hope this book will be a valuable contribution to the progress of the field.

Editor

1

Dietary Flaxseed as a Strategy for Improving Human Health

Mihir Parikh [1,2,3], Thane G. Maddaford [1,2,3], J. Alejandro Austria [1,2,3], Michel Aliani [2,4], Thomas Netticadan [1,2,5] and Grant N. Pierce [1,2,3,*]

1. Department of Physiology and Pathophysiology, College of Medicine, Faculty of Health Sciences, University of Manitoba, Winnipeg, MB R3E 0W3, Canada; mparikh@sbrc.ca (M.P.); tmaddaford@sbrc.ca (T.G.M.); aaustria@sbrc.ca (J.A.A.); tnetticadan@sbrc.ca (T.N.)
2. Canadian Centre for Agri-Food Research in Health and Medicine (CCARM), Albrechtsen Research Centre, St Boniface Hospital, 351 Taché Avenue, Winnipeg, MB R2H 2A6, Canada; maliani@sbrc.ca
3. Institute of Cardiovascular Sciences, Albrechtsen Research Centre, St. Boniface Hospital, 351 Taché Avenue, Winnipeg, MB R2H 2A6, Canada
4. Department of Human Nutritional Sciences, Faculty of Agricultural and Food Sciences, University of Manitoba, Winnipeg, MB R3T 2N2, Canada
5. Morden Research and Development Centre, Agriculture and Agri-Food Canada, Morden, MB R6M 1Y5, Canada

* Correspondence: gpierce@sbrc.ca

Abstract: Flaxseed is a rich source of the omega-3 fatty acid, alpha linolenic acid, the lignan secoisolariciresinol diglucoside and fiber. These compounds provide bioactivity of value to the health of animals and humans through their anti-inflammatory action, anti-oxidative capacity and lipid modulating properties. The characteristics of ingesting flaxseed or its bioactive components are discussed in this article. The benefits of administering flaxseed or the individual bioactive components on health and disease are also discussed in this review. Specifically, the current evidence on the benefits or limitations of dietary flaxseed in a variety of cardiovascular diseases, cancer, gastro-intestinal health and brain development and function, as well as hormonal status in menopausal women, are comprehensive topics for discussion.

Keywords: flaxseed; cancer; cardiovascular; microbiome; diabetes; menopause; nutraceutical; functional food

1. Introduction

Dietary flaxseed has an impressive and growing research literature supporting its use in a variety of health conditions. Whereas in the late 20th century, little was known of the health-related benefits of flaxseed as well as how to consume flaxseed to achieve any health benefits, today is an entirely different time. Research information on the effects of dietary flaxseed has increased dramatically. We now know what diseases flaxseed can treat or prevent, the health impacts dietary flaxseed can provide, the bioactives within flaxseed that provide these health-related effects in many cases and the forms of flaxseed that are required to provide these bioactives to the body. Data on the impact of dietary flaxseed on disease have been translated, albeit in limited amounts, from animal research studies to human trials. Many of these trials have been conducted with the highest standards of control available in order to provide solid, reliable information on its value to the general public and, more specifically, to those in a disease compromised condition. These data have sparked the food processing industry to create a greater variety of foods that contain flaxseed, giving the public an increased opportunity to incorporate flaxseed into their everyday diet. With this growing availability of flaxseed in the marketplace and the increasing awareness of the public to its impact on human health when supplemented into the diet on a daily basis, it would be expected that flaxseed will also grow in the coming years in economic importance to the farmer, the food processer and the retailer in the marketplace [1].

We now know that environmental factors like diet can have a profound effect on the maintenance of health and the appearance of disease [2]. It is also increasingly apparent that the treatment of disease is not only achieved through pharmacological therapy, but through dietary interventions as well. The purpose of this review is to provide a broad summary of the highlights of the research that have supported the growth of flaxseed as a commodity with significance in the fields of health and medicine.

2. Flaxseed and Its Use in the Diet

The main bioactive compounds in flaxseed include alpha-linolenic acid (ALA), lignans and fiber. Four common forms of flaxseed available for human consumption include whole flaxseed, ground flaxseed, flaxseed oil and partially defatted flaxseed meal [3]. A new form available in the marketplace is flax "milk" (Pizzey Ingredients Inc, Manitoba, Canada). An alternative to "milks" like almond milk, flax milk is finely milled flaxseed mixed with filtered water and other minor compounds. Flax milk is high in ALA and is an excellent alternative to dairy milk, as it has no cholesterol or lactose. It is suitable for people allergic to soy, nuts and gluten, and it contains more health benefits than almond milk.

However, no matter how good a food is for the general public to consume, if that food does not have acceptable taste, texture, appearance, colour and aroma qualities, then the majority of people will not eat it. Flaxseed has several characteristics that could negatively affect its flavour profile and that are cause for concern. The two most important are the potential for the very high omega-3 fatty acid content in flaxseed to become rancid through oxidation, and the propensity for bitterness. The high content of alpha linolenic acid (ALA) renders it highly susceptible to oxidation. The oxidation and subsequent rancidity will lead to off flavours and a musty aroma that would be rejected in taste tests. The antioxidant content in flaxseed, provided in turn by its secoisolariciresinol diglucoside (SDG) content, is of great value in curtailing any oxidation process. In addition, flaxseed has been described as possessing a "nice nutty smell and aroma" [4], and is potentially ideal for the incorporation into a variety of foods. In research studies, flaxseed has been incorporated successfully into snack bars, muffins, bagels, bread, buns, tea biscuits, cinnamon rolls and pasta [5,6]. The concentration of flaxseed in the food will, of course, influence its flavour characteristics. Flaxseed has been incorporated into foods for human consumption at concentrations of 5–28% of total ingredients (by weight) before baking [7]. The amount of flaxseed ingested daily over an extended period of time has been as much as 40 to 50 g [8]. Clinical trials having patients ingesting a food each day for up to one year have been successfully completed with drop-out rates of approximately 20% in both placebo and flax groups [5]. This demonstrates that it is not the flaxseed that induces non-compliance *per se*, but instead a great number of different flax-containing foods are needed to allow variety in the daily choices if one is to maintain subjects in a trial with an extended duration.

The most common foods in which to have flaxseed are baked goods. The process of baking even up to 178 °C for two hours does not alter the composition or content of ALA in a baked muffin, for example [9]. The addition of flavouring to the baked good also makes it possible to disguise any less than optimal flavour profile induced by the bitterness of flaxseed or any minor rancidity. Flavourings like banana and nuts, banana chocolate chip, cinnamon apple raisin, cinnamon raisin, cinnamon spice, gingerbread raisin, cappuccino chocolate chip, sunflower sesame and cranberry orange have been used in research studies [7,10]. The public will have preferences to these flavourings and matrices for the flaxseed. In a study of the daily preferences of the ingestion of food products containing 30 g of milled flaxseed over one year, bagels were consumed > muffins > snack bars > sprinkles > tea biscuits > pasta > sundried tomato buns [11]. Cinnamon raisin flavourings were preferred > cranberry orange > apple spiced > sunflower sesame [11]. The recent development of flax "milk" provides an even more convenient way to consume flaxseed and preserve it as well.

Each of these different food matrices can influence the stability of the flaxseed. Processing of the seed, storage temperature and duration as well as the form of flaxseed (milled flaxseed versus whole seed versus flax oil) will also influence the stability of the product. Milling, grinding or crushing flaxseed will destroy the hard protective seed coat on flaxseed, exposing the ALA and SDG to oxidation [12]. However, this process is required to render these bioactive ingredients bioavailable [13]. ALA is more bioavailable to the body if it is in oil or milled form [13]. The incorporation of milled flaxseed into baked products may actually protect the ALA and SDG from degradation [12]. Cooler storage temperatures and a shortened storage duration, particularly for flax oil, will also result in a better preservation of the ALA and SDG [12].

Recently, a concern was raised about the presence of components in flaxseed that may have undesirable effects that could affect the bioavailability and bioaccessibility of essential nutrients [14]. These include the presence of protease inhibitors, phytic acids, linatine and cyanogenic glycosides in flaxseed. However, there are no deleterious effects reported of these components in human studies. The concentrations of these components delivered through dietary flaxseed may be below that needed to induce any biological actions. Nevertheless, it is prudent to take into account the raised concern. Plant bio-breeding and/or food processing methods may be considered to reduce the levels of these components in flaxseed.

3. Dietary Flaxseed and Cardiovascular Disease

The effects of flaxseed on parameters of cardiovascular disease have become one of the most intensely studied areas with regard to the health-related benefits of dietary flaxseed (Figure 1).

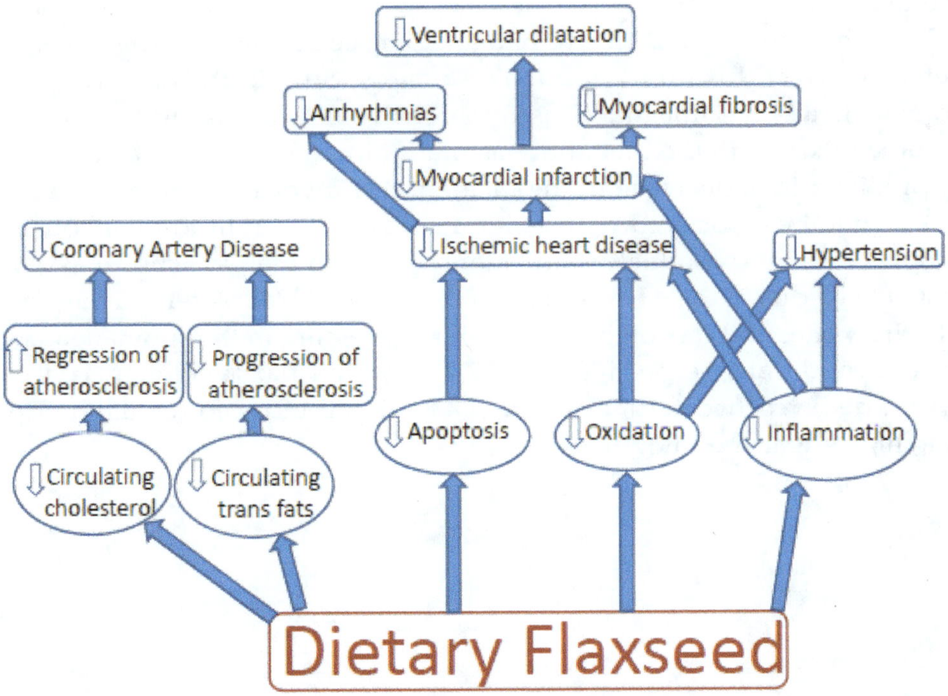

Figure 1. The effect of dietary flaxseed on the various types of cardiovascular disease. Arrows going up denote an increase in a specific parameter whereas arrows going down denote a decrease in a specific parameter.

In animal models of heart disease, dietary flaxseed has decreased the progression of atherosclerosis induced by high dietary cholesterol or high dietary trans fat content [15–17], likely via an anti-inflammatory action provided through its ALA content [15,16,18]. Depending upon the animal species, flaxseed may (mice and rats) or may not (rabbits) lower circulating cholesterol levels [15,16,18]. Flaxseed can also lower circulating trans fats levels [17]. In a stable, established atherosclerotic plaque, supplementation of the diet with flaxseed can also regress atherosclerosis [19].

Ischemic reperfusion challenge to isolated hearts can induce arrhythmias. Rabbits on a flaxseed supplemented diet prior to being subjected to the ischemic reperfusion insult are protected from ventricular fibrillation [20]. If rats are placed on a flaxseed supplemented diet prior to and after the induction of a myocardial infarction, they exhibit smaller infarcts, less arrhythmias and a reduction in left ventricular dilation [18]. The mechanism once again is likely to involve the ALA content of flaxseed [18]. ALA has shown a capacity to alter arrhythmogenic ionic currents in the heart [21]. However, the metabolism of SDG into enterolignans within the circulation may also have a cardioprotective role [18,22].

In humans exhibiting symptoms of cardiovascular disease, dietary flaxseed has displayed powerfully protective effects. The most impressive involves the decrease in both systolic and diastolic blood pressure in patients with peripheral arterial disease (PAD) [5]. Both brachial and central blood pressures were significantly reduced by dietary flaxseed in this trial [5,23]. In the double-blinded, placebo-controlled, randomized FlaxPAD Trial [24], PAD patients fed 30 g of milled flaxseed every day for 6 months exhibited significant decreases in both systolic and diastolic blood pressure [5]. As shown in Figure 2, not all patients responded to the flaxseed diet with decreases in systolic blood pressure (SBP). In the placebo group, fifteen subjects showed a decrease in SBP over the 6 months, whereas twenty-one exhibited an increase in SBP. In the flax-fed group, twenty-seven subjects exhibited a decrease in SBP over the 6 months and twelve had an increase in SBP over this time. The SBP in two subjects was unchanged over this time period. The average drop in the flax group was substantial (10 mm Hg) and statistically significant. This hypotensive effect was shown as early as 1 month after commencing the flaxseed in the diet and was maintained for up to one year [5]. The decrease was sufficient to predict a 50% decrease in the incidence of myocardial infarctions and strokes [5]. This action was shown to be associated with a significant change in lipid metabolism such that the generation of oxylipins with less vasodilatory and more pro-inflammatory action was blocked [25]. This action was suggested to be due to the ALA content of the flaxseed [25]. Alternatively, in animal studies, flaxseed protein hydrolysates and flax oil decreased blood pressure in the spontaneously hypertensive rat in acute or chronic conditions, respectively [26,27]. As well, a flaxseed lignan concentrate reduced blood pressure in the deoxycorticosterone acetate (DOCA-salt) induced renal hypertensive rats [28] and in the high fat, high sugar-fed rat [29].

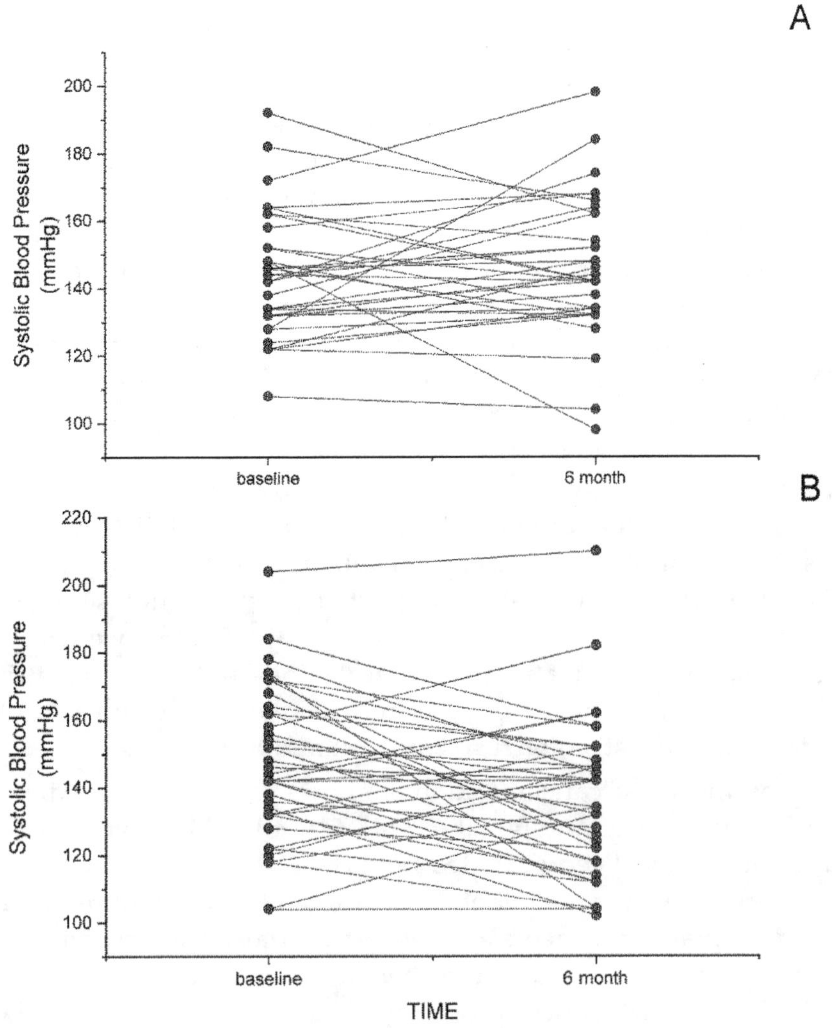

Figure 2. Individual values of systolic blood pressure at baseline or after 6 months of dietary supplementation with a placebo (**A**) or 30 g of milled flaxseed per day (**B**). Baseline systolic blood pressures in the placebo group were 143.5 ± 2.88 at baseline and 144.8 ± 3.33 after 6 months (n = 36). Baseline systolic blood pressures in the flax group were 146.6 ± 3.37 at baseline and 136.5 ± 3.53 after 6 months (n = 41). Results are obtained from Rodriguez-Leyva et al, 2013 [5].

4. Dietary Flaxseed and Diabetes

Flaxseed also impacts another major disease that is growing in incidence across the globe: diabetes. Flaxseed supplementation reduced blood glucose in subjects with type 2 diabetes [30,31] and lowered blood glucose in subjects with prediabetes [32]. Flaxseed derived gum and lignan supplement also decreased blood glucose in subjects with Type 2 diabetes [33,34]. Pre-clinical studies have reported anti-hyperglycemic effects of the flaxseed lignan SDG in animals with Type I diabetes [35]. Whether SDG or flaxseed supplementation improves glycemic control in human subjects with Type 1 diabetes remains unknown and could be a topic of experimentation in the future.

5. Dietary Flaxseed and Cancers

Flaxseed is already used extensively in animal studies to treat a variety of cancers [36]. Perhaps the most studied cancer with respect to the impact of dietary flaxseed is breast cancer. In both experimental animal studies [36,37] and in human trials [36–38], dietary flaxseed has significant protective effects against breast cancer. A systematic review of 10 human trials led to the conclusion that flaxseed reduced tumour growth in women with breast cancer [36,38]. They also found evidence in support of flax-associated protection against primary breast cancer as well as a reduced risk of mortality in women living with breast cancer [38]. Beneficial effects were observed with 25 g doses of milled flaxseed [38].

Flaxseed lignans are nonsteroidal phytoestrogens that have a chemical structure that resembles mammalian estrogens, and hence produce estrogen-like effects in mammals. Flax lignans are metabolized by intestinal bacteria to become bioavailable in the plasma [39]. Lignans derived from food occur mainly as glucosides and undergo deglycosylation by β-glucosidases from gut microbiota before their intestinal absorption. Secoisolariciresinol diglucoside (SDG) is hydrolyzed in this way to release secoisolariciresinol (SECO). Deglycosylation of SECO is followed by demethylation by microbiota to produce dihydroxyenterodiol, which further results in the formation of enterodiol through dehydroxylation. Finally, dehydrogenation of enterodiol produces enterolactone. Enterodiol and enterolactone are absorbed from the large intestine, and ultimately appear as glucuronide and sulfate conjugates in body fluid and are excreted in urine [40]. The metabolism of SDG to enterolactone occurs in all subjects irrespective of gender [39]. A pharmacokinetic study in humans demonstrated the appearance of enterolignans in the plasma 8–10 h after ingestion of SDG, with the mean maximum plasma concentrations of enterodiol and enterolactone attaining ~14.8 h and ~19.7 h, respectively, after consumption [40]. The mean elimination half-life reported for enterodiol is ~4.4 h, and enterolactone is ~12.6 h [40]. Epidemiological studies in postmenopausal breast cancer patients have reported an association of higher blood concentrations of enterolactone with a reduced risk of breast cancer, decreased mortality rate and better survival. Clinical evidence also supports the protective effect of enterolactone in cancers of the breast, colon, prostate, gut and lung [41].

Breast cancer is not the only cancer that has shown sensitivity to dietary flaxseed or its components. Cancer of the prostate gland [42], lung [43,44], colon [45], ovary [41], endometrium [41], hepatocellular [41] and cervix have been inhibited by flaxseed.

The mechanisms responsible for the beneficial anti-oncotic action of milled flaxseed have been studied in cell culture, in animal experiments and in human trials. The rich compositions of both SDG and ALA have been postulated to play a role in the beneficial action of flaxseed on cancer [37,38,45,46]. Lignans like SDG reduce the breast cancer mortality by 33–70% and reduce all-cause mortality by 40–53% [36]. Doses of 50 mg of SDG will reduce tumours [38]. However, it is unlikely that SDG is itself responsible for the anti-tumour activity. SDG is restricted to the gastro-intestinal space and does not enter the blood stream. It is metabolized within the gastrointestinal tract to the enterolignans: enterolactone and enterodiol [47]. These compounds have estrogenic and antioxidative properties [36]. Enterolactone and enterodiol can bind to estrogen receptors and alter cell growth [37]. It is likely that these metabolites of SDG are ultimately responsible for the anti-tumour capacity of SDG [41]. The anti-inflammatory action of ALA may also play a role [41]. Flaxseed oil (enriched in ALA) also potentiates the anti-tumour action of drugs used in oncotic therapy. Flax oil administered with trastuzumab for epidermal growth factor receptor 2 positive breast cancer enhanced the anti-tumour effects of trastuzumab and significantly lowered the concentrations of trastuzumab needed to kill tumours in athymic mice [48]. Similar results have been observed using flaxseed with tamoxifen, another anti-tumour drug [37].

The cellular oncotic pathways affected by flaxseed and its bioactive components include a modulation of estrogen metabolism [36], an inhibition of cellular proliferation, angiogenesis, metastasis and inflammation, as well as a stimulation of apoptosis within the tumour [36,38,41–43,45,46]. The molecular targets for the anti-tumour actions of flaxseed and its bioactive components include a suppression of the phosphorylation of p-AKT, p-ERK and p-JNK kinases (resulting in a general slowing of the MAPK pathways) [43,46], inhibition of CDK4 [45], down regulation of multiple miRNAs [44], decreased expression of mRNAs for Bcl2, cell cycle proteins, ERalpha and beta and epidermal and insulin-like growth factor receptors [46].

It would appear that increasing our understanding of the value of dietary flaxseed, flax oil and SDG in this field and its efficacy in human trials may be a profitable avenue of future study. As in the case of the effects of flaxseed and its bioactive constituents in cardiovascular disease, it would appear that sufficient data already exists for the institution of these dietary therapies in specific cases of cancer prevention and treatment.

6. Dietary Flaxseed and the Brain

The critical role that omega-3 fatty acids obtained from marine sources play in brain development is well known [49]. This work has focused in the past primarily on the omega-3 fatty acids docosahexaenoic acid (DHA) and eicosapentaenoic acid (EPA). Whereas research has established an essential role for DHA in pre- and post-natal brain development [49,50], EPA appears to modulate behaviour and mood [50]. A loss of brain DHA content has been associated with poorer performance in spatial and learning tasks [51].

These data suggest that another omega-3 fatty acid, ALA, which is enriched in flaxseed, may have similar functional significance for the brain. When mothers of rats were fed flaxseed during pregnancy, the brains of newborn pups were heavier and contained significantly greater amounts of both ALA and DHA [52]. In pups given milled flaxseed or flaxseed oil soon after birth, these pups showed higher brain mass, demonstrating the value of milled flaxseed particularly in contributing to early postnatal brain development [53]. However, although dietary flaxseed may improve brain development and spatial memory, research has cautioned that the diet may depress body growth due to an imbalance between omega-3 and omega-6 fatty acid levels [54].

Dietary flaxseed may also improve aspects of brain function during conditions of neural disease. Maternal intake of flaxseed prevented depressive symptoms in offspring and demonstrated neuroprotection during experimental neonatal hypoxic-ischemic encephalopathy by lessening brain mass loss together with improvements in motor hyperactivity and spatial memory [55]. In mice exposed to chronic mild stress, dietary flaxseed reduced all parameters of chronic stress [56]. Supplementation to the diet with flaxseed lignans like SDG have shown anti-depressant-like effects in mice subjected to chronic stress [57] and demonstrated protective effects in cortical neurons against NMDA-induced neurotoxicity [58].

7. Dietary Flaxseed and Female Hormonal Status

Dietary flaxseed may also exhibit a protective effect against menopausal symptoms [59]. Several studies have examined the effects of flaxseed or its bioactive ingredients on the quality of life and the frequency and severity of hot flashes in post-menopausal women. The estrogenic action of certain metabolites of flaxseed suggested a potentially positive effect on these post-menopausal symptoms. In a study of 140 postmenopausal women, menopausal symptoms decreased and the quality of life increased in women who ingested a flaxseed supplemented diet [60]. A particularly large trial (199 women) of an unusually long duration (1 year) on a high dose of flaxseed (40 g per day) reported a significant decrease in menopausal symptoms, but this effect did not differ from the control group that ingested a wheat germ placebo [8]. Another study reported similar inconclusive evidence of a positive effect of flaxseed on menopausal symptoms with up to 90 g of flaxseed per day [61]. Further randomized controlled trials and systematic reviews of clinical trials found no significant effect of flaxseed on quality of life or hot flashes during menopause [62–65]. It is concluded that randomized, placebo-controlled trials are necessary to determine conclusive effects on menopausal symptoms. When carefully controlled trials are carried out in this manner, it would appear that flaxseed does not induce a significant effect on quality of life or the incidence and severity of hot flashes in menopausal women.

Caution has been advised for flaxseed consumption during pregnancy and lactation. SDG and flaxseed oil given to pregnant rats have shown opposite effects on total fat mass of the body. SDG administration resulted in higher fat mass, whereas flaxseed oil lowered fat mass. Furthermore, flax oil also reduced serum and milk triglyceride and cholesterol levels in female rats during lactation [66,67]. Similarly, male and female pups of mothers supplemented with flaxseed oil exhibited lower body fat mass and triglyceride levels [66,67]. With such changes in maternal and offspring biochemical parameters, it may be prudent to exercise caution when using flaxseed or its components in pregnancy.

However, as no other studies have reported similar changes, randomized, placebo-controlled trials in pregnant subjects are warranted to provide any conclusive evidence.

Postmenopausal women are at an increased risk of osteoporosis. In a short 6 weeks study by Arjmandi et al [68], a slightly lower bone resorption marker (tartrate-resistant acid phosphatase) was observed in postmenopausal women receiving flaxseed. However, no influence was reported when using anabolic bone agents. Conversely, most studies have shown no effect of flaxseed consumption on bone mineral density, bone mineral content or bone turnover in postmenopausal women [69]. In an animal model, flaxseed supplementation resulted in an additional benefit when combined with estrogen therapy. Flax oil rich in ALA showed a positive effect on bone health, particularly in pathological conditions such as obesity and kidney disease. ALA may be more responsible for this improvement in osteoporotic bone conditions than the estrogenic lignan content of flaxseed [69].

8. Dietary Flaxseed and Skin Health

A 12 week, randomized, double-blinded study on healthy female volunteers with sensitive skin reported a positive improvement in skin properties with the ingestion of flaxseed oil. A significant decrease was noted in skin sensitivity, transepidermal water loss, skin roughness and scaling, with an increase in skin hydration and smoothness [70]. ALA was identified as the main bioactive responsible for these effects on skin and aging. Compared to a younger population, older individuals have higher concentrations of proinflammatory oxylipins including 5-HETE, 9,10,13-TriHOME and 9,12-13-TriHOME, which could explain higher levels of inflammation in this older demographic [71]. Dietary supplementation of flaxseed has been shown to correct the balance of pro- and anti-inflammatory oxylipins and thus may exert a healthy effect on aging [71].

9. Dietary Flaxseed and Gastro-Intestinal Health

The influence of the microbiome on human and animal health is receiving increasing attention from the research community [72]. However, our understanding of the impact of dietary flaxseed on the gut microbiome in either healthy or diseased populations is limited. It was known that the lignans that are unusually high in content within flaxseed need to be metabolized by intestinal bacteria in order to gain access to the systemic circulation in humans. The production of enterolignans like enterodiol and enterolactone from SDG is best generated from milled flaxseed and defatted flaxseed meal, in comparison to a variety of other foods that contain SDG [73]. This intestinal metabolism is accomplished via the biotransformative action of specific intestinal bacteria [74] including *Ruminococcus bromii* and *Ruminococcus lactaris* [75]. Others have found *Lactobacillus casei* and *Lactobacillus acidophilus* were important for the digestion of whole flaxseed in order to increase enterodiol bioaccessibility [76].

Early studies have shown the capacity of flaxseed supplementation in the diet to alter the bacterial flora in the intestines of animals. For example, flaxseed supplemented to the diet of mice will alter *Enterobacteriaceae* diversity and prevalence in the feces and cecum [77]. Power and colleagues [78] showed that a flaxseed supplemented diet will alter the microbial microenvironment in the colon with a 20-fold increase in *Prevotella* spp. and a 30-fold decrease in *Akkermansia muciniphila* abundance. Others have shown that a combined high fat, flaxseed and fish oil supplemented diet increased the abundance of intestinal *Bifidobacterium* [79].

Changes in specific bacteria in the microbiome may have implications on disease progression (Figure 3). Dietary flax oil consumption can, under some conditions, reduce the presence of *Proteobacteria* and *Porphyromonadaceae* in the gut microbiome, which may have a positive impact on alcoholic liver disease [80]. Defatted flaxseed meal (which is a partially delipidated form of flaxseed) reduced the appearance of aberrant crypt foci in the colon of mice through an increase in the expression of *Bifidobacterium* [81]. Daily intake of flaxseed mucilage resulted in changes in the abundance of 33 different metagenomics species in the gut microbiota, including eight different species of *Faecalibacterium*. This altered insulin sensitivity in these women [82]. These data contrast with those of Lagkouvardos et al [75], who found that flaxseed did not significantly change the fecal microbiome nor the abundance of the dominant bacterial species present. Others have also challenged the efficacy of dietary flaxseed to alter the appearance of disease based upon a change in the gut microbiome. For example, a 5% flaxseed supplemented diet had no protective effect against the development of intestinal tumours [83]. Caution in the use of flaxseed in the diet has also been introduced by the results of Maatanen and co-workers, who showed that whereas a reduced fat diet could protect against colitis, the high levels of PUFAs provided by flaxseed supplementation to the diet diminished these beneficial effects [84].

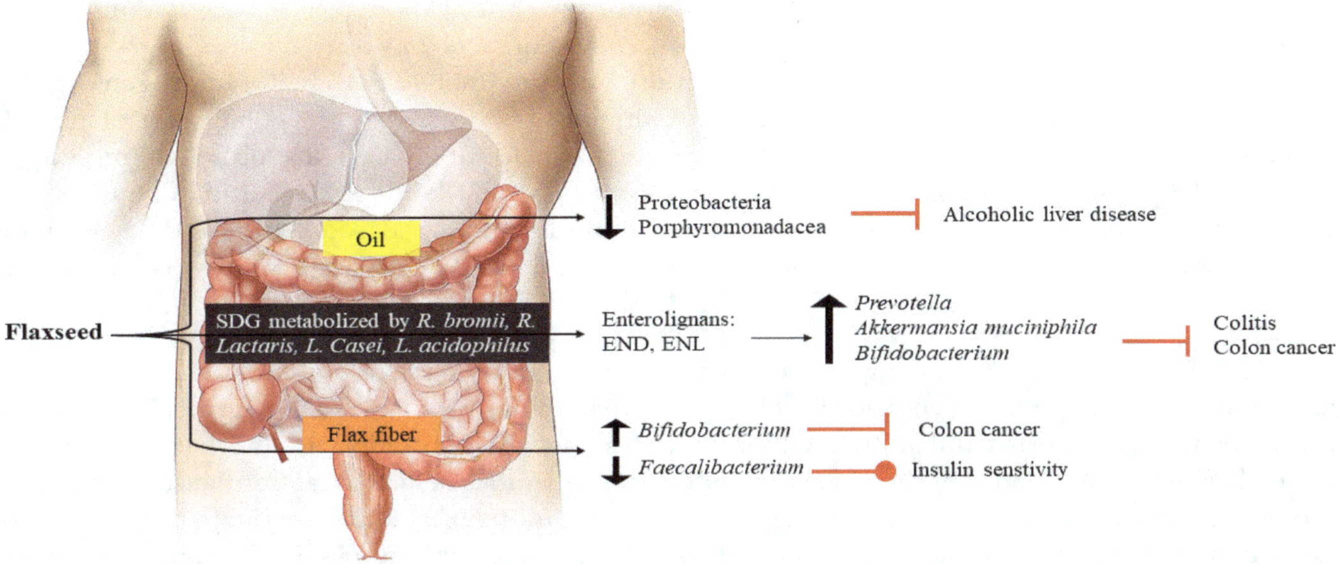

Figure 3. The effect of dietary flaxseed on the gastrointestinal health.

The potential for dietary flaxseed to replace or reduce the use of constipation medication in different populations at risk (the elderly, the ill, in personal health care homes, etc.) and the reduction in side-effects associated with conventional constipation medication is worthy of study. Two recent randomized trials have generated results of great interest for the introduction of flaxseed into diets for relief from constipation. In the first trial [30], flaxseed baked into cookies was ingested in constipated patients with Type 2 diabetes. They found the flaxseed reduced constipation symptoms, weight, fasting plasma glucose, triglycerides and LDL and HDL cholesterol levels. In a subsequent trial using the same type of patient population, flaxseed affected all of these parameters once again and, importantly, was superior in its capacity to reduce constipation symptoms to psyllium [85]. Flaxseed may also be of use in reducing the symptoms of irritable bowel syndrome; however, further research is required [86]. Flaxseed oil was also beneficial in reducing experimental diarrhea [87].

The mechanism of action of flaxseed in stimulating fecal output during constipation clearly lies largely with its high fiber content. It is not surprising, therefore, that even partially defatted flaxseed meal was a valuable laxative in both normal and constipated condition [78]. However, flaxseed oil has been shown to act on intestinal muscarinic receptors and blocks K+ channels [77], actions that would both lead to modifications of intestinal motility.

10. Toxicity of Flaxseed

Although no toxicity has ever been reported in clinical studies with dietary supplementation of flaxseed, some compounds within flaxseed such as cyanogenic glycosides and linatine have been identified as potential toxic compounds. Cyanogenic glycosides such as linamarin, linustatin, neolinustatin, lotaustralin and amygdalin are nitrogenous secondary plant metabolites [3]. These compounds are not exclusively found in flaxseed, but are also present in other food items including apples, spinach and cassavas [88–90]. The glycoside is converted by intestinal β-glycosidase to cyanohydrin, which then decomposes to hydrogen cyanide [90]. In flaxseed, this process is catalyzed by two distinct enzymes: linustatinase and linamarase β-glucosidase [90]. Hydrogen cyanide could cause acute cyanide poisoning, which may place the respiratory and nervous system at risk [3]. However, no increase in plasma cyanide levels above baseline have been observed with the consumption of 15–100 g of flaxseed [90]. The linustatin and neolinustatin found in flaxseed are thought to be the lowest cyanide producers compared to other cyanogenic glycosides. This is because flaxseed glycosides have a gentiobiose moiety that needs to be hydrolyzed to glucose. The cyanohydrin formed by metabolism is highly stable [90], which, therefore, resists any spontaneous decomposition to hydrogen cyanide. Theoretically, 1–2 tablespoons of flaxseed will produce approximately 5–10 mg of hydrogen cyanide after ingestion. This is highly unlikely to cause toxicity for three reasons: a) 50–60 mg dose of cyanide is required to cause acute toxicity; b) the human body can routinely detoxify up to 100 mg/day of cyanide [3,89] and c) cooking destroys cyanide (cyanide is heat labile [91]). Human studies with 50 g/day flaxseed did not increase urinary thiocyanate levels [3]. Based on these data, humans would need to consume the unrealistic amount of 1 kg of flaxseed daily for cyanide toxicity to ever manifest itself.

Another potentially toxic compound is linatine (antipyridoxin factor), which has been identified as a vitamin B6 antagonist in chicks [89]. However, flaxseed has never been shown to induce vitamin B6 deficiency in clinical studies [91]. Other compounds such as phytic acid and trypsin inhibitor have also been suggested to induce negative effects on the nutritional status after flaxseed ingestion. However, once again, no studies have reported any alterations in zinc status due to phytic acid, or any difference in trypsin inhibitor activity in flaxseed compared with canola or soybean seeds [89,91]. In conclusion, it is important to recognize that no definitive scientific data have been produced to support the concept of toxicity from dietary flaxseed because of any of these compounds.

11. Conclusions

Supplementation of the diet with milled flaxseed has many healthy benefits to the body. Although cardiovascular disease and canceer are probably the best researched areas that have shown convincing evidence of a beneficial action for dietary flaxseed, other areas like gastro-intestinal health and diabetes have also been receptive to the beneficial effects of dietary flaxseed. Other areas in human health require further research to make definitive conclusions but the preliminary data is encouraging. With little or no evidence of toxicity for dietary supplementation with flaxseed, there appears to be a clear argument to support its inclusion in the daily diet and little reason to oppose it.

Author Contributions: For conceptualization, T.N., M.P. and G.N.P.; resources, T.N. and G.N.P.; writing—original draft preparation, M.P. and G.N.P.; data processing for figures, M.P., T.G.M. and J.A.A.; writing—review and editing, M.P., T.G.M., J.A.A., M.A., T.N., and G.N.P.; supervision, G.N.P.; funding acquisition, G.N.P.

References

1. Brown, L.; Caligiuri, S.P.B.; Brown, D.; Pierce, G.N. Clinical trials using functional foods provide unique challenges. *J. Funct. Foods* **2018**, *45*, 233–238. [CrossRef]
2. Caligiuri, S.P.B.; Pierce, G.N. A review of the relative efficacy of dietary, nutritional supplements, lifestyle and drug therapies in the management of hypertension. *Crit. Rev. Food Sci. Nutr.* **2017**, *57*, 3508–3527. [CrossRef] [PubMed]
3. Parikh, M.; Netticadan, T.; Pierce, G.N. Flaxseed: Its bioactive components and their cardiovascular benefits. *Am. J. Physiol. Heart Circ. Physiol.* **2018**, *314*, H146–H159. [CrossRef] [PubMed]

4. Ramicharitrar, A.; Badrie, N.; Mattfeldt-Beman, M.; Matsuo, H.; Ridley, C. Consumer acceptability of muffins with flaxseed (*Linum usitatissimum*). *J. Food Sci.* **2005**, *70*, 5504–5507.
5. Rodriguez-Leyva, D.; Weighell, W.; Edel, A.L.; La Vallee, R.; Dibrov, E.; Pinneker, R.; Maddaford, T.G.; Ramjiawan, B.; Aliani, M.; Guzman, R.; et al. Potent anti-hypertensive action of dietary flaxseed in hypertensive patients. *Hypertension* **2013**, *62*, 1081–1089. [CrossRef]
6. Pohjanheimo, T.A.; Hakala, M.A.; Tahvonen, R.L.; Salminen, S.J.; Kallio, H.P. Flaxseed in breadmaking: Effects on sensory quality, aging, and composition of bakery products. *J. Food Sci.* **2006**, *71*, S343–S348. [CrossRef]
7. Aliani, M.; Ryland, D.; Pierce, G.N. Effect of flax addition on the flavor profile of muffins and snack bars. *Food Res. Int.* **2011**, *44*, 2489–2496. [CrossRef]
8. Dodin, S.; Lemay, A.; Jacques, H.; Légaré, F.; Forest, J.C.; Mâsse, B. The effects of flaxseed dietary supplement on lipid profile, bone mineral density, and symptoms in menopausal women; a randomized, double-blind, wheat germ placebo-controlled clinical trial. *J. Clin. Endocrinol. Metab.* **2005**, *90*, 1390–1397. [CrossRef]
9. Chen, Z.Y.; Ratnayake, W.M.N.; Cunnane, S.C. Oxidative stability of flaxseed lipids during baking. *J. Am. Oil Chem. Soc.* **1994**, *71*, 629–632. [CrossRef]
10. Aliani, M.; Ryland, D.; Pierce, G.N. Effect of flax addition on the flavor profile and acceptability of bagels. *J. Food Sci.* **2012**, *71*, S62–S79. [CrossRef]
11. Austria, J.A.; Aliani, M.; Malcolmson, L.J.; Dibrov, E.; Blackwood, E.P.; Maddaford, T.G.; Guzman, R.; Pierce, G.N. Daily food choices over one year when patient diets are supplemented with milled flaxseed. *J. Funct. Foods* **2016**, *26*, 772–780. [CrossRef]
12. Edel, A.E.; Aliani, M.; Pierce, G.N. Stability of bioactives in flaxseed and flaxseed-fortified foods. *Food Res. Int.* **2015**, *77*, 140–155. [CrossRef]
13. Austria, J.A.; Richard, M.N.; Chahine, M.N.; Edel, A.L.; Malcolmson, L.J.; Dupasquier, C.M.C.; Pierce, G.N. Bioavailability of alpha linolenic acid in subjects after ingestion of three different forms of flaxseed. *J. Am. Coll. Nutr.* **2008**, *27*, 214–221. [CrossRef] [PubMed]
14. Dzuvor, C.K.O.; Taylor, J.T.; Acquah, C.; Pan, S.; Agyei, D. Bioprocessing of functional ingredients from flaxseed. *Molecules* **2018**, *23*, 2444. [CrossRef] [PubMed]
15. Dupasquier, C.M.C.; Weber, A.-M.; Ander, B.P.; Rampersad, P.P.; Steigerwald, S.; Wigle, J.T.; Mitchell, R.W.; Kroeger, E.A.; Gilchrist, J.S.C.; Moghadasian, M.M.; et al. The effects of dietary flaxseed on vascular contractile function and atherosclerosis in rabbits during prolonged hypercholesterolemia. *Am. J. Physiol.* **2006**, *291*, H2987–H2996.
16. Dupasquier, C.M.C.; Dibrov, E.; Kneesh, A.L.; Cheung, P.K.M.; Lee, K.G.Y.; Alexander, H.K.; Yeganeh, B.; Moghadasian, M.H.; Pierce, G.N. Dietary flaxseed inhibits atherosclerosis in the LDL receptor deficient mouse in part through anti-proliferative and anti-inflammatory actions. *Am. J. Physiol.* **2007**, *293*, H2394–H2402.
17. Bassett, C.M.C.; McCullough, R.S.; Edel, A.L.; Patenaude, A.; La Vallee, R.; Pierce, G.N. The alpha linolenic acid content of flaxseed can prevent the atherogenic effects of dietary trans-fat. *Am. J. Physiol.* **2011**, *301*, H2220–H2226.
18. Parikh, M.; Raj, P.; Austria, J.A.; Yu, L.; Garg, B.; Netticadan, T.; Pierce, G.N. Dietary flaxseed protects against ventricular arrhythmias and left ventricular dilation after a myocardial infarction. *J. Nutr. Biochem.* **2019**, in press.
19. Francis, A.A.; Austria, J.A.; La Vallee, R.K.; Deniset, J.F.; Maddaford, G.G.; Dibrov, E.; Pierce, G.N. The effects of dietary flaxseed on atherosclerotic plaque regression. *Am. J. Physiol. Heart Circ. Physiol.* **2013**, *304*, H1743–H1751. [CrossRef]
20. Ander, B.P.; Weber, A.R.; Rampersad, P.; Gilchrist, J.S.C.; Pierce, G.N.; Lukas, A. Dietary flaxseed protects against ventricular fibrillation induced by ischemia- reperfusion in normal and hypercholesterolemic rabbits. *J. Nutr.* **2004**, *134*, 3250–3256. [CrossRef]
21. Ander, B.P.; Hurtado, C.; Raposo, C.S.; Maddaford, T.G.; Deniset, J.F.; Hryshko, L.V.; Pierce, G.N.; Lukas, A. Differential sensitivities of the NCX 1.1 and NCX 1.3 isoforms of the Na^{+}-Ca^{2+} exchanger to alpha-linolenic acid. *Cardiovasc. Res.* **2007**, *73*, 395–403. [CrossRef]
22. Prasad, K. Flax lignan complex slows down the progression of atherosclerosis in hyperlipidemic rabbits. *J. Cardiovasc. Pharmacol. Ther.* **2009**, *14*, 38–48. [CrossRef]

23. Caligiuri, S.P.B.; Rodriguez-Leyva, D.; Aukema, H.; Ravandi, A.; Weighell, W.; Guzman, R.; Pierce, G.N. Dietary flaxseed reduces central aortic blood pressure without cardiac involvement but through changes in plasma oxylipins. *Hypertension* **2016**, *68*, 1031–1038. [CrossRef]
24. Rodriguez-Leyva, D.; Zahradka, P.; Ramjiawan, B.; Guzman, R.; Aliani, M.; Pierce, G.N. The effect of dietary flaxseed on improving symptoms of cardiovascular disease in patients with peripheral arterial disease: The rationale and design of the FlaxPAD randomized controlled trial. *Contemp. Clin. Trials* **2011**, *32*, 724–730. [CrossRef]
25. Caligiuri, S.P.B.; Aukema, H.M.; Ravandi, A.; Guzman, R.; Dibrov, E.; Pierce, G.N. Flaxseed consumption reduces blood pressure in hypertensive patients by altering circulating oxylipins via an alpha linolenic acid-induced inhibition of soluble epoxide hydrolase. *Hypertension* **2014**, *64*, 53–59. [CrossRef]
26. Ogawa, A.; Suzuki, Y.; Aoyama, T.; Takeuchi, H. Dietary α-linolenic acid inhibits angiotensin-converting enzyme activity and mRNA expression levels in the aorta of spontaneously hypertensive rats. *J. Oleo Sci.* **2009**, *58*, 355–360. [CrossRef]
27. Udenigwe, C.C.; Adebiyi, A.P.; Doyen, A.; Li, H.; Bazinet, L.; Aluko, R.E. Low molecular weight flaxseed protein-derived arginine-containing peptides reduced blood pressure of spontaneously hypertensive rats faster than amino acid form of arginine and native flaxseed protein. *Food Chem.* **2012**, *132*, 468–475. [CrossRef]
28. Sawant, S.H.; Bodhankar, S.L. Flax lignan concentrate reverses alterations in blood pressure, left ventricular functions, lipid profile and antioxidant status in DOCA-salt induced renal hypertension in rats. *Renal Fail.* **2016**, *38*, 411–423. [CrossRef]
29. Park, J.B.; Velasquez, M.T. Potential effects of lignan-enriched flaxseed powder on bodyweight, visceral fat, lipid profile, and blood pressure in rats. *Fitoterapia.* **2012**, *83*, 941–946. [CrossRef]
30. Soltanian, N.; Janghorbani, M. A randomized trial of the effects of flaxseed to manage constipation, weight, glycemia, and lipids in constipated patients with type 2 diabetes. *Nutr. Metab.* **2018**, *15*, 36. [CrossRef]
31. Mani, U.V.; Mani, I.; Biswas, M.; Kumar, S.N. An open-label study on the effect of flax seed powder (Linum usitatissimum) supplementation in the management of diabetes mellitus. *J. Diet. Suppl.* **2011**, *8*, 257–265. [CrossRef]
32. Hutchins, A.M.; Brown, B.D.; Cunnane, S.C.; Domitrovich, S.G.; Adams, E.R.; Bobowiec, C.E. Daily flaxseed consumption improves glycemic control in obese men and women with pre-diabetes: A randomized study. *Nutr. Res.* **2013**, *33*, 367–375. [CrossRef]
33. Thakur, G.; Mitra, A.; Pal, K.; Rousseau, D. Effect of flaxseed gum on reduction of blood glucose and cholesterol in type 2 diabetic patients. *Int. J. Food Sci. Nutr.* **2009**, *60* (Suppl. 6), 126–136. [CrossRef]
34. Pan, A.; Sun, J.; Chen, Y.; Ye, X.; Li, H.; Yu, Z.; Wang, Y.; Gu, W.; Zhang, X.; Chen, X.; et al. Effects of a flaxseed-derived lignan supplement in type 2 diabetic patients: A randomized, double-blind, cross-over trial. *PLoS ONE* **2007**, *2*, e1148. [CrossRef]
35. Prasad, K.; Mantha, S.V.; Muir, A.D.; Westcott, N.D. Protective effect of secoisolariciresinol diglucoside against streptozotocin-induced diabetes and its mechanism. *Mol. Cell. Biochem.* **2000**, *206*, 141–149. [CrossRef]
36. Mason, J.K.; Thompson, L.U. Flaxseed and its lignan and oil components: Can they play a role in reducing the risk of and improving the treatment of breast cancer? *Appl. Physiol. Nutr. Metab.* **2014**, *39*, 663–678. [CrossRef]
37. Calado, A.; Neves, P.M.; Santos, T.; Ravasco, P. The effect of flaxseed in breast cancer: A Literature Review. *Front. Nutr.* **2018**, *5*, 4. [CrossRef]
38. Flower, G.; Fritz, H.; Balneaves, L.G.; Verma, S.; Skidmore, B.; Fernandes, R.; Kennedy, D.; Cooley, K.; Wong, R.; Sagar, S.; et al. Flax and Breast Cancer: A systematic review. *Integr. Cancer Ther.* **2014**, *13*, 181–192. [CrossRef]
39. Gaya, P.; Medina, M.; Sánchez-Jiménez, A.; Landete, J.M. Phytoestrogen metabolism by adult human gut microbiota. *Molecules* **2016**, *21*, 1034. [CrossRef]
40. Kuijsten, A.; Arts, I.C.W.; Vree, T.B.; Hollman, P.C.H. Pharmacokinetics of enterolignans in healthy men and women consuming a single dose of secoisolariciresinol diglucoside. *J. Nutr.* **2005**, *135*, 795–801. [CrossRef]
41. Mali, A.V.; Padhye, S.B.; Anant, S.; Hegde, M.V.; Kadam, S.S. Anticancer and antimetastatic potential of enterolactone: Clinical, preclinical and mechanistic perspectives. *Eur. J. Pharmacol.* **2019**, *852*, 107–124. [CrossRef] [PubMed]
42. Lin, X.; Gingrich, J.R.; Bao, W.; Li, J.; Haroon, Z.A.; Demark-Wahnefried, W. Effect of flaxseed supplementation on prostatic carcinoma in transgenic mice. *Urology* **2002**, *60*, 919–924. [CrossRef]

43. Chikara, S.; Mamidi, S.; Sreedasyam, A.; Chittem, K.; Pietrofesa, R.; Zuppa, A.; Moorthy, G.; Dyer, N.; Christofidou-Solomidou, M.; Reindl, K.M. Flaxseed consumption inhibits chemically induced lung tumorigenesis and modulates expression of Phase II enzymes and inflammatory cytokines in A/J mice. *Cancer Prev. Res.* **2018**, *11*, 27–37. [CrossRef] [PubMed]
44. Christofidou-Solomidou, M.; Pietrofesa, R.; Arguiri, E.; McAlexander, M.A.; Witwer, K.W. Dietary flaxseed modulates the miRNA profile in irradiated and non-irradiated murine lungs: a novel mechanism of tissue radioprotection by flaxseed. *Cancer Biol. Ther.* **2014**, *15*, 930–937. [CrossRef]
45. Shah, N.R.; Patel, B.M. Secoisolariciresinol diglucoside rich extract of L. usitatissimum prevents diabetic colon cancer through inhibition of CDK4. *Biomed. Pharmacother.* **2016**, *83*, 733–739. [CrossRef]
46. Chen, J.; Saggar, J.K.; Corey, P.; Thompson, L.U. Flaxseed and pure secoisolariciresinol diglucoside, but not flaxseed hull, reduce human breast tumor growth (MCF-7) in athymic mice. *J. Nutr.* **2009**, *139*, 2061–2066. [CrossRef]
47. Edel, A.L.; Patenaude, A.F.; Richard, M.N.; Dibrov, E.; Austria, J.A.; Aukema, H.M.; Pierce, G.N.; Aliani, M. The effect of flaxseed dose on circulating concentrations of alpha-linolenic acid and secoisolariciresinol diglucoside derived enterolignans in young healthy adults. *Eur. J. Nutr.* **2016**, *55*, 651–663. [CrossRef]
48. Mason, J.K.; Chen, J.; Thompson, L.U. Flaxseed oil-trastuzumab interaction in breast cancer. *Food Chem. Toxicol.* **2010**, *48*, 2223–2226. [CrossRef]
49. Lauritzen, L.; Brambilla, P.; Mazzocchi, A.; Harsløf, L.B.; Ciappolino, V.; Agostoni, C. DHA effects in brain development and function. *Nutrients* **2016**, *8*, 6. [CrossRef]
50. Kidd, P.M. Omega-3 DHA and EPA for cognition, behavior, and mood: clinical findings and structural-functional synergies with cell membrane phospholipids. *Altern. Med. Rev.* **2007**, *12*, 207–227.
51. Salem, N., Jr.; Moriguchi, T.; Greiner, R.S.; McBride, K.; Ahmad, A.; Catalan, J.N.; Slotnick, B. Alterations in brain function after loss of docosahexaenoate due to dietary restriction of n-fatty acids. *J. Mol. Neurosci.* **2001**, *16*, 299–307. [CrossRef]
52. Lenzi Almeida, K.C.; Teles Boaventura, G.; Guzman Silva, M.A. Influence of omega-3 fatty acids from the flaxseed (*Linum usitatissimum*) on the brain development of newborn rats. *Nutr. Hosp.* **2011**, *26*, 991–996.
53. Pessanha, C.R.; da Camara Boueri, B.F.; da Costa, L.R.; Ferreira, M.R.; Melo, H.S.; de Abreu, M.D.; Pessoa, L.R.; da Silva, P.C.; Pereira, A.D.; Ribeiro, D.C.; et al. Brain development in male rats subjected to early weaning and treated with diet containing flour or flaxseed oil after 21 days until 60 days. *J. Dev. Orig. Health Dis.* **2015**, *6*, 268–271. [CrossRef]
54. Fernandes, F.S.; de Souza, A.S.; do Carmo, M.; Boaventura, G.T. Maternal intake of flaxseed-based diet (*Linum usitatissimum*) on hippocampus fatty acid profile: implications for growth, locomotor activity and spatial memory. *Nutrition* **2011**, *27*, 1040–1047. [CrossRef]
55. Mucci Dde, B.; Fernandes, F.S.; Souza Ados, S.; Sardinha, F.L.; Soares-Mota, M.; Tavares do Carmo, M. Flaxseed mitigates brain mass loss, improving motor hyperactivity and spatial memory, in a rodent model of neonatal hypoxic-ischemic encephalopathy. *Prostaglandins Leukot. Essent. Fatty Acids* **2015**, *97*, 13–19. [CrossRef]
56. Naveen, S.; Siddalingaswamy, M.; Singsit, D.; Khanum, F. Anti-depressive effect of polyphenols and omega-3 fatty acid from pomegranate peel and flax seed in mice exposed to chronic mild stress. *Psychiatry Clin. Neurosci.* **2013**, *67*, 501–508. [CrossRef]
57. Ma, X.; Wang, R.; Zhao, X.; Zhang, C.; Sun, J.; Li, J.; Zhang, L.; Shao, T.; Ruan, L.; Chen, L.; et al. Antidepressant-like effect of flaxseed secoisolariciresinol diglycoside in ovariectomized mice subjected to unpredictable chronic stress. *Metab. Brain Dis.* **2013**, *28*, 77–84. [CrossRef]
58. Li, X.B.; Yang, Z.X.; Yang, L.; Chen, X.L.; Zhang, K.; Yang, Q.; Wu, Y.M.; Liu, S.B.; Tao, K.S.; Zhao, M.G. Neuroprotective effects of flax lignan against NMDA-induced neurotoxicity in vitro. *CNS Neurosci. Ther.* **2012**, *18*, 927–933. [CrossRef]
59. Landete, J.M.; Arqués, J.; Medina, M.; Gaya, P.; de Las Rivas, B.; Munoz, R. Bioactivation of phytoestrogens: Intestinal bacteria and health. *Crit. Rev. Food Sci. Nutr.* **2016**, *56*, 1826–1843. [CrossRef] [PubMed]
60. Cetisli, N.E.; Saruhan, A.; Kivcak, B. The effects of flaxseed on menopausal symptoms and quality of life. *Holist. Nurs. Pract.* **2015**, *29*, 151–157.
61. Colli, M.C.; Bracht, A.; Soares, A.A.; de Oliveira, A.L.; Bôer, C.G.; de Souza, C.G.; Peralta, R.M. Evaluation of the efficacy of flaxseed meal and flaxseed extract in reducing menopausal symptoms. *J. Med. Food.* **2012**, *15*, 840–845. [CrossRef] [PubMed]

62. Lewis, J.E.; Nickell, L.A.; Thompson, L.U.; Szalai, J.P.; Kiss, A.; Hilditch, J.R. A randomized controlled trial of the effect of dietary soy and flaxseed muffins on quality of life and hot flashes during menopause. *Menopause* **2006**, *13*, 631–642. [CrossRef] [PubMed]
63. Dew, T.P.; Williamson, G. Controlled flax interventions for the improvement of menopausal symptoms and postmenopausal bone health: A systematic review. *Menopause* **2013**, *20*, 1207–1215. [CrossRef] [PubMed]
64. Lethaby, A.; Marjoribanks, J.; Kronenberg, F.; Roberts, H.; Eden, J.; Brown, J. Phytoestrogens for menopausal vasomotor symptoms. *Cochrane Database Syst. Rev.* **2013**, *12*, CD001395. [CrossRef] [PubMed]
65. Pruthi, S.; Qin, R.; Terstreip, S.A.; Liu, H.; Loprinzi, C.L.; Shah, T.R.; Tucker, K.F.; Dakhil, S.R.; Bury, M.J.; Carolla, R.L.; et al. A phase III, randomized, placebo-controlled, double-blind trial of flaxseed for the treatment of hot flashes: North Central Cancer Treatment Group N08C7. *Menopause* **2012**, *1*, 48–53. [CrossRef] [PubMed]
66. Guarda, D.S.; Lisboa, P.C.; de Oliveira, E.; Nogueira-Neto, J.F.; de Moura, E.G.; Figueiredo, M.S. Flaxseed oil during lactation changes milk and body composition in male and female suckling pups rats. *Food Chem. Toxicol.* **2014**, *69*, 69–75. [CrossRef] [PubMed]
67. Troina, A.A.; Figueiredo, M.S.; Passos, M.C.F.; Reis, A.M.; Oliveira, E.; Lisboa, P.C.; Moura, E.G. Flaxseed bioactive compounds change milk, hormonal and biochemical parameters of dams and offspring during lactation. *Food Chem. Toxicol.* **2012**, *50*, 2388–2396. [CrossRef] [PubMed]
68. Arjmandi, B.; Juma, S.; Lucas, E.; Wei, L.; Venkatesh, S.; Khan, D. Flaxseed supplementation positively influences bone metabolism in postmenopausal women. *JANA* **1998**, *1*, 27–32.
69. Kim, Y.; Ilich, J.Z. Implications of dietary α-linolenic acid in bone health. *Nutrition* **2011**, *27*, 1101–1107. [CrossRef] [PubMed]
70. Neukam, K.; De Spirt, S.; Stahl, W.; Bejot, M.; Maurette, J.M.; Tronnier, H.; Heinrich, U. Supplementation of flaxseed oil diminishes skin sensitivity and improves skin barrier function and condition. *Skin Pharmacol. Physiol.* **2011**, *24*, 67–74. [CrossRef]
71. Caligiuri, S.P.B.; Aukema, H.M.; Ravandi, A.; Pierce, G.N. Elevated levels of pro-inflammatory oxylipins in older subjects are normalized by flaxseed consumption. *Exp. Gerontol.* **2014**, *59*, 51–57. [CrossRef]
72. Ettinger, G.; MacDonald, K.; Reid, G.; Burton, J.P. The influence of the human microbiome and probiotics on cardiovascular health. *Gut Microbes* **2014**, *5*, 719–728. [CrossRef]
73. Thompson, L.U.; Robb, P.; Serraino, M.; Cheung, F. Mammalian lignan production from various foods. *Nutr. Cancer* **1991**, *16*, 43–52. [CrossRef]
74. Wang, C.Z.; Ma, X.Q.; Yang, D.H.; Guo, Z.R.; Liu, G.R.; Zhao, G.X.; Tang, J.; Zhang, Y.N.; Ma, M.; Cai, S.Q.; et al. Production of enterodiol from defatted flaxseeds through biotransformation by human intestinal bacteria. *BMC Microbiol.* **2010**, *10*, 115. [CrossRef]
75. Lagkouvardos, I.; Kläring, K.; Heinzmann, S.S.; Platz, S.; Scholz, B.; Engel, K.H.; Schmitt-Kopplin, P.; Haller, D.; Rohn, S.; Skurk, T. Gut metabolites and bacterial community networks during a pilot intervention study with flaxseeds in healthy adult men. *Mol. Nutr. Food Res.* **2015**, *59*, 1614–1628. [CrossRef]
76. Munoz, O.; Fuentealba, C.; Ampuero, D.; Figuerola, F.; Estévez, A.M. The effect of Lactobacillus acidophilus and Lactobacillus casei on the in vitro bioaccessibility of flaxseed lignans (*Linum usitatissimum* L.). *Food Funct.* **2018**, *9*, 2426–2432. [CrossRef]
77. Pulkrabek, M.; Rhee, T.; Gibbs, P.; Hall, C. Flaxseed- and Buckwheat-supplemented diets altered enterobacteriaceae diversity and prevalence in the cecum and feces of obese mice. *J. Diet. Suppl.* **2017**, *14*, 667–678. [CrossRef]
78. Power, K.A.; Lepp, D.; Zarepoor, L.; Monk, J.M.; Wu, W.; Tsao, R.; Liu, R. Dietary flaxseed modulates the colonic microenvironment in healthy C57Bl/6 male mice which may alter susceptibility to gut-associated diseases. *J. Nutr. Biochem.* **2016**, *28*, 61–69. [CrossRef]
79. Patterson, E.; O'Doherty, R.M.; Murphy, E.F.; Wall, R.; O'Sullivan, O.; Nilaweera, K.; Fitzgerald, G.F.; Cotter, P.D.; Ross, R.P.; Stanton, C. Impact of dietary fatty acids on metabolic activity and host intestinal microbiota composition on C57BL/6J mice. *Br. J. Nutr.* **2014**, *111*, 1905–1917. [CrossRef]
80. Zhang, X.; Wang, H.; Yin, P.; Fan, H.; Sun, L.; Liu, Y. Flaxseed oil ameliorates alcoholic liver disease via anti-inflammation and modulating gut microbiota in mice. *Lipids Health Dis.* **2017**, *16*, 44. [CrossRef]
81. Gomides, A.F.; Concalves, R.V.; de Paula, S.O.; Ferreira, C.L.; Comastri, D.S.; Peluzio Mdo, C. Defatted flaxseed meal prevents the appearance of aberrant crypt foci in the colon of mice increasing the gene expression of p53. *Nutr. Hosp.* **2015**, *31*, 1675–1681.

82. Brahe, L.K.; Le Chatelier, E.; Prifti, E.; Pons, N.; Kennedy, S.; Blaedel, T.; Håkansson, J.; Dalsgaard, T.K.; Hansen, T.; Pedersen, O.; et al. Dietary modulation of the gut microbiota—A randomized controlled trial in obese postmenopausal women. *Br. J. Nutr.* **2015**, *114*, 406–417. [CrossRef]
83. van Kranen, H.J.; Mortensen, A.; Sørensen, I.K.; van den Berg-Wijnands, J.; Beems, R.; Nurmi, T.; Adlercreutz, H.; van Kreijl, C.F. Lignan precursors from flaxseed or rye bran do not protect against the development of intestinal neoplasia in ApcMin mice. *Nutr.Cancer* **2003**, *45*, 203–210. [CrossRef]
84. Määttänen, P.; Lurz, E.; Botts, S.R.; Wu, R.Y.; Yeung, C.W.; Li, B.; Abiff, S.; Johnson-Henry, K.C.; Lepp, D.; Power, K.A.; et al. Ground flaxseed reverses protection of a reduced-fat diet against Citrobacter rodentium-induced colitis. *Am. J. Physiol. Gastrointest. Liver Physiol.* **2018**, *315*, G788–G798. [CrossRef]
85. Soltanian, N.; Janghorbani, M. Effect of flaxseed or psyllium vs. placebo on management of constipation, weight, glycemia, and lipids: A randomized trial in constipated patients with type 2 diabetes. *Clin. Nutr. ESPEN* **2019**, *29*, 41–48. [CrossRef]
86. Cockerell, K.M.; Watkins, A.S.; Reeves, L.B.; Goddard, L.; Lomer, M.C. Effects of linseeds on the symptoms of irritable bowel syndrome: A pilot randomized controlled trial. *J. Hum. Nutr. Diet.* **2012**, *5*, 435–443. [CrossRef]
87. Hanif, P.A.; Gilani, A.H. Dual effectiveness of flaxseed in constipation and diarrhea: possible mechanism. *J. Ethnopharmacol.* **2015**, *169*, 60–68. [CrossRef]
88. Bolarinwa, I.F.; Orfila, C.; Morgan, M.R. Determination of amygdalin in apple seeds, fresh apples and processed apple juices. *Food Chem.* **2015**, *170*, 437–442. [CrossRef]
89. Touré, A.; Xueming, X. Flaxseed lignans: Source, biosynthesis, metabolism, antioxidant activity, bio-active components, and health benefits. *Comp. Rev. Food Sci. Food Saf.* **2010**, *9*, 261–269.
90. Cressey, P.; Reeve, J. Metabolism of cyanogenic glycosides: A review. *Food Chem. Toxicol.* **2019**, *125*, 225–232. [CrossRef]
91. Kajla, P.; Sharma, A.; Sood, D.R. Flaxseed-a potential functional food source. *J. Food Sci. Technol.* **2015**, *52*, 1857–1871. [CrossRef]

2

Consumption of Stilbenes and Flavonoids is Linked to Reduced Risk of Obesity Independently of Fiber Intake

Olatz Mompeo [1], Tim D. Spector [1,*], Marisa Matey Hernandez [1], Caroline Le Roy [1], Geoffrey Istas [2], Melanie Le Sayec [2], Massimo Mangino [1,3], Amy Jennings [4], Ana Rodriguez-Mateos [2], Ana M. Valdes [1,5,†] and Cristina Menni [1,*,†]

1. Department of Twin Research & Genetic Epidemiology, King's College London, St Thomas' Hospital Campus, Westminster Bridge Road, London SE1 7EH, UK; olatz.mompeo@kcl.ac.uk (O.M.); mateyhernandezm@gmail.com (M.M.H.); caroline.le_roy@kcl.ac.uk (C.L.R.); massimo.mangino@kcl.ac.uk (M.M.); Ana.Valdes@nottingham.ac.uk (A.M.V.)
2. Department of Nutritional Sciences, King's College London, Franklin-Wilkins Building, Stamford St, London SE1 9NH, UK; geoffrey.istas@gmail.com (G.I.); melanie.le_sayec@kcl.ac.uk (M.L.S.); ana.rodriguez-mateos@kcl.ac.uk (A.R.-M.)
3. NIHR Biomedical Research Centre at Guy's and St Thomas' Foundation Trust, London SE1 9RT, UK
4. Norwich Medical School, University of East Anglia, Norwich NR4 7TJ, UK; amy.jennings@uea.ac.uk
5. Academic Rheumatology, University of Nottingham, Hucknall Road, Nottingham NG5 1PB, UK

* Correspondence: tim.spector@kcl.ac.uk (T.D.S.); cristina.menni@kcl.ac.uk (C.M.)

† Equal contribution.

Abstract: Background: Polyphenol consumption is implicated in gut microbiome composition and improved metabolic outcomes, but it is unclear whether the effect is independent of dietary fiber. Methods: We investigated the links between (poly)phenol intake, gut microbiome composition (16s RNA) and obesity independently of fiber intake in UK women ($n = 1810$) and in a small group of UK men ($n = 64$). Results: (Poly)phenol intakes correlated with microbiome alpha diversity (Shannon Index) after adjusting for confounders and fiber intake. Moreover, flavonoid intake was significantly correlated with the abundance of *Veillonella*, (a genus known to improve physical performance), and stilbene intake with that of butyrate-producing bacteria (*Lachnospira* and *Faecalibacterium*). Stilbene and flavonoid intake also correlated with lower odds of prevalent obesity (*Stilbenes:* Odds Ratio (95% Confidence Interval) (OR(95%CI)) = 0.80 (0.73, 0.87), $p = 4.90 \times 10^{-7}$; *Flavonoids*: OR(95%CI) = 0.77 (0.65, 0.91), $p = 0.002$). Formal mediation analyses revealed that gut microbiome mediates ~11% of the total effect of flavonoid and stilbene intake on prevalent obesity. Conclusions: Our findings highlight the importance of (poly)phenol consumption for optimal human health.

Keywords: polyphenol intake; obesity; gut microbiome diversity; gut microbiome composition; fiber intake; stilbene intake; flavonoid intake

1. Introduction

Many of the gut microbiome's effects on health parameters are the result of microbes metabolising diverse compounds from our diet [1]. Dietary (poly)phenols, which include flavonoids (such as flavan-3-ols, flavonols, anthocyanins, flavanones, flavones and isoflavones) and non-flavonoids (such as stilbenes, ellagitannins, lignans and phenolic acids), are actively studied for their potential health benefits in chronic diseases, such as cardiovascular diseases (CVD) and age-related cognitive decline [2].

Common (poly)phenol-rich foods include fruits, berries, nuts, tea, cocoa products, coffee, vegetables, olive oil, soy products and red wine [3].

Studies have shown that diets based on a high intake of plant (poly)phenols and fermentable fibers alter microbial activities within the gut [4]. Indeed, the gut microbiome converts (poly)phenols and fibers into biologically active compounds, thereby regulating energy and lipids metabolism [5] with potential impact on metabolic diseases [6]. (Poly)phenols, for instance, exert a protective effect on vascular endothelial cells by preventing the oxidation of low-density lipoprotein [7]. In animal studies, supplementation with high concentrations of polyphenols inhibits the growth of detrimental species, such as *Clostridia* and *Enterobacteria*, and increases the abundance of Lactic acid bacteria and *Akkermansia* [8].

Small interventional studies have shown that (poly)phenol consumption (e.g., from wine, cocoa, tea, blueberries or aronia berries) results in increases in specific beneficial bacterial communities in the gut, particularly *Bifidobacterium*, *Lactobacillus* and *Anaerostipes* [9–13], while the relative abundance of *Bacteroides* increases in subjects consuming red wine or aronia berry (poly)phenols [10,13,14]. A recent study from our group found that red wine consumption was associated with an increase in gut microbial alpha diversity, potentially mediating host body mass index (BMI) reduction in two cohorts [15]. (Poly)phenols have also been implicated in the reduced abundance of pathogenic bacterial species in the gut microbiome. A study examining the antibacterial activity of fruit (poly)phenols found a high sensitivity to these compounds in the enteropathogens *Staphylococcus aureus* and *Salmonella typhimurium* [16], while reductions in pathogenic *Clostridium* species (*C. perfringens* and *C. histolyticum*) have been reported following consumption of fruit, seed, wine and tea polyphenols [17–20].

(Poly)phenols are well known antioxidants [21], and the pivotal role of oxidative stress as a key pathway in weight gain has been highlighted before [22]. It has therefore been hypothesized that both flavonoids, such as curcumin, and stilbenes such as resveratrol, have beneficial effects on adipose tissue by alleviating intracellular oxidative stress, reducing chronic low-grade inflammation, inhibiting adipogenesis and lipogenesis, and suppressing the differentiation of preadipocytes to mature adipocytes [23].

However, it is not clear whether polyphenols and fermentable fibers act in tandem (or synergistically) through the gut microbiota to improve different physiological processes linked to metabolic disease risk, or whether they have independent effects [4].

Here we assess the association between (poly)phenol intake, as measured by food frequency questionnaires (FFQs), and gut microbial diversity and abundances, independently of fiber intake (measured as non-starch polysaccharides) in a large-population cohort. We then investigate whether the gut microbiome mediates part of the benefits of (poly)phenols intake on obesity. This can help prioritize interventions.

2. Methods

2.1. Study Populations

Discovery cohort: The Discovery cohort included female twins enrolled in the TwinsUK registry, a national register of adult twins recruited as volunteers without selecting for any particular disease or traits [24]. Here we analyzed data from 1810 female twins aged 62.03 (Standard Deviation (SD) = 11.58), 71.4% of them post-menopausal, with 16s microbiome data and (poly)phenol intake measured within 1.59 (SD = 1.08) years (Table 1). A subset of 508 study participants also had concurrent fecal lactate measured by mass spec (Metabolon inc) [25]. The TwinsUK study was approved by St Thomas' Hospital Research Ethics Committee, and all twins provided written informed consent.

Table 1. Demographic characteristics of the study population.

Phenotype	TwinsUK	Aronia
n	1810	64
Females, *n* (%)	1810 (100%)	0
Post-Menopausal, *n* (%)	1287 (71.4%)	0
Hypertension, *n* (%)	601 (49.71%)	0
Obesity, *n* (%)	320 (17.68%)	0
Type 2 diabetes, *n* (%)	73 (4.33%)	0
	Mean (SD)	
Age, yrs	61.31 (11.27)	23.61 (0.59)
BMI, kg/m^2	25.83 (4.77)	22.77 (2.12)
Energy intake, kcal	1806.88 (527.45)	
Fiber intake, g/day	19.88 (7.26)	14.33 (6.94)
(Poly)phenol intake, mg/day		
Total (poly)phenol intake	1488.36 (585.19)	432.40 (421.55)
Flavonoids	724.68 (385.46)	NA
Lignans	85.70 (49.89)	NA
Phenolic acids	637.80 (491.36)	NA
Stilbenes	0.81 (0.96)	NA
Other (poly)phenols	39.37 (31.51)	NA
Measure of alpha diversity		
Shannon Diversity	5.16 (0.72)	2.61 (0.59)
Observed number OTUs	348.10 (102.23)	NA

Validation cohort: We also included a small validation cohort, the Aronia study, of 64 helthy male volunteers aged 18–45 y, recruited from King's College London and the nearby areas [13] (Table 1). This replication cohort was chosen given the very different pattern from polyphenol cohort, to enable assessing the generalizability of associations between gut microbiome and (poly)phenol intake. The study was a double blind randomized controlled trial, with the main aim of investigating the effects of aronia berries on vascular function and gut microbiota composition in a healthy population. The study was approved by King's College London Ethics Committee (HR-15/16–3739) and the trial was registered at clinicaltrials.gov as NCT03041961. The main findings of this study have been previously published [13]. For the purposes of this work, baseline clinical characteristics, dietary data on (poly)phenol and fiber intake, and 16s microbiome data are presented here.

(Poly)phenols and fiber intake: A validated 131-item semi-quantitative FFQ established for the European Prospective Investigations into Cancer and Nutrition (EPIC)-Norfolk study [26] was used to assess dietary intake in both the TwinsUK and the Aronia study. Estimated intakes of fiber (non-starch polysaccharides, in grams per day) were derived from the UK Nutrient Database [27] and were adjusted for energy intake using the residual method prior to analysis [28]. Estimated intakes of total (poly)phenols (in mg per day) were derived from the Phenol-Explorer Database [29]. The main sources of (poly)phenol intake are reported in Table S1.

Obesity: Measurements of weight and height were used to calculate body mass index (BMI), calculated as weight in kilograms divided by the square of height in meters. Participants were classified as obese if their BMI was greater than 30.

2.2. Microbiota Analysis

Gut microbiome composition was determined by sequencing of the 16s rRNA gene, as previously described [30]. Fecal samples were brought to clinical visit or posted in sealed ice packs and frozen at −80 °C, before being sent on dry ice to Cornell University where DNA was amplified. Amplicons were sequenced on an Illumina MiSeq platform and samples read. Paired ends were merged following demultiplexing. Operational taxonomic units(OTUs) were generated from the 16s rRNA gene sequencing and collapsed under taxonomic units at the genus level as previously described [31]. Residuals for genera were generated via regression against technical covariates including sequencing depth, sequencing run, sequencing technician and sample collection method. These residuals were inverse normalized, as they were not normally distributed, and used in downstream analyses. In order to calculate alpha diversity, the complete OTU count table was rarefied to 10,000 sequences per sample 50 times. Alpha diversity metrics were calculated for each sample in each of the rarefied tables, and final diversity measures taken as the mean score across all 50. Alpha diversities were quantified as observed OTU counts and Shannon diversity index. Alpha diversity indexes were standardized to have mean 0 and SD 1.

Regarding fecal samples from the Aronia study, gut microbiota composition was also determined via 16s RNA sequencing as previously described [13].

2.3. Availability of Data and Materials

16s sequencing data used for this study is deposited in the European Nucleotide Archive (ERP015317). All other TwinsUK data are available upon request on the department website.

2.4. Statistical Analysis

Statistical analysis was carried out using R studio version 3.5.1. We normalized measures of (poly)phenol intake by taking the log. We assessed the association between alpha diversity indexes (outcome) and measures of (poly)phenol intake (exposure) by using a linear mixed model with family as a random intercept, adjusting for age, BMI, dietary fiber and daily energy intake. Linear/logistic mixed models, adjusting for age, BMI, dietary fiber and daily energy intake, and family relatedness were also employed to investigate the association between (i) taxa (outcome: genus with an abundance > 0.001) and (poly)phenol intake (stilbenes/flavonoids—exposure), adjusting for multiple testing using false discovery rate (FDR < 0.05); and (ii) obesity and (poly)phenol (stilbenes/flavonoids—exposure) intake, adjusting for the aforementioned variables but BMI.

We further employed mediation analysis as implemented in the R package "mediation" [32] to test the mediation effects of Shannon diversity (indirect effect) on the total effect of (poly)phenol intake (stilbene/flavonoid) on obesity (BMI > 30 kg/m^2), adjusting for age, fiber, daily energy intake and family structure. We constructed a mediation model to quantify both the direct effect of (poly)phenols intake on obesity, and the indirect (mediated) effects mentioned above. The variance accounted for (VAF) score, which represents the ratio of indirect-to-total effect and determines the proportion of the variance explained by the mediation process, was further used to determine the significance of mediation effect [33].

3. Results

The demographic characteristics of the study population are presented in Table 1.

Correlations between dietary (poly)phenol intake and gut microbiome diversity and composition.

In 1810 female twins from the TwinsUK cohort, with microbiome data available and (poly)phenol intake from FFQs measured within 1.59 years (SD = 1.08), we find that both Shannon diversity and the number of observed OTUs were significantly associated with total (poly)phenol intake (*Shannon*: Beta (SE) = 0.19 (0.05), $p = 3.77 \times 10^{-4}$, *Observed number of OTUs*: 0.21 (0.05), $p = 2.99 \times 10^{-5}$), stilbene (*Shannon*: 0.06 (0.02), $p = 5.42 \times 10^{-5}$, *Observed number of OTUs*: 0.07 (0.01), $p = 6.51 \times 10^{-3}$) and flavonoid intake (*Shannon*: 0.09 (0.03), $p = 9.67 \times 10^{-3}$, *Observed number of OTUs*: 0.14 (0.03), $p = 2.31 \times 10^{-5}$) after adjusting for age, BMI, fiber intake, energy intake and family relatedness (Figure 1). We validated the association between Shannon diversity and total (poly)phenol intake, adjusting for fiber intake, age and BMI, in a small independent cohort of 64 men from the Aronia study [13] (Beta (SE) = 0.25 (0.11), $p = 0.02$).

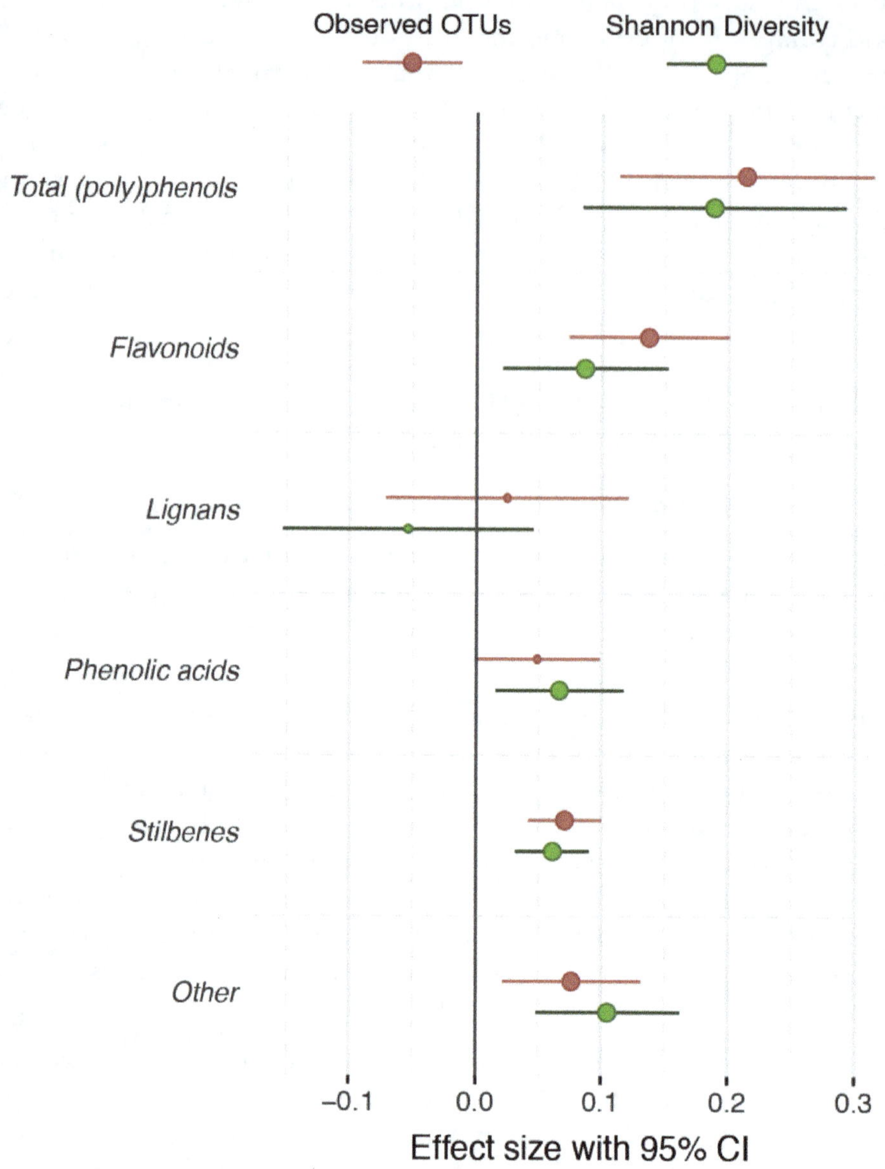

Figure 1. Dietary (poly)phenols and measures of gut microbiome alpha diversity in the TwinsUK cohort.

Analyses were adjusted by age, BMI, dietary fiber intake, total energy intake and family relatedness. CI indicates confidence interval.

We then examined, in the TwinsUK cohort, the association between stilbene and flavonoid intakes and bacterial abundances (genus with abundance > 0.001). We identified five genera significantly associated with stilbene intake and three genera associated with flavonoid intake, after adjusting for age, BMI, fiber intake, energy intake, family relatedness and multiple testing using FDR correction (FDR < 0.05) (Figure 2). These include (i) the positive correlation of flavonoid intake and *Veillonella* a performance-enhancing microbe that functions via its metabolic conversion of exercise-induced lactate into the short-chain fatty acid propionate [34], and (ii) the positive correlation of stilbene intake with some known butyrate-producing bacteria, such as *Lachnospira* and *Faecalibacterium*.

In addition, we found that *Veillonella* abundances were positively correlated with fecal abundance of lactate (Beta (SE) = 0.27 (0.04), $p = 1.45 \times 10^{-10}$) in TwinsUK.

Correlations between dietary stilbene and flavonoid intakes, obesity and gut microbiome diversity.

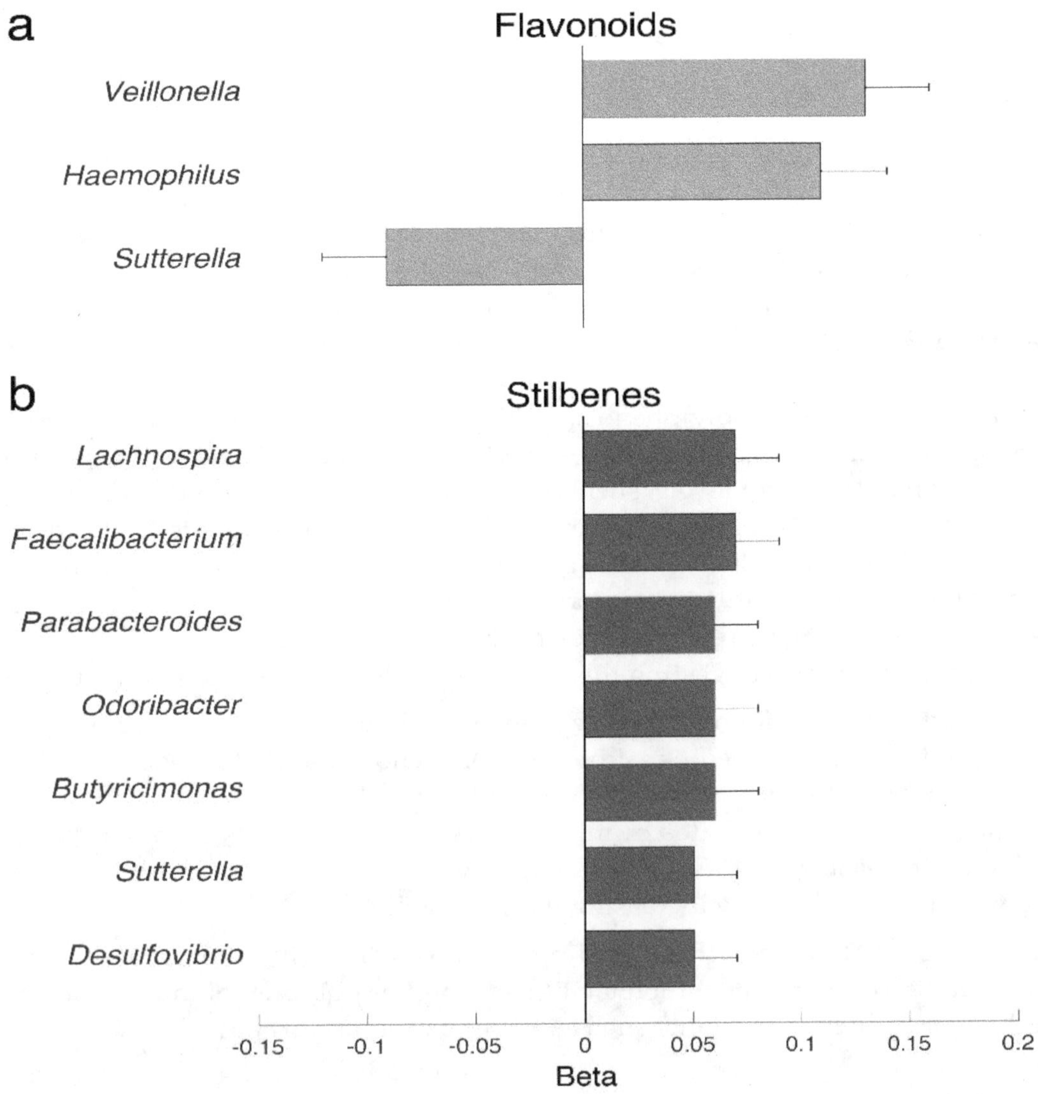

Figure 2. (**a**) Genus–flavonoid intake association. (**b**) Genus–stilbene intake association. Analyses are adjusted for age, BMI, fiber intake, energy intake and multiple testing (FDR < 0.05).

We next investigated, in the TwinsUK cohort, the associations between stilbene and flavonoid intake and obesity, adjusting for covariates, fiber intake and family structure. We found that both stilbene and flavonoid intake (in the log scale) were also associated with a significantly lower prevalence of obesity. (*Stilbenes*: OR(95%CI) = 0.80 (0.73,0.87), $p = 4.90 \times 10^{-7}$; *Flavonoids*: OR(95%CI) = 0.77 (0.65,0.91), $p = 0.002$) (Table 2).

Table 2. Obesity–(poly)phenol intake (stilbenes and flavonoids) association.

	Stilbenes			Flavonoids		
	OR	SE	*P*	OR	SE	*P*
Obesity	0.80	0.04	4.90×10^{-7}	0.77	0.07	0.002

Analyses are adjusted for age, fiber intake, total daily energy intake and family relatedness.

We therefore conducted a formal mediation analysis with TwinsUK to determine the indirect effect of the gut microbiome (Shannon index) on the relationship between (poly)phenol intake (stilbene- and flavonoid-high versus -low) and obesity. The analysis found that the Shannon diversity acted as a potential partial mediator in the negative association between stilbene intake and obesity (VAF

= 11.16% (8.13%, 16.66%) $p < 0.001$), and in the negative association between flavonoids intake and obesity (11.11% (4.71%, 93.80%)).

4. Discussion

In the largest study to date, we report that (poly)phenol intake, and particularly stilbenes and flavonoids, are associated with higher gut microbiota diversity and lower prevalence of obesity, independent of fiber intake. Furthermore, gut microbial diversity mediated the association between stilbene and flavonoid intakes and obesity. In addition, we identified a positive correlation between flavonoid intake and *Veillonella,* the energy-enhancing bacteria, and a positive association between stilbene intake and *Faecalibacterium,* a key marker of a healthy gut.

Stilbenes are non-flavonoid (poly)phenols, characterized by the presence of a 1,2-diphenylethylene nucleus in their structure, and include resveratrol and its derivatives [35]. They are present in different foods and plants at high levels, such as red grapes, red wine, some kinds of tea, berries and peanuts [36], though their levels are very low in foods overall. Because of this, the association between gut microbiome diversity and stilbene intake may be a marker of other factors, such as consumption of red wine and berries, which are also very rich in other (poly)phenols, such as anthocyanins and flavan-3-ols. However, when we repeated the analyses adjusting for anthocyanins and flavan-3-ols, the results remained the same, suggesting that the effect of stilbenes is independent.

Several small studies have found that polyphenols might be effective in preventing small increases in weight during periods of overfeeding, although there is no evidence for them reducing weight [37 Our finding of a 20–23% lower prevalence of obesity with higher intakes of total flavonoids and stilbenes, of which up to 11% is mediated by microbial diversity, highlights the public health importance of these results. By increasing the dietary intake of polyphenols, it may be possible to prevent some of the weight gain which is constantly increasing worldwide [38].

The intakes associated with these findings could be readily incorporated into the diet by encouraging a Mediterranean diet, which facilitates a higher polyphenol intake than the traditional western diet [39], or by including plants such as Hibiscus [21] as part of the diet.

The flavonoid class embraces the largest and most widely studied group of (poly)phenols, with a structure characterized by two phenyl rings and a heterocyclic ring. The main food sources of flavonoids in the TwinsUK cohort are tea, dark chocolate, cocoa and fruit (Table S1). Previous studies have suggested that (poly)phenols and fiber may provide complementary health benefits [40]. Only a small percentage (<10%) of the (poly)phenols ingested is absorbed in the small intestine. The rest accumulates in the lumen, and is subjected to the catabolic reactions of the gut microbial community, which breaks them down into a series of low molecular weight phenolic metabolites that, being absorbable, may be responsible for the health benefits of (poly)phenols [41].

According to current UK dietary guidelines, the recommended average fiber intake for adults is 30g per day [42]. However, though the dietary guidelines suggest that adults should consume five portions of fruits and vegetables per day [43], and though the newly published Cardiovascular disease risk Reduction (CRESSIDA) study shows that adherence to UK dietary guidelines is associated with higher dietary intake of total and specific (poly)phenols [44], there is no indication as to the amount of total and specific (poly)phenols that should be ingested. We found that (poly)phenols, and in particular stilbenes and flavonoids, are associated with microbiome diversity independently of fiber intake. Our results in both the TwinsUK and Aronia cohorts indicate that even moderate consumption of (poly)phenols in the diet may have a positive impact on gut microbiome diversity. As the range of (poly)phenols in fruits and vegetables is highly variable [45], our results could inform new guidelines for increasing awareness of the beneficial effects of (poly)phenol consumption. More importantly, our study highlights that different types of phenolic compounds have different links to gut microbiome composition, which may in turn have different effects on human health. Future studies are needed to look at more specific sub-classes of polyphenols, and the food sources of these polyphenols, as they will have structurally diverse polyphenol profiles, which is likely to lead to differing interactions with the gut microbiome.

In our exploratory study, we also report a link between flavonoid dietary intake and the abundance of *Veillonella*. A recent study by Schelman and coworkers [34] found that not only is the abundance of this bacterium linked to improved exercise performance, but that this is due to a transformation of lactate into propionate. Moreover, in our data, we find a significant positive association between *Veillonella* and the fecal abundance of lactate. The association between *Veillonella* and flavonoid intake then suggests one of the mechanisms whereby flavonoids may improve metabolic health, as up to certain doses, propionate is expected to improve energy metabolism. It also suggests that there may be scope for investigating the role of flavonoid supplementation or dietary interventions in improving athletic performance.

Another interesting aspect to come out of our study is the higher abundance of *Faecalibacterium* in individuals with higher stilbene intakes. *Faecalibacterium prausnitzii* is known to be a major butyrate producer [46], and it has been widely claimed that among the main benefits of prebiotic fibers, such as inulin, is the increase in butyrate production [47], a powerful anti-inflammatory and histone deacetylase regulator [48] shown to be protective against colon cancer [49]. This suggests that some of the health benefits commonly associated with stilbenes, such as resveratrol, may be due to their link to butyrate production, and this is an aspect that deserves further investigation.

We note some study limitations. First, we have used FFQs rather than other methods for assessing nutrient intake. FFQs have become a well-accepted method for the quantitative assessment of usual nutrient intake [50], but being recalled, the data are subject to some bias. However, the value of FFQs for assessing dietary composition has been documented objectively, by correlations with biochemical indicators and the prediction of outcomes in prospective studies [51,52]. Second, the discovery cohort was based on middle-aged white female twins. However, we replicated our main results in a small independent study of males, suggesting that the results are generalizable to both sexes. Thirdly, the cross-sectional and observational nature of this study does not allow us to determine causal relationships between (poly)phenol intake, gut microbiome composition and health, where ideally randomized control trials are needed. It does not allow us to understand some associations, which go in the opposite direction for flavonoids and stilbenes, such as the one with *Sutterellla*. Moreover, we here investigated the distinct impact of polyphenols on the microbiome using only bio-informatics tools. Additional investigations, involving diets with omitted polyphenols or dietary fibers, are recommended to validate the current findings. Further, an important future avenue for research will be investigating whether any of these interactions between (poly)phenols and gut microbes are different in men vs women, or young vs old, and if the type and amount of polyphenol intake can be optimized based on demographic considerations. On the other hand, we note several strengths, including the sample size of the study and the detailed clinical and molecular phenotyping of the study subjects, which has allowed us to test the relative contributions of (poly)phenol intake to metabolic phenotypes.

5. Conclusions

In conclusion, stilbene, flavonoid and total (poly)phenol intake was associated with higher gut microbiome diversity independently of fiber intake, suggesting that polyphenols provide complementary health benefits to fiber, and may be included in an expanded prebiotics group. Our results also suggest that gut microbiome diversity mediates the reverse association of (poly)phenols with obesity, increasing our understanding of how they interact with the gut microbiota. Our results indicate that the beneficial impact of (poly)phenol consumption on metabolic health may be partially driven by the interaction between the type of phenolic compound in the diet and the gut microbiota. Additional studies, including dietary intervention studies, exploring these associations in relation to health and diseases, are required to provide a sustainable basis for dietary recommendations.

Author Contributions: Conceptualization: T.D.S., A.M.V., C.M. Formal Analysis: O.M., M.M.H., C.M. Resources: C.L.R., G.I., M.L.S., M.M., A.J. Writing—Original Draft Preparation: O.M., A.R.-M., A.M.V., C.M. Writing—Review & Editing: T.D.S., C.L.R., M.M., A.J. All authors have read and agreed to the published version of the manuscript.

Acknowledgments: We thank all the participants for contributing and supporting our research.

References

1. Forkosh, E.; Ilan, Y. The heart-gut axis: New target for atherosclerosis and congestive heart failure therapy. *Open Hear.* **2019**, *6*, e000993. [CrossRef] [PubMed]
2. Del Rio, D.; Rodriguez-Mateos, A.; Spencer, J.P.; Tognolini, M.; Borges, G.; Crozier, A. Dietary (poly)phenolics in human health: Structures, bioavailability, and evidence of protective effects against chronic diseases. *Antioxid. Redox Signal.* **2012**, *18*, 1818–1892. [CrossRef] [PubMed]
3. Pérez-Jiménez, J.; Neveu, V.; Voß, F.; Scalbert, A. Identification of the 100 richest dietary sources of polyphenols: An application of the Phenol-Explorer database. *Eur. J. Clin. Nutr.* **2010**, *64*, S112–S120. [CrossRef]
4. Tuohy, K.; Fava, F.; Viola, R.E. 'The way to a man's heart is through his gut microbiota'—Dietary pro- and prebiotics for the management of cardiovascular risk. *Proc. Nutr. Soc.* **2014**, *73*, 172–185. [CrossRef]
5. Fava, F.; Lovegrove, J.A.; Gitau, R.; Jackson, K.G.; Tuohy, K.M. The gut microbiota and lipid metabolism: Implications for human health and coronary heart disease. *Curr. Med. Chem.* **2006**, *13*, 3005–3021.
6. Marques, F.Z.; Nelson, E.; Chu, P.-Y.; Horlock, D.; Fiedler, A.; Ziemann, M.; Tan, J.; Kuruppu, S.; Rajapakse, N.; El-Osta, A.; et al. High-Fiber Diet and Acetate Supplementation Change the Gut Microbiota and Prevent the Development of Hypertension and Heart Failure in Hypertensive Mice. *Circulation* **2017**, *135*, 964–977. [CrossRef]
7. Tuso, P.; Stoll, S.; Li, W.W. A Plant-Based Diet, Atherogenesis, and Coronary Artery Disease Prevention. *Perm. J.* **2015**, *19*, 62–67. [CrossRef] [PubMed]
8. Anhê, F.F.; Roy, D.; Pilon, G.; Dudonné, S.; Matamoros, S.; Varin, T.V.; Garofalo, C.; Moine, Q.; Desjardins, Y.; Levy, E.; et al. A polyphenol-rich cranberry extract protects from diet-induced obesity, insulin resistance and intestinal inflammation in association with increased Akkermansia spp. population in the gut microbiota of mice. *Gut* **2015**, *64*, 872–883. [CrossRef]
9. Tzounis, X.; Rodriguez-Mateos, A.; Vulevic, J.; Gibson, G.R.; Kwik-Uribe, C.; Spencer, J.P. Prebiotic evaluation of cocoa-derived flavanols in healthy humans by using a randomized, controlled, double-blind, crossover intervention study. *Am. J. Clin. Nutr.* **2010**, *93*, 62–72. [CrossRef]
10. Moreno-Indias, I.; Sánchez-Alcoholado, L.; Pérez-Martínez, P.; Andres-Lacueva, C.; Cardona, F.; Tinahones, F.J.; Queipo-Ortuño, M.I. Red wine polyphenols modulate fecal microbiota and reduce markers of the metabolic syndrome in obese patients. *Food Funct.* **2016**, *7*, 1775–1787. [CrossRef]
11. Rodriguez-Mateos, A.; Rendeiro, C.; Bergillos-Meca, T.; Tabatabaee, S.; George, T.; Heiss, C.; Spencer, J.P. Intake and time dependence of blueberry flavonoid–induced improvements in vascular function: A randomized, controlled, double-blind, crossover intervention study with mechanistic insights into biological activity. *Am. J. Clin. Nutr.* **2013**, *98*, 1179–1191. [CrossRef] [PubMed]
12. Rodriguez-Mateos, A.; Feliciano, R.; Boeres, A.; Weber, T.; Santos, C.; Ventura, M.R.; Heiss, C. Cranberry (poly)phenol metabolites correlate with improvements in vascular function: A double-blind, randomized, controlled, dose-response, crossover study. *Mol. Nutr. Food Res.* **2016**, *60*, 2130–2140. [CrossRef] [PubMed]
13. Istas, G.; Wood, E.; Le Sayec, M.; Rawlings, C.; Yoon, J.; Dandavate, V.; Cera, E.D.; Rampelli, S.; Costabile, A.; Fromentin, E.; et al. Effects of aronia berry (poly)phenols on vascular function and gut microbiota: A double-blind randomized controlled trial in adult men. *Am. J. Clin. Nutr.* **2019**, *110*, 316–329. [CrossRef] [PubMed]
14. Barroso, E.; Muñoz-Gonzalez, I.; Jiménez, E.; Bartolomé, B.; Moreno-Arribas, M.V.; Peláez, C.; Martínez-Cuesta, M.D.C.; Requena, T.; Martínez-Cuesta, M.C. Phylogenetic profile of gut microbiota in healthy adults after moderate intake of red wine. *Mol. Nutr. Food Res.* **2016**, *61*, 1600620. [CrossRef]
15. Le Roy, C.I.; Wells, P.M.; Si, J.; Raes, J.; Bell, J.T.; Spector, T.D. Red Wine Consumption Associated With Increased Gut Microbiota α-diversity in 3 Independent Cohorts. *Gastroenterology* **2020**, *158*, 270–272. [CrossRef]

16. Parkar, S.G.; Stevenson, D.E.; Skinner, M. The potential influence of fruit polyphenols on colonic microflora and human gut health. *Int. J. Food Microbiol.* **2008**, *124*, 295–298. [CrossRef]
17. Kemperman, R.; Gross, G.; Mondot, S.; Possemiers, S.; Marzorati, M.; Van De Wiele, T.; Dore, J.; Vaughan, E.E. Impact of polyphenols from black tea and red wine/grape juice on a gut model microbiome. *Food Res. Int.* **2013**, *53*, 659–669. [CrossRef]
18. Etxeberria, U.; Fernández-Quintela, A.; Milagro, F.I.; Aguirre, L.; Martínez, J.A.; Portillo, M.P. Impact of Polyphenols and Polyphenol-Rich Dietary Sources on Gut Microbiota Composition. *J. Agric. Food Chem.* **2013**, *61*, 9517–9533. [CrossRef]
19. Cardona, F.; Andres-Lacueva, C.; Tulipani, S.; Tinahones, F.J.; Queipo-Ortuño, M.I. Benefits of polyphenols on gut microbiota and implications in human health. *J. Nutr. Biochem.* **2013**, *24*, 1415–1422. [CrossRef]
20. Dueñas, M.; Muñoz-González, I.; Cueva, C.; Jiménez-Girón, A.; Sánchez-Patán, F.; Santos-Buelga, C.; Moreno-Arribas, M.V.; Bartolomé, B. A survey of modulation of gut microbiota by dietary polyphenols. *BioMed Res. Int.* **2015**, *2015*, 850902. [CrossRef]
21. Herranz-López, M.; Olivares-Vicente, M.; Encinar, J.A.; Barrajón-Catalán, E.; Segura-Carretero, A.; Joven, J.; Micol, V. Multi-Targeted Molecular Effects of Hibiscus sabdariffa Polyphenols: An Opportunity for a Global Approach to Obesity. *Nutrients* **2017**, *9*, 907. [CrossRef]
22. Menni, C.; Migaud, M.; Kastenmuller, G.; Pallister, T.; Zierer, J.; Peters, A.; Mohney, R.P.; Spector, T.D.; Bagnardi, V.; Gieger, C.; et al. Metabolomic Profiling of Long-Term Weight Change: Role of Oxidative Stress and Urate Levels in Weight Gain. *Obesity* **2017**, *25*, 1618–1624. [CrossRef]
23. Zhao, Y.; Chen, B.; Shen, J.; Wan, L.; Zhu, Y.; Yi, T.; Xiao, Z. The Beneficial Effects of Quercetin, Curcumin, and Resveratrol in Obesity. *Oxidative Med. Cell. Longev.* **2017**, *2017*, 1459497. [CrossRef]
24. Moayyeri, A.; Hammond, C.J.; Valdes, A.; Spector, T. Cohort Profile: TwinsUK and healthy ageing twin study. *Int. J. Epidemiol.* **2012**, *42*, 76–85. [CrossRef]
25. Zierer, J.; Jackson, M.A.; Kastenmüller, G.; Mangino, M.; Long, T.; Telenti, A.; Mohney, R.P.; Small, K.S.; Bell, J.T.; Steves, C.; et al. The fecal metabolome as a functional readout of the gut microbiome. *Nat. Genet.* **2018**, *50*, 790–795. [CrossRef]
26. Bingham, S.A.; Welch, A.A.; McTaggart, A.; Mulligan, A.A.; Runswick, S.A.; Luben, R.; Oakes, S.; Khaw, K.T.; Wareham, N.; Day, N.E. Nutritional methods in the European Prospective Investigation of Cancer in Norfolk. *Public Heal. Nutr.* **2001**, *4*, 847–858. [CrossRef]
27. Holland, B.; Welch, A.; Buss, D.H. *McCance and Widdowson's the Composition of Foods*; The Royal Society of Chemistry: Cambridge, UK, 1992.
28. Englyst, H.N.; Cummings, J.H. Improved Method for Measurement of Dietary Fiber as Non-Starch Polysaccharides in Plant Foods. *J. Assoc. Off. Anal. Chem.* **1988**, *71*, 808–814. [CrossRef]
29. Neveu, V.; Pérez-Jiménez, J.; Vos, F.; Crespy, V.; Du Chaffaut, L.; Mennen, L.; Knox, C.; Eisner, R.; Cruz, J.; Wishart, D.; et al. Phenol-Explorer: An online comprehensive database on polyphenol contents in foods. *Database* **2010**, *2010*, bap024. [CrossRef]
30. Goodrich, J.K.; Davenport, E.; Beaumont, M.; Jackson, M.A.; Knight, R.; Ober, C.; Spector, T.D.; Bell, J.T.; Clark, A.G.; Ley, R.E. Genetic Determinants of the Gut Microbiome in UK Twins. *Cell Host Microbe* **2016**, *19*, 731–743. [CrossRef]
31. Jackson, M.A.; Bell, J.T.; Spector, T.D.; Steves, C. A heritability-based comparison of methods used to cluster 16S rRNA gene sequences into operational taxonomic units. *PeerJ* **2016**, *4*, e2341. [CrossRef]
32. Imai, K.; Keele, L.; Tingley, D.; Yamamoto, T. Causal Mediation Analysis Using R. In *Advances in Social Science Research Using R.*; Vinod, H.D., Ed.; Springer: New York, NY, USA, 2010; pp. 129–154.
33. Tingley, D.; Yamamoto, T.; Hirose, K.; Keele, L.; Imai, K. Mediation: R Package for Causal Mediation Analysis. *J. Stat. Softw.* **2014**, *59*, 1–38. [CrossRef]
34. Scheiman, J.; Luber, J.M.; Chavkin, T.A.; MacDonald, T.; Tung, A.; Pham, L.-D.; Wibowo, M.C.; Wurth, R.C.; Punthambaker, S.; Tierney, B.T.; et al. Meta-omics analysis of elite athletes identifies a performance-enhancing microbe that functions via lactate metabolism. *Nat. Med.* **2019**, *25*, 1104–1109. [CrossRef]
35. Sirerol, J.A.; Rodríguez, M.L.; Mena, S.; Asensi, M.A.; Estrela, J.M.; Ortega, A.L. Role of natural stilbenes in the prevention of cancer. *Oxid. Med. Cell. Longev.* **2016**, *2016*, 3128951. [CrossRef]
36. Zamora-Ros, R.; Andres-Lacueva, C.; Lamuela-Raventós, R.M.; Berenguer-Llergo, A.; Jakszyn, P.; Martínez, C.;

Sanchez, M.J.; Navarro-Mateu, F.; Chirlaque, M.D.; Tormo, M.-J.; et al. Concentrations of resveratrol and derivatives in foods and estimation of dietary intake in a Spanish population: European Prospective Investigation into Cancer and Nutrition (EPIC)-Spain cohort. *Br. J. Nutr.* **2008**, *100*, 188–196. [CrossRef]

37. Farhat, G.; Drummond, S.; Al-Dujaili, E.A. Polyphenols and Their Role in Obesity Management: A Systematic Review of Randomized Clinical Trials. *Phytotherapy Res.* **2017**, *31*, 1005–1018. [CrossRef]
38. Ng, M.; Fleming, T.; Robinson, M.; Thomson, B.; Graetz, N.; Margono, C.; Mullany, E.C.; Biryukov, S.; Abbafati, C.; Abera, S.F.; et al. Global, regional, and national prevalence of overweight and obesity in children and adults during 1980-2013: A systematic analysis for the Global Burden of Disease Study 2013. *Lancet* **2014**, *384*, 766–781. [CrossRef]
39. Castro-Barquero, S.; Lamuela-Raventos, R.M.; Doménech, M.; Estruch, R. Relationship between Mediterranean Dietary Polyphenol Intake and Obesity. *Nutrients* **2018**, *10*, 1523. [CrossRef]
40. Edwards, C.A.; Havlik, J.; Cong, W.; Mullen, W.; Preston, T.; Morrison, D.J.; Combet, E. Polyphenols and health: Interactions between fibre, plant polyphenols and the gut microbiota. *Nutr. Bull.* **2017**, *42*, 356–360. [CrossRef]
41. Taguri, T.; Tanaka, T.; Kouno, I. Antimicrobial activity of 10 different plant polyphenols against bacteria causing food-borne disease. *Boil. Pharm. Bull.* **2004**, *27*, 1965–1969. [CrossRef]
42. Evans, C.E.L. Dietary fibre and cardiovascular health: A review of current evidence and policy. *Proc. Nutr. Soc.* **2020**, *79*, 61–67. [CrossRef]
43. Castiglione, C.; Mazzocchi, M. Ten years of five-a-day policy in the UK: Nutritional outcomes and environmental effects. *Ecol. Econ.* **2019**, *157*, 185–194. [CrossRef]
44. Castro-Acosta, M.L.; Sanders, T.; Reidlinger, D.P.; Darzi, J.; Hall, W.L. Adherence to UK dietary guidelines is associated with higher dietary intake of total and specific polyphenols compared with a traditional UK diet: Further analysis of data from the Cardiovascular risk REduction Study: Supported by an Integrated Dietary Approach (CRESSIDA) randomised controlled trial. *Br. J. Nutr.* **2018**, *121*, 402–415.
45. Knaze, V.; Rothwell, J.A.; Zamora-Ros, R.; Moskal, A.; Kyrø, C.; Jakszyn, P.; Skeie, G.; Weiderpass, E.; Santucci de Magistris, M.; Agnoli, C.; et al. A new food-composition database for 437 polyphenols in 19,899 raw and prepared foods used to estimate polyphenol intakes in adults from 10 European countries. *Am. J. Clin. Nutr.* **2018**, *108*, 517–524. [CrossRef]
46. Ferreira-Halder, C.V.; Faria, A.V.d.; Andrade, S.S. Action and function of Faecalibacterium prausnitzii in health and disease. *Best Pract. Res. Clin. Gastroenterol.* **2017**, *31*, 643–648. [CrossRef]
47. Holscher, H.D. Dietary fiber and prebiotics and the gastrointestinal microbiota. *Gut Microbes* **2017**, *8*, 172–184. [CrossRef]
48. Steliou, K.; Boosalis, M.S.; Perrine, S.P.; Sangerman, J.; Faller, D.V. Butyrate histone deacetylase inhibitors. *BioResearch Open Access* **2012**, *1*, 192–198. [CrossRef]
49. McNabney, S.M.; Henagan, T.M. Short chain fatty acids in the colon and peripheral tissues: A focus on butyrate, colon cancer, obesity and insulin resistance. *Nutrients* **2017**, *9*, 12. [CrossRef]
50. Sempos, C.T. Invited commentary: Some limitations of semiquantitative food frequency questionnaires. *Am. J. Epidemiol.* **1992**, *135*, 1127–1132. [CrossRef]
51. Willett, W.C.; Sampson, L.; Stampfer, M.J.; Rosner, B.; Bain, C.; Witschi, J.; Hennekens, C.H.; Speizer, F.E. Reproducibility and validity of a semiquantitative food frequency questionnaire. *Am. J. Epidemiol.* **1985**, *122*, 51–65. [CrossRef]
52. Pallister, T.; Jennings, A.; Mohney, R.P.; Yarand, D.; Mangino, M.; Cassidy, A.; MacGregor, A.; Spector, T.D.; Menni, C. Characterizing Blood Metabolomics Profiles Associated with Self-Reported Food Intakes in Female Twins. *PLoS ONE* **2016**, *11*, e0158568. [CrossRef]

3

Bioactive Compounds of Strawberry and Blueberry and their Potential Health Effects based on Human Intervention Studies

Katharina Miller [1], Walter Feucht [2] and Markus Schmid [1,*]

1 Faculty of Life Sciences, Albstadt-Sigmaringen University, Anton-Günther-Str. 51, 72488 Sigmaringen, Germany

2 Unit of Fruit Science, TUM School of Life Sciences Weihenstephan, Technical University of Munich, Dürnast 2, 85354 Freising, Germany

* Correspondence: schmid@hs-albsig.de

Abstract: Strawberries and blueberries are two of the most commonly consumed berries. Berries, in general, are characterized by their highly nutritive compounds, including minerals, vitamins, fatty acids, and dietary fiber, as well as their high content and wide diversity of bioactive compounds, such as phenolic compounds and organic acids. These bioactive compounds have been associated with protective effects against chronic diseases, such as cardiovascular disease, cancer, Alzheimer's and other disorders. In this paper 16 human intervention studies investigating the beneficial health effects of dietary strawberry or blueberry consumption on inflammation, cardiovascular disease or cognitive function and mental health are reviewed.

Keywords: anthocyanidins; polyphenols; berries; cardiovascular disease; inflammation

---

1. Introduction

Cardiovascular disease (CVD) is still the leading cause of death and disability in the world. CVDs describe numerous diseases involving the heart, brain, and blood vessels. Coronary heart disease (heart attack) and cerebrovascular disease (stroke) are two major CVDs caused by arteriosclerosis, the pathological process in the walls of blood vessels. In arteriosclerosis, deposits of fatty material and cholesterol (plaques) in blood vessels lead to narrow vessels and decreased blood flow. A blood clot can occur when the plaque ruptures. Depending on the place of development, in a coronary artery or in the brain, a blood clot can cause a heart attack or a stroke. The major metabolic risk factors for CVDs are overweight/obesity, raised blood pressure (hypertension), raised blood sugar (diabetes) and raised blood lipids (e.g., cholesterol). The occurrence and extent of these metabolic risk factors highly depend on behavioral risk factors like physical activity and diet. Overweight (BMI ≥ 25 kg/m^2) and obesity (BMI ≥ 30 kg/m^2) are the result of an imbalanced energy intake/usage and strongly related to the other metabolic risk factors. With increasing body mass index, the risk of coronary heart disease, ischaemic stroke, and type 2 diabetes mellitus increases [1].

A major contributing factor to the development, progression, and complication of chronic diseases, such as type 2 diabetes, CVD and Alzheimer's, is a sustained pro-inflammatory state. Inflammation is known as the common, protective, and temporary response of the innate immune system to pathogens and injury stimuli, characterized by the production of pro- and anti-inflammatory cytokines. Cytokines are small soluble proteins, which act as signals between immune cells to coordinate the inflammatory response. Among cytokines, interleukin 1β (IL-1 β), interleukin-6 (IL 6) and tumor necrosis factor-alpha (TNF-α) are commonly induced together and act as pro-inflammatory and alarm cytokines [2–4]. In addition to the production of TNF-a, IL-1 and IL-6, endothelial dysfunction, oxidative stress in vascular endothelial cells, macrophage accumulation and formation of inflammasome characterize the inflammatory process, leading to atherogenesis, the plaque forming process [5]. Other biomarkers of inflammatory status, which are measured in humans, are acute phase proteins (i.e., C-reactive protein (CRP), fibrinogen, serum amyloid A), chemokines (i.e., monocyte chemoattractant protein (MCP)-1) and adhesion molecules (i.e., E-selectin, P-selectin, sVCAM-1). In addition to classic inflammatory stimuli, acute inflammatory stress can be induced by a single energy-dense meal providing a surplus of readily available carbohydrates and fat. In the long term, poor diet can lead to obesity, which is known as a chronic, low-grade inflammatory state [4]. A chronic, low-grade inflammatory state can lead to, for instance, tissue damage, endothelial dysfunction, thrombosis, insulin resistance, and high blood pressure, which can result in cardiovascular disease, diabetes, some forms of cancer, arthritis, neurodegenerative diseases, and many others [6].

Over 350 million people worldwide are affected by a major depressive disorder. Impaired cognitive and executive function are two common symptoms of depression. Executive function describes cognitive processes such as working memory, planning, problem-solving, cognitive flexibility, inhibitory control, directing attention, thoughts and, therefore, behaviors. Depressive symptoms, such as negative self-perception and low mood, are believed to be maintained by impaired executive function via perseveration and rumination. Consumption of flavonoids is associated with a decreased risk of developing depression [7].

Berries are characterized by their highly nutritive compounds, including minerals, vitamins, fatty acids, and dietary fiber. They also contain high contents and wide diversity of nonessential biologically active components, such as organic acids or polyphenols, with their subclasses, tannins and flavonoids [3,4,8]. Anthocyanins, a subclass of flavonoids, are important bioactive compounds in berries, which are responsible for the red-blue-purple coloring of berries [3,4]. Bioactive compounds are believed to have the ability to provide and activate cellular antioxidant protection, scavenge free radicals, inhibit inflammatory gene expression, and consequently protect against oxidant-induced and inflammatory cell damage and cytotoxicity. Therefore, bioactive compounds have been associated with protective effects against chronic diseases, such as cardiovascular disease (CVD), cancer, Alzheimer's, depression, and other disorders [4,7–9].

Strawberries (*Fragaria*) and blueberries (*Vaccinium*) are two of the most demanded berries in fresh and frozen forms, as well as in processed and derived products like dried and canned forms, yogurts, beverages, jams, and jellies [3,10–13]. Numerous in vitro and in vivo studies demonstrated that amongst other foods strawberries and blueberries aid in providing and reducing the risk of developing several chronic diseases [2,13]. Strawberry and blueberry highly differ in the amount of different subclasses of bioactive compounds. The chemical compositions of strawberry and blueberry are compared in Table 1.

Table 1. Chemical composition of strawberry and blueberry [14].

	Strawberry	(Highbush) Blueberry
Flavonoids		
Anthocyanidins (mg/kg FW)	73.0	134
Flavanols (mg/kg FW)	9.1	1.1
Flavonols (mg/kg FW)	2.3	38.7
Phenolic acids		
Hydroxybenzoic acids (mg/kg FW)	5.7	1.5
Hydroxycinnamic acids (mg/kg FW)	7.1	135.0

Literature research was carried out in June 2018. To review most current research, google scholar and the database Food Science and Technology Abstracts (FSTA) were used to identify topic related articles published later than January 2011. The searches used the following terms and text words alone and in combination: "strawberry", "blueberry", "berries", "bioactive compounds", "health effects", "human intervention", "inflammation", "cardiovascular disease, "cognitive function" and "cancer".

In vitro studies, as well as in vivo studies conducted with animals, were excluded. In this paper 16 human intervention studies investigating the beneficial health effects of dietary strawberry or blueberry consumption are reviewed.

2. Strawberry

2.1. Composition

With about 60 mg per 100 g fresh fruit, strawberries are especially known for their high content of vitamin C. Strawberries also provide several other vitamins in lower extent, such as thiamine, riboflavin, niacin and vitamin B6 and contain fat-soluble vitamins, including carotenoids, vitamin A, vitamin E and vitamin K. Among fruits, strawberries are one of the richest natural folate sources (43 μg per 100 g fresh fruit) and show a remarkably high antioxidant activity. Strawberries are also a good source of manganese, iodine, magnesium, copper, iron, and phosphorus [3,15,16]. In addition, strawberries are rich in bioactive compounds, mainly represented by flavonoids, especially anthocyanidins, followed by phenolic acids like hydroxycinnamic, and hydroxybenzoic acids [14].

2.2. Inflammation

Seven clinical trials investigating the effects of strawberry intervention on inflammatory markers were identified. Among those seven studies, three tested postprandial effects and four long-term feeding effects on inflammation. Two studies were conducted with overweight participants, three with abdominally obese subjects, one with type two diabetic participants, and one with obese subjects with osteoarthritis.

In a cross-over design, the effect of strawberry antioxidants in beverage form on meal-induced postprandial inflammatory and insulin responses over a 6 h period has been investigated. Therefore, 24 overweight adults consumed a high-carbohydrate, moderate-fat meal, to increase markers of oxidative stress and insulin resistance, accompanied by either a single serving strawberry or a placebo beverage. The results showed a significant decrease in high sensitivity c-reactive protein (hs-CRP) and a reduction in postprandial insulin response (IL-6) by the strawberry beverage, but not by the placebo. No significant differences for plasminogen activator inhibitor (PAI)-1, IL-1 β and TNF- α concentrations were found among treatments [17]. In contrast, a similar study with the same 24 overweighed adults was conducted over six weeks and showed a significant attenuation of PAI-1 concentration and IL-1β response in the strawberry group, but no differences for platelet aggregation, hs-CRP, TNF-α, IL-6, insulin or glucose were found among treatments [18]. Despite a similar experimental set-up, Edirisinghe et al. [17] and Ellis et al. [18] reported different effects on postprandial PAI-1, IL-1β, IL-6, and hs-CRP concentrations by strawberry intake over different time periods. However, in both studies, an anti-inflammatory effect was found, though represented in a decrease of different biomarkers of inflammation.

On the other hand, two of the seven identified studies, conducted with abdominally obese subjects, observed no significant influence of strawberry consumption on tested inflammatory markers. In another 6-h postprandial study, 21 abdominally obese subjects with insulin resistance received a standard high-fat breakfast with one of four beverages containing 0, 10, 20 or 40 g freeze-dried strawberry (FDS). In this four-arm, placebo-controlled, 6-h postprandial, crossover study, Park et al. reported some effects on CVD related biomarker, as described in Section 2.3, but no influence on the measured inflammatory biomarker IL-6 was found [19]. In a seven-week double-blind, randomized, cross-over trial, 20 obese subjects received a prepared diet and either the strawberry powder (equivalent to four servings of 80 g frozen strawberry) or a placebo in form of a beverage. Zunino et al. reported no influence on cytokine concentrations of IL-1 β, IL-6, and TNF-α in the clinical trial [20]. The two studies of this section, showing no significant effects on inflammatory markers, primally investigated the effect of strawberry intervention on CVD and are therefore also listed in Section 2.3.

Basu et al. [21] (also listed in Section 2.3), Moazen et al. [22] and Shell et al. [23] reported anti-inflammatory effects of strawberry consumption in subjects with type II diabetes mellitus and obese subjects with osteoarthritis or elevated serum lipids. In a 12-week randomized, dose-response controlled trial, 60 subjects with abdominal adiposity and elevated serum lipids were assigned to consume one of four beverages: a low or high dose FDS beverage (25 g/day or 50 g/day) or a low or high dose calorie- and fiber-matched beverage. No effects on hs-CRP and adhesion molecules were observed among treatments. A significant decrease in serum malondialdehyde, a biomarker for oxidative stress, was found by both FDS-groups compared to control groups [21]. Thirty-six subjects with type II diabetes mellitus daily consumed either 50 g FDS beverage or a matched placebo beverage in a randomized, double-blind, controlled trial for six weeks. The results showed a significant increase of markers of total serum antioxidant status while serum malondialdehyde, glycated hemoglobin (Hb)A1c and hs-CRP concentrations significantly decreased. Serum glucose concentrations and anthropometric indices did not change significantly [22]. In double-blind crossover study 17 obese adults with osteoarthritis were randomly assigned to consume either an FDS beverage (50 g/day) or a control beverage daily for 12 weeks, respectively, with a two-week washout phase in between, to examine the effects of dietary strawberries on pain, markers of inflammation and quality of life indicators. The study showed a decrease in IL-6, IL-1, and matrix metalloproteinase, which are serum biomarkers of inflammation and cartilage degradation, after FDS beverage, but not after control beverage consumption. Moreover, constant, intermittent, and total pain were only significantly reduced by the FDS beverage consumption, but no differences for hs-CRP, nitrite, glucose, and lipid profiles were found [23].

Collectively, in five out of seven studies, an anti-inflammatory effect was presented by a decrease in some cytokine or acute phase protein concentrations or a decrease in oxidative stress. In two studies, no significant anti-inflammatory effect was observed.

2.3. Cardiovascular Disease

Several intervention studies provide a suggestion that berry fruit consumption has significant potential in the prevention and treatment of most risk factors mentioned above [6]. Coherent to the studies presented in Section 2.2, five human intervention studies investigating the effect of strawberry consumption on CVD-related markers were identified. Among those five studies, four were conducted with abdominal obese subjects and one with postmenopausal women. The major metabolic risk factors for CVDs are overweight/obesity, raised blood pressure (hypertension), raised blood sugar (diabetes), and raised blood lipids (e.g., cholesterol). Biomarkers for CVD, which are measured in humans, are, i.e., systolic and diastolic blood pressure, insulin, and glucose concentrations, distribution and size of blood lipids and antioxidant markers like plasma antioxidant capacity, whole blood glutathione, superoxide dismutase levels and serum catalase activity.

In addition to the results presented in Section 2.2, Park et al. reported a significant reduction in postprandial plasma insulin concentrations, insulin:glucose ratio, and rate of glucose and insulin increase in 21 abdominally obese subjects with insulin resistance, receiving a 40 g FDS beverage. A significant reduction in oxidized low-density lipoprotein was shown by the 20 g FDS beverage compared to all other beverages [19]. In addition to IL-1 β, IL-6, TNF-α concentrations, the seven-week double-blind, randomized, cross-over trial with 20 obese subjects, receiving a prepared diet and either the strawberry powder (equivalent to four servings of 80 g frozen strawberry) or a placebo observed no differences in blood pressure and medium and large HDL-cholesterol particles. However, a reduction in plasma concentrations of small HDL particles and small HDL-cholesterol, as well as an increase in LDL particle size was observed after the three-week strawberry intervention, but not the placebo intervention [20]. LDL and HDL particle distribution and size have been linked in previous studies to health status, in detail, to the metabolic syndrome and insulin resistance [20,24–26].

In a 12-week randomized, dose-response controlled trial, 60 subjects with abdominal adiposity and elevated serum lipids were assigned to consume one of four beverages: a low or high dose FDS beverage (25 g/day or 50 g/day) or a low or high dose calorie- and fiber-matched beverage. The results showed a significant reduction in serum total and LDL-cholesterol, and NMR-derived small LDL particles by the high FDS-dose compared to the low FDS-dose and the placebo beverages. No effects on any measures of adiposity, blood pressure, glycemia, and serum concentrations of HDL cholesterol and triglycerides were found [21]. In a similar study with the same experimental setup, Basu et al. reported a significant increase in plasma antioxidant capacity and whole blood glutathione at the end of the intervention by both FDS doses vs. controls. Other than the plasma antioxidant capacity, blood glutathione was significantly higher in the HD-FDS versus LD-FDS. Serum catalase activity was increased only in the LD-FDS compared to the controls. No effects on glutathione peroxidase and glutathione reductase enzyme activities, plasma copper, iron, selenium, and zinc, which also play an important role in antioxidant and pro-oxidant activities, were shown [27].

In an eight-week, randomized, double-blind, placebo-controlled, parallel intervention 60 postmenopausal women were either assigned to consume one of three beverages twice a day containing in total 0 g, 25 g or 50 g FDS. A decrease of systolic blood pressure and brachial- and femoral-ankle pulse wave velocity, a measured marker for arterial stiffness, was shown by 25 g FDS beverage compared to baseline but not to the other groups. An increase of plasma nitric oxide metabolite levels was shown by the 50 g FDS beverage but not the other beverages. In all three groups (0 g, 25 g or 50 g FDS) serum levels of superoxide dismutase increased at four weeks returning to baseline levels at eight weeks. No significant effect on diastolic blood pressure and metabolites were observed in all groups [28].

Collectively, the effect of strawberry consumption on cardiovascular disease has been examined in five intervention studies. Park et al. [19] and Basu et al. [27] reported anti-oxidant effects and Zunino et al. [20] and Basu et al. [21] reported some positive effects on distribution and size of blood lipids of strawberry consumption in obese subjects. In 60 postmenopausal women, a decrease in systolic blood pressure, arterial stiffness, and antioxidant effects were reported after eight-week strawberry intervention [28].

2.4. *Cognitive Function and Mental Health*

No studies investigating the effect of strawberry intervention on cognitive functions were identified during literature research.

3. Blueberry

3.1. *Composition*

Blueberries are nutritious fruits, as they are high in dietary fibers (3–3.5% of their fruit weight) and antioxidants, such as vitamin C, B complex, E, and A. Blueberries also provide high amounts of selenium, zinc, iron, and manganese and contain b-carotene, lutein, and zeaxanthin [9,12,13,29]. In addition, blueberries are rich in bioactive compounds, mainly represented by flavonoids, especially anthocyanidins and flavonols, as well as by phenolic acids like hydroxycinnamic acids [14].

3.2. *Inflammation*

Three clinical trials investigating the effects of blueberry intervention on markers, which are associated with inflammation, were identified. One study was conducted with subjects with metabolic syndrome, one with males with cardiovascular risk factors and one with women with at least two risk factors for type 2 diabetes.

In a double-blind, placebo-controlled study, 44 subjects with metabolic syndrome, consumed either a blueberry smoothie (yogurt and a milk-based smoothie with 22.5 g of freeze-dried blueberry powder added) or a placebo smoothie (identical smoothie without the blueberry powder) twice a day for six weeks. In the blueberry group, the endothelial function, expressed as reactive hyperemia index, was improved significantly more versus the placebo group [30]. On the other hand, no significant differences for markers of endothelial function and total plasma nitric oxide and soluble vascular adhesion molecule-were detected in a six-week randomized, placebo-controlled, crossover intervention with 18 male volunteers with cardiovascular risk factors receiving a wild blueberry drink (25 g freeze-dried powder, providing 375 mg of ACNs) or a placebo drink. However, in contrast to the placebo drink intake, the wild blueberry drink intake significantly reduced the levels of endogenously oxidized DNA bases, and the levels of H_2O_2-induced DNA damage in this study [31]. No influence on inflammatory markers, adhesion molecules, oxidative stress, and endothelial function were found in a single-blind, randomized, placebo-controlled, crossover design trial, 19 women with at least two risk factors for type 2 diabetes, who consumed 240 mL of wild blueberry juice or a placebo beverage for seven days [32].

Whereas Stull et al. [30] demonstrated an improvement in endothelial function after six-weeks blueberry consumption, Riso et al. [31] and Stote et al. [32] reported no significant influence on endothelial function and other inflammatory-related markers, with the exception of an antioxidant effect. The absence of an effect of blueberry intervention on inflammation studied by Stote et al. [32] could be based on the comparatively short intervention period of one week. Whereas Stull et al. and Riso et al. both conducted clinical trials over six weeks, the 44 subjects with metabolic syndrome received 45 g of freeze-dried blueberry powder per day (2 × 22.5 g) [30] and the 18 male subjects with cardiovascular risk factors received 25 g freeze-dried wild blueberry powder per day [31]. The different dose and type of blueberry powder intake, providing different amounts of bioactive compounds, could relate to the influence on endothelial function.

3.3. *Cardiovascular Disease*

In addition to markers of inflammation, the three clinical trials examined in Section 3.2 also investigated the influence of blueberry intervention on other CVD related markers like blood pressure, blood lipids, insulin sensitivity, etc. In addition to those three studies, a fourth study, conducted with postmenopausal women with pre- and stage 1- hypertension, has been identified for this section.

Besides the improvement of endothelial function in 44 subjects with metabolic syndrome consuming 22.5 g freeze-dried blueberry powder twice a day over six weeks, Stull et al. reported no difference in blood pressure and insulin sensitivity between the blueberry and placebo groups [30]. No influence on blood pressure (systolic and diastolic), as well as Framingham reactive hyperemia index and augmentation index were also found by Riso et al., where 18 male subjects with cardiovascular risk factors consumed 25 g wild blueberry freeze-dried powder for six weeks [31]. Stote et al. observed a trend for lowering systolic blood pressure and increased serum concentrations of nitrates and nitrites, an index of nitric oxide production, in 19 women with at least two risk factors for type 2 diabetes after one week 240 mL of wild blueberry juice. No significant changes in glucose, insulin, insulin sensitivity, triglycerides or blood pressure were detected [32]. In an eight-week, randomized, double-blind, placebo-controlled clinical trial, 48 postmenopausal women with pre- and stage 1- hypertension were randomly assigned to receive either 22 g freeze-dried blueberry powder or 22 g control powder in the form of a 480 mL drink. At the end of the intervention systolic blood pressure, diastolic blood pressure and brachial-ankle pulse wave velocity were significantly lower and Nitric oxide levels greater in the blueberry powder group compared with baseline values, whereas there were no changes in the group receiving the control powder [33].

In conclusion, these four intervention studies documented partially contrary findings on the effect of blueberry consumption on blood pressure, insulin sensitivity and oxidative stress. Three of four investigated clinical trials showed no significant effects of blueberry consumption on measured CVD related markers. Other than Stull et al. [30], Riso et al. [31] (six-week periods) and Stote et al. [32] (one-week period), Johnson et al. [33] reported a significant decrease in systolic and diastolic blood pressure after eight-week daily blueberry consumption.

3.4. *Cognitive Function and Mental Health*

Relating to epidemiological evidence, the consumption of flavonoids is associated with a decreased risk of developing depression, an attenuated rate of cognitive decline, and a reduced risk of dementia [7,34]. Three studies investigating the effects of blueberry intervention on cognitive function or mental health were identified. Two studies were conducted with healthy older adults and one with healthy young adults and children.

Two randomized, double-blind, placebo-controlled trials with twenty-one young adults (age: 20.1 ± 1.0 years) and fifty-two children (age: 8.2 ± 1.0 years) showed that the blueberry intervention (30 g freeze-dried wild blueberry with 30 mL low-flavonoid Rocks Orange Squash and 220 mL of water) increased post-consumption positive affect scores but had no effect on negative affect scores (PANS-NOW and PANS-C) compared to placebo intervention. There was also a significant main effect of session reduction of negative affect scores after both blueberry and placebo consumption [7]. Bowtell et al. investigated whether blueberry consumption improved brain perfusion, task-related activation, and cognitive function. Favorable effects on cerebrovascular and cognitive function in healthy older adults were shown in a randomized, double-blind, placebo-controlled trial after 12 weeks of blueberry concentrate supplementation (30 mL/day containing 387 mg anthocyanidins per day). Specifically, brain activation responses in several task related different areas and resting-state perfusion in the gray matter of the parietal and occipital lobes increased from baseline levels after 12 weeks of blueberry supplementation but not after placebo supplementation. A significant decrease in serum glutathione concentration was found in blueberry and placebo supplementation. No significant differences between the groups and no significant changes to baseline were found in brain activity, resting state perfusion in the frontal lobes, protein carbonylation HNE adduct or malonaldehyde formation and serum hs-CRP or BDNF concentration [34]. In a randomized, double-blind, placebo-controlled trial, 37 participants were asked to consume either freeze-dried blueberry beverage (24 g/day FDB, equivalent to one cup of fresh blueberries) or a blueberry placebo beverage for 90 days. Participants in the blueberry group showed significantly fewer repetition errors in a learning test and reduced switch cost in a task-switching test across study visits, relative to controls, but no improvement was observed in gait or balance. Moreover, in this study, no significant effect of blueberry consumption was observed on either the Geriatric Depression Scale or the Profile of Mood States [35].

The effect of blueberry consumption on cognitive function and mental health has been investigated in three studies. Whereas Miller et al. [35] reported no significant effect on the mood of the participants, Khalid et al. [7] reported a positive effect on the mood of both subject groups, referring to better positive affect scores. In contrast to the post consumption effect observed by Khalid et al., no long-term effect on mood was observed by Miller et al. after 45- and 90-days blueberry intervention. Bowtell et al. and Miller et al. also reported positive effects on cognitive function, referring to improvement in several tests.

4. Final Remarks

Strawberries (*Fragaria*) and Blueberries (*Vaccinium*) contain a wide variety of bioactive compounds, including many antioxidants with specific biochemical functions and beneficial health effects. The beneficial health effects are associated as protective effects against chronic diseases, such as cardiovascular disease, cancer, Alzheimer's and other disorders. In this paper, nine studies investigating the effects of strawberry intervention and seven studies investigating the effect of blueberry intervention on inflammation, cardiovascular disease and cognitive function and mental health have been reviewed. The intervention type, the characteristics of participants, the format of berry and placebo consumption, the dose of berries and the main findings of the sixteen reviewed studies are summarized in Tables 2 and 3

Table 2. Effect of strawberry consumption on inflammation, cardiovascular disease and metabolic syndrome.

Intervention	Subjects	Format	Dose/day	Main findings	References
Post-prandial, randomized, single-blind, placebo-controlled, cross-over intervention	24 overweight males and females (BMI: 29.2 ± 2.3 kg/m^2; age: 50.9 ± 15.0 year)	High-carbohydrate, moderate-fat meal + Berry group: Strawberry powder, water-based beverage Control group: Placebo drink	10 g powder	1. Attenuation of the postprandial inflammatory response 2. Reduction in postprandial insulin response 3. No differences for PAL-1, IL-1β and TNF-α	[17]
6-week, randomized, single-blind, placebo-controlled, parallel intervention + post-prandial high carbohydrates fat meal	24 overweight and obese males and females (BMI: 29.2 ± 2.3 kg/m^2; age: 50.9 ± 15.0 year)	High-carbohydrate, moderate-fat meal + Berry group: Strawberry powder, water-based beverage Control group: Placebo powder, water-based beverage	10 g powder	1. Attenuation of the postprandial PAL-1 concentration and IL-1β response 2. No differences for platelet aggregation, hsCRP, TNF-α, insulin or glucose	[18]
Post-prandial, randomized, controlled, 4-arm, crossover intervention	21 males and females with abdominal obesity and insulin resistance (BMI 40.2 ± 7.2 kg/m^2; age 39.8 ± 13.8 year)	High-fat breakfast + freeze-dried strawberry powder, beverage	Berry group: Group 1: 10 g Group 2: 20 g Group 3: 40 g Control group: 0 g powder (10 g powder is equivalent to 110 g fresh strawberries)	1. Reduction in postprandial plasma insulin concentrations, insulin: glucose ratio, and rate of glucose and insulin increase by 40 g FDS 2. Reduction in Oxidized low-density lipoprotein by 20 g FDS 3. IL-6 was not different among treatments	[19]
7-week, randomized, double-blind, placebo-controlled, cross-over intervention	20 obese males and females (13 Females: BMI, 35.6 ± 3.0 kg/m^2; age, 31.8 ± 11.4 year; 7 Males: BMI, 32.3 ± 2.1 kg/m^2; age, 29.4 ± 6.6 year)	Berry group: Strawberry powder, water-based beverage Control group: Placebo powder, water-based beverage	Powder equivalent to 320 g frozen strawberries	1. Reduction in serum cholesterol, small HDL particles, small HDL-cholesterol and Na and CO_2 concentrations in the blood 2. Increase in mean particle size of LDL 3. No difference in blood pressure	[20]
12-week, randomized, controlled, parallel intervention	60 males and females with abdominal adiposity and elevated serum lipids LD-FDS: 15 subjects (BMI, 34.5 ± 4.4 kg/m^2; age, 50 ± 10 year) HD-FDS: 15 subjects (BMI, 38.0 ± 7.1 kg/m^2; age, 49 ± 11 year) LD-C: 15 subjects (BMI, 37.0 ± 4.4 kg/m^2; age, 48 ± 10 year) HD-C: 15 subjects (BMI, 35.0 ± 5.2 kg/m^2; age 48 ± 10 year)	Berry group: Freeze-dried strawberry powder, water-based beverage Control group: Placebo powder, calorie- and fiber-matched water-based beverage	Berry group: Group 1 (LD-FDS): 25 g (equivalent to 250 g fresh strawberries); Group 2 (HD-FDS): 50 g (equivalent to 500 g fresh strawberries)	1. Reduction in serum total and LDL-cholesterol, and NMR-derived small LDL particles by HD-FDS 2. Increase in Serum catalase activity by LD-FDS 3. Decrease in serum malondialdehyde by LD-FDS and HD-FDS 4. No effects on adiposity, blood pressure, glycemia, and serum concentrations of HDL cholesterol and triglycerides, C-reactive protein and adhesion molecules	[21]
6-week, randomized, double-blind, placebo-controlled, parallel intervention	36 males and females with type 2 diabetes (berry group: n = 19; BMI, 27.36 ± 4.23 kg/m^2; age 51.9 ± 8.2 year; control group: n = 17; BMI, 28.58 ± 4.7 kg/m^2; age 51.1 ± 13.8 year)	Berry group: Freeze-dried strawberry powder, water-based beverage Control group: Iso-caloric drink with strawberry flavoring	50 g powder	1. Increase of total serum antioxidant status 2. Decrease of serum malondialdehyde, glycated hemoglobin HbA1c, and hs-CRP concentrations 3. No effects on serum glucose concentrations and anthropometric indices	[22]
12-week, randomized, double-blind, placebo-controlled, cross-over intervention	17 males and females with radiographic evidence of knee OA (BMI: 39.1 ± 1.5 kg/m^2; age: 57 ± 7 year)	Berry group: Freeze-dried strawberry powder, water-based beverage Control group: Placebo powder, water-based beverage	2 × 50 g powder	1. Decrease in interleukin (IL)-6, IL-1 and matrix metalloproteinase 2. Reduction in constant, intermittent, and total pain 3. No differences for hs-CRP, nitrite, glucose, and lipid profiles	[23]

Table 2. *Cont.*

Intervention	Subjects	Format	Dose/day	Main findings	References
12-week, randomized, controlled, parallel intervention	60 males and females with abdominal adiposity and elevated serum lipids (Age and BMI of subjects are identical to those in [21])	Berry group: Freeze-dried strawberry powder, water-based beverage Control group: Placebo powder, calorie- and fiber-matched water-based beverage	Berry group: Group 1 (LD-FDS): 25 g (equivalent to 250 g fresh strawberries); Group 2 (HD-FDS): 50 g (equivalent to 500 g fresh strawberries)	1. Increase in plasma antioxidant capacity 2. Increase in whole blood glutathione by LD-FDS and much higher by HD-FDS 3. No effects on glutathione peroxidase and glutathione reductase enzyme activities, plasma copper, iron, selenium and zinc	[27]
8-week, randomized, double-blind, placebo-controlled, parallel intervention	60 postmenopausal women (berry group 25 g FDS: n = 20; BMI, 31.0 ± 1.0 kg/m^2; age 61 ± 1 year; 50 g FDS: n = 20; BMI, 32.7 ± 1.1 kg/m^2; age 59 ± 1 year; control group: n = 20; BMI, 32.1 ± 0.7 kg/m^2; age 58 ± 1 year)	Berry groups: Freeze-dried strawberry powder, water-based beverage Control group: Iso-caloric drink with strawberry flavoring	Berry group: Group 1: 2 × 25 g FDS (equivalent to three cups of sliced fresh strawberries); Group 2: 25 g FDS + 25 g placebo powder (equivalent to 1.5 cups of sliced fresh strawberries)	1. Decrease of systolic BP and brachial- and femoral-ankle pulse wave velocity by 25 g FDS 2. Increase of plasma nitric oxide metabolite levels by 50 g FDS 3. No effect on diastolic blood pressure and metabolites	[28]

Table 3. Effect of blueberry consumption on cardiovascular disease, metabolic syndrome, cognitive function, mood and associated risk factors.

Intervention	Subjects	Format	Dose/day	Main findings	References
6-week randomized, double-blind, placebo-controlled, parallel intervention	44 males and females with metabolic syndrome (Blueberry group: BMI 35.2 ± 0.8 kg/m^2; age 55 ± 2 year; Control group: BMI 36.0 ± 1.1 kg/m^2; age 59 ± 2 year)	Berry group: Blueberry powder, Smoothie Control group: Identical smoothie without blueberry bioactives	45 g powder	1. Improved reactive hyperemia index (endothiel function) 2. No difference in blood pressure and insulin sensitivity	[30]
6-week, randomized, placebo-controlled, crossover intervention	18 males with CVD risk factors (BMI 24.8 ± 2.6 kg/m^2; age 47.8 ± 9.7 year)	Berry group: Wild blueberry (WB) powder, water-based beverage Control group: Placebo drink	25 g powder (equivalent to 148 g fresh wild blueberry)	1. Reduction of levels of endogenously oxidized DNA bases and levels of H2O2-induced DNA damage 2. No significant differences for markers of endothelial function and the other variables	[31]
1-week, randomized, single-blind, placebo-controlled, crossover intervention	19 females with at least two risk factors for type 2 diabetes (BMI: 31.4 ± 2.9 kg/m^2, age: 53 ± 6.3 year)	Berry group: Wild blueberry juice Control group: Placebo beverage	240 mL juice	1. Trend for lowering systolic blood pressure and increased serum concentrations of nitrates and nitrites 2. No changes in glucose, insulin, insulin sensitivity, triglycerides, inflammatory markers, adhesion molecules, oxidative stress, endothelial function or blood pressure	[32]
8-week, randomized, double-blind, placebo-controlled, parallel intervention	48 postmenopausal women with pre- and stage 1-hypertension (Blueberry group: BMI 30.1 ± 5.94 kg/m^2; age 59.7 ± 4.58 year; Control group: BMI 32.7 ± 6.79 kg/m^2; age 57.3 ± 4.76 year)	Berry group: Freeze-dried blueberry powder, water-based beverage Control group: Placebo drink	22 g powder (equivalent to one fresh cup blueberries)	1. Decrease in systolic blood pressure, diastolic blood pressure and brachial-ankle pulse wave velocity 2. Increase in Nitric oxide levels	[33]

Table 3. *Cont.*

Intervention	Subjects	Format	Dose/day	Main findings	References
1: Randomized, double-blind, placebo-controlled, crossover intervention 2: Randomized, double-blind, placebo-controlled intervention	1:21 males and females (age: 20.1 ± 1.0) 2:52 males and females (age: 8.2 ± 1.0)	Berry group: Freeze-dried WB powder + low-flavonoid Rocks Orange Squash, water-based beverage Control group: Vitamin C and sugar matched placebo drink + 30 mL low-flavonoid Rocks Orange Squash, water-based beverage	30 g powder 30 mL Orange Squash	1. Increase in post-consumption positive affect score 2. No effect on negative affect score 3. Session reduction of NA after both blueberry and placebo consumption	[7]
12-week, randomized, double-blind, placebo-controlled intervention	26 males and females(Blueberry group: BMI 25.9 ± 3.3 kg/m^2, age 67.5 ± 3.0 year; Control group: BMI 27.1 ± 4.0 kg/m^2, age 69.0 ± 3.3 year)	Berry group: Blueberry concentrate Control group: Placebo concentrate	30 mL concentrate (providing 387 mg anthocyanidins)	1. Increase in brain activation responses and resting-state perfusion in the gray matter of the parietal and occipital lobes 2. Decrease in serum glutathione concentration 3. No differences in brain activity, resting state perfusion in the frontal lobes, protein carbonylation HNE adduct or malonaldehyde formation and serum hsCRP or BDNF concentration	[34]
90 days, randomized, double-blind, placebo-controlled intervention	37 males and females with English fluency, ability to walk 20 min unassisted, and >12 months postmenopausal (Blueberry group: BMI 24.1 ± 3.7, age 67.8 ± 4.6 year, Placebo group: BMI 24.0 ± 2.5, age 67.3 ± 4.8 year)	Berry group: Freeze-dried blueberry powder Control group: Placebo powder	24 g powder (equivalent to one cup of fresh blueberries)	1. Decrease in repetition errors and reduction in switch cost 2. No improvement in gait or balance 3. No effect of Geriatric Depression Scale or the Profile of Mood States	[35]

Collectively, the sixteen investigated human intervention studies provide tendencies for an improvement in health by daily strawberry or blueberry consumption. In some studies, strawberry intervention selectively showed favorable effects on inflammation, insulin sensitivity, antioxidant status, insulin response and distribution or size of blood lipids, whereas some studies showed no effect on those attributes. Blueberry intervention showed positive effects in some cognitive tests and in some cases, selectively positive effects on blood pressure, endothelial function, insulin sensitivity or oxidative stress. However, several authors discussed the need for larger subject groups and longer trial periods to obtain more precise and consistent findings. Dose of anthocyanins, as well as age, overall health and predominantly sex of participants may have also influenced the results of the reviewed studies. It was also suggested to use fresh berries instead of powder. Most authors concluded that daily strawberry or blueberry consumption may have a positive effect on health., which should be investigated in further intervention studies.

Author Contributions: K.M. conceived the focus of the review, conducted the literature search, and drafted the manuscript. W.F. reviewed and contributed to the manuscript. M.S. reviewed and edited the manuscript upon critical revision of the text.

References

1. World Health Organization. *Global Atlas on Cardiovascular Disease Prevention and Control*; World Health Organization: Geneva, Switzerland, 2011.

2. Forbes-Hernandez, T.Y.; Gasparrini, M.; Afrin, S.; Bompadre, S.; Mezzetti, B.; Quiles, J.L.; Giampieri, F.; Battino, M. The healthy effects of strawberry polyphenols: Which strategy behind antioxidant capacity? *Crit. Rev. Food Sci. Nutr.* **2016**, *56* (Suppl. 1), 46–59. [CrossRef] [PubMed]
3. Giampieri, F.; Forbes-Hernandez, T.Y.; Gasparrini, M.; Alvarez-Suarez, J.M.; Afrin, S.; Bompadre, S.; Quiles, J.L.; Mezzetti, B.; Battino, M. Strawberry as a health promoter: An evidence based review. *Food Funct.* **2015**, *6*, 1386–1398. [CrossRef] [PubMed]
4. Joseph, S.V.; Edirisinghe, I.; Burton-Freeman, B.M. Berries: Anti-inflammatory effects in humans. *J. Agric. Food Chem.* **2014**, *62*, 3886–3903. [CrossRef] [PubMed]
5. Katsiari, C.G.; Bogdanos, D.P.; Sakkas, L.I. Inflammation and cardiovascular disease. *WJTM* **2019**, *8*, 1–8. [CrossRef]
6. Vendrame, S.; Del Bo, C.; Ciappellano, S.; Riso, P.; Klimis-Zacas, D. Berry fruit consumption and metabolic syndrome. *Antioxidants* **2016**, *5*, 34. [CrossRef] [PubMed]
7. Khalid, S.; Barfoot, K.L.; May, G.; Lamport, D.J.; Reynolds, S.A.; Williams, C.M. Effects of Acute Blueberry Flavonoids on Mood in Children and Young Adults. *Nutrients* **2017**, *9*, 158. [CrossRef]
8. Jimenez-Garcia, S.N.; Guevara-Gonzalez, R.G.; Miranda-Lopez, R.; Feregrino-Perez, A.A.; Torres-Pacheco, I.; Vazquez-Cruz, M.A. Functional properties and quality characteristics of bioactive compounds in berries: Biochemistry, biotechnology, and genomics. *Food Res. Int.* **2013**, *54*, 1195–1207. [CrossRef]
9. Shi, M.; Loftus, H.; McAinch, A.J.; Su, X.Q. Blueberry as a source of bioactive compounds for the treatment of obesity, type 2 diabetes and chronic inflammation. *J. Funct. Foods* **2017**, *30*, 16–29. [CrossRef]
10. Caruso, G.; Villari, G.; Melchionna, G.; Conti, S. Effects of cultural cycles and nutrient solutions on plant growth, yield and fruit quality of alpine strawberry (*Fragaria vesca* L.) grown in hydroponics. *Sci. Hortic.* **2011**, *129*, 479–485. [CrossRef]
11. Conti, S.; Villari, G.; Faugno, S.; Melchionna, G.; Somma, S.; Caruso, G. Effects of organic vs. conventional farming system on yield and quality of strawberry grown as an annual or biennial crop in southern Italy. *Sci. Hortic.* **2014**, *180*, 63–71. [CrossRef]
12. Michalska, A.; Łysiak, G. Bioactive Compounds of Blueberries: Post-Harvest Factors Influencing the Nutritional Value of Products. *Int. J. Mol. Sci.* **2015**, *16*, 18642–18663. [CrossRef] [PubMed]
13. Nile, S.H.; Park, S.W. Edible berries: Bioactive components and their effect on human health. *Nutrition* **2014**, *30*, 134–144. [CrossRef] [PubMed]
14. Rothwell, J.A.; Perez-Jimenez, J.; Neveu, V.; Medina-Remón, A.; M'Hiri, N.; García-Lobato, P.; Manach, C.; Knox, C.; Eisner, R.; Wishart, D.S.; et al. Phenol-Explorer 3.0: A major update of the Phenol-Explorer database to incorporate data on the effects of food processing on polyphenol content. *Database* **2013**, *2013*. [CrossRef] [PubMed]
15. Nour, V.; Trandafir, I.; Cosmulescu, S. Antioxidant compounds, nutritional quality and colour of two strawberry genotypes from Fragaria × Ananassa. *Erwerbs-Obstbau* **2017**, *59*, 123–131. [CrossRef]
16. Souci, S.W.; Fachmann, W.; Kraut, H. *Food Composition and Nutrition Tables: Die Zusammensetzung der Lebensmittel, Nährwert-Tabellen = La composition des Aliments, Tableaux des Valeurs Nutritives*, 8th ed.; MedPharm Scientific Publishers: Stuttgart, Germany, 2016.
17. Edirisinghe, I.; Banaszewski, K.; Cappozzo, J.; Sandhya, K.; Ellis, C.L.; Tadapaneni, R.; Kappagoda, C.T.; Burton-Freeman, B.M. Strawberry anthocyanin and its association with postprandial inflammation and insulin. *Br. J. Nutr.* **2011**, *106*, 913–922. [CrossRef]
18. Ellis, C.L.; Edirisinghe, I.; Kappagoda, T.; Burton-Freeman, B. Attenuation of meal-induced inflammatory and thrombotic responses in overweight men and women after 6-week daily strawberry (Fragaria) intake. *JAT* **2011**, *18*, 318–327. [CrossRef] [PubMed]
19. Park, E.; Edirisinghe, I.; Wei, H.; Vijayakumar, L.P.; Banaszewski, K.; Cappozzo, J.C.; Burton-Freeman, B. A dose-response evaluation of freeze-dried strawberries independent of fiber content on metabolic indices in abdominally obese individuals with insulin resistance in a randomized, single-blinded, diet-controlled crossover trial. *Mol. Nutr. Food Res.* **2016**, *60*, 1099–1109. [CrossRef]
20. Zunino, S.J.; Parelman, M.A.; Freytag, T.L.; Stephensen, C.B.; Kelley, D.S.; Mackey, B.E.; Woodhouse, L.R.; Bonnel, E.L. Effects of dietary strawberry powder on blood lipids and inflammatory markers in obese human subjects. *Br. J. Nutr.* **2012**, *108*, 900–909. [CrossRef]

21. Basu, A.; Betts, N.M.; Nguyen, A.; Newman, E.D.; Fu, D.; Lyons, T.J. Freeze-dried strawberries lower serum cholesterol and lipid peroxidation in adults with abdominal adiposity and elevated serum lipids. *J. Nutr.* **2014**, *144*, 830–837. [CrossRef]
22. Moazen, S.; Amani, R.; Homayouni Rad, A.; Shahbazian, H.; Ahmadi, K.; Taha Jalali, M. Effects of freeze-dried strawberry supplementation on metabolic biomarkers of atherosclerosis in subjects with type 2 diabetes: A randomized double-blind controlled trial. *Ann. Nutr. Metab.* **2013**, *63*, 256–264. [CrossRef]
23. Schell, J.; Scofield, R.H.; Barrett, J.R.; Kurien, B.T.; Betts, N.; Lyons, T.J.; Zhao, Y.D.; Basu, A. Strawberries improve pain and inflammation in obese adults with radiographic evidence of knee osteoarthritis. *Nutrients* **2017**, *9*, 949. [CrossRef] [PubMed]
24. Bhalodkar, N.C.; Blum, S.; Rana, T.; Bhalodkar, A.; Kitchappa, R.; Kim, K.-S.; Enas, E. Comparison of levels of large and small high-density lipoprotein cholesterol in Asian Indian men compared with Caucasian men in the Framingham Offspring Study. *Am. J. Cardiol.* **2004**, *94*, 1561–1563. [CrossRef] [PubMed]
25. Cheung, C.M.; Brown, G.B.; Wolf, A.C.; Albers, J.J. Altered particle size distribution of apoA-I-containing lipoproteins in subjects with coronary heart disease. *J. Lipid Res.* **1991**, *32*, 383–394. [PubMed]
26. Zeljkovic, A.; Vekic, J.; Spasojevic-Kalimanovska, V.; Jelic-Ivanovic, Z.; Bogavac-Stanojevic, N.; Gulan, B.; Spasic, S. LDL and HDL subclasses in acute ischemic stroke: Prediction of risk and short-term mortality. *Atherosclerosis* **2010**, *210*, 548–554. [CrossRef] [PubMed]
27. Basu, A.; Morris, S.; Nguyen, A.; Betts, N.M.; Fu, D.; Lyons, T.J. Effects of dietary strawberry supplementation on antioxidant biomarkers in obese adults with above optimal serum lipids. *J. Nutr. Metab.* **2016**. [CrossRef] [PubMed]
28. Feresin, R.G.; Johnson, S.A.; Pourafshar, S.; Campbell, J.C.; Jaime, S.J.; Navaei, N.; Elam, M.L.; Akhavan, N.S.; Alvarez-Alvarado, S.; Tenenbaum, G.; et al. Impact of daily strawberry consumption on blood pressure and arterial stiffness in pre- and stage 1-hypertensive postmenopausal women: A randomized controlled trial. *Food Funct.* **2017**, *8*, 4139–4149. [CrossRef] [PubMed]
29. Liu, S.-X.; Yang, H.-Y.; Li, S.-Y.; Zhang, J.-Y.; Li, T.; Zhu, B.-Q.; Zhang, B.-L. Polyphenolic Compositions and Chromatic Characteristics of Bog Bilberry Syrup Wines. *Molecules* **2015**, *20*, 19865–19877. [CrossRef] [PubMed]
30. Stull, A.J.; Cash, K.C.; Champagne, C.M.; Gupta, A.K.; Boston, R.; Beyl, R.A.; Johnson, W.D.; Cefalu, W.T. Blueberries improve endothelial function, but not blood pressure, in adults with metabolic syndrome: A randomized, double-blind, placebo-controlled clinical trial. *Nutrients* **2015**, *7*, 4107–4123. [CrossRef]
31. Riso, P.; Klimis-Zacas, D.; Del Bo', C.; Martini, D.; Campolo, J.; Vendrame, S.; Møller, P.; Loft, S.; de Maria, R.; Porrini, M. Effect of a wild blueberry (*Vaccinium angustifolium*) drink intervention on markers of oxidative stress, inflammation and endothelial function in humans with cardiovascular risk factors. *Eur. J. Nutr.* **2013**, *52*, 949–961. [CrossRef]
32. Stote, K.S.; Sweeney, M.I.; Kean, T.; Baer, D.J.; Novotny, J.A.; Shakerley, N.L.; Chandrasekaran, A.; Carrico, P.M.; Melendez, J.A.; Gottschall-Pass, K.T. The effects of 100% wild blueberry (*Vaccinium angustifolium*) juice consumption on cardiometablic biomarkers: A randomized, placebo-controlled, crossover trial in adults with increased risk for type 2 diabetes. *BMC Nutr.* **2017**, *3*, 524. [CrossRef]
33. Johnson, S.A.; Figueroa, A.; Navaei, N.; Wong, A.; Kalfon, R.; Ormsbee, L.T.; Feresin, R.G.; Elam, M.L.; Hooshmand, S.; Payton, M.E.; et al. Daily blueberry consumption improves blood pressure and arterial stiffness in postmenopausal women with pre- and stage 1-hypertension: A randomized, double-blind, placebo-controlled clinical trial. *J. Acad. Nutr. Diet.* **2015**, *115*, 369–377. [CrossRef] [PubMed]
34. Bowtell, J.L.; Aboo-Bakkar, Z.; Conway, M.E.; Adlam, A.-L.R.; Fulford, J. Enhanced task-related brain activation and resting perfusion in healthy older adults after chronic blueberry supplementation. *Appl. Physiol. Nutr. Metab. Physiol. Appl. Nutr. Et Metab.* **2017**, *42*, 773–779. [CrossRef] [PubMed]
35. Miller, M.G.; Hamilton, D.A.; Joseph, J.A.; Shukitt-Hale, B. Dietary blueberry improves cognition among older adults in a randomized, double-blind, placebo-controlled trial. *Eur. J. Nutr.* **2018**, *57*, 1169–1180. [CrossRef] [PubMed]

4

Prebiotic Effects of Partially Hydrolyzed Guar Gum on the Composition and Function of the Human Microbiota—Results from the PAGODA Trial

Simon J. Reider [1,2], Simon Moosmang [3], Judith Tragust [1], Lovro Trgovec-Greif [4], Simon Tragust [5], Lorenz Perschy [4], Nicole Przysiecki [1,2], Sonja Sturm [3], Herbert Tilg [2], Hermann Stuppner [3], Thomas Rattei [4] and Alexander R. Moschen [1,2,*]

1 Christian Doppler Laboratory for Mucosal Immunology, Medical University Innsbruck, 6020 Innsbruck, Austria; simon.reider@i-med.ac.at (S.J.R.); Judith.Tragust@hotmail.de (J.T.); Nicole.Przysiecki@i-med.ac.at (N.P.)

2 Department of Internal Medicine I, Gastroenterology, Hepatology, Endocrinology & Metabolism, Medical University Innsbruck, 6020 Innsbruck, Austria; herbert.tilg@i-med.ac.at

3 Institute of Pharmacy/Pharmacognosy & Center for Molecular Biosciences Innsbruck, Leopold-Franzens Universität, 6020 Innsbruck, Austria; Simon-Moosmang@web.de (S.M.); sonja.sturm@uibk.ac.at (S.S.); hermann.stuppner@i-med.ac.at (H.S.)

4 Division of Computational Systems Biology, Department of Microbiology, University of Vienna, 1010 Vienna, Austria; lovro.lovro@hotmail.com (L.T.-G.); lorenz.perschy@icloud.com (L.P.); thomas.rattei@univie.ac.at (T.R.)

5 General Zoology Institute of Biology, University Halle, 06108 Halle, Germany; simon.tragust@zoologie.uni-halle.de

* Correspondence: alexander.moschen@i-med.ac.at

Abstract: (1) Background: Alterations in the structural composition of the human gut microbiota have been identified in various disease entities along with exciting mechanistic clues by reductionist gnotobiotic modeling. Improving health by beneficially modulating an altered microbiota is a promising treatment approach. Prebiotics, substrates selectively used by host microorganisms conferring a health benefit, are broadly used for dietary and clinical interventions. Herein, we sought to investigate the microbiota-modelling effects of the soluble fiber, partially hydrolyzed guar gum (PHGG). (2) Methods: We performed a 9 week clinical trial in 20 healthy volunteers that included three weeks of a lead-in period, followed by three weeks of an intervention phase, wherein study subjects received 5 g PHGG up to three times per day, and concluding with a three-week washout period. A stool diary was kept on a daily basis, and clinical data along with serum/plasma and stool samples were collected on a weekly basis. PHGG-induced alterations of the gut microbiota were studied by 16S metagenomics of the V1–V3 and V3–V4 regions. To gain functional insight, we further studied stool metabolites using nuclear magnetic resonance (NMR) spectroscopy. (3) Results: In healthy subjects, PHGG had significant effects on stool frequency and consistency. These effects were paralleled by changes in α- (species evenness) and β-diversity (Bray–Curtis distances), along with increasing abundances of metabolites including butyrate, acetate and various amino acids. On a taxonomic level, PHGG intake was associated with a bloom in *Ruminococcus*, *Fusicatenibacter*, *Faecalibacterium* and *Bacteroides* and a reduction in *Roseburia*, *Lachnospiracea* and *Blautia*. The majority of effects disappeared after stopping the prebiotic and most effects tended to be more pronounced in male participants. (4) Conclusions: Herein, we describe novel aspects of the prebiotic PHGG on compositional and functional properties of the healthy human microbiota.

Keywords: prebiotics; fiber; partially hydrolyzed guar gum; PHGG; microbiota; short-chain fatty acids; SCFA

---

1. Introduction

The human intestinal tract is populated by a complex microbial community, providing essential metabolic and immunological functions to the host, influencing normal physiology as well as disease susceptibility [1]. Using metagenomic techniques, more than 2000 bacterial species have been detected in the intestinal tract and approximately 100–1000 different bacterial taxa are present in a given individual [2,3]. The majority of these bacteria are members of the phyla Bacteroidetes and Firmicutes, while others belong to Proteobacteria, Actinobacteria and Verrucomicrobia [4,5]. The composition of the microbiota in the steady state is characterized by high diversity and marked inter-individual variability. On a functional level, however, different species share metabolic properties, resulting in set of core metabolic functions that are shared by the healthy microbiota. Bacterial communities are stabilized by microbe–microbe interactions and exhibit a remarkable resilience to perturbations. In spite of these mechanisms, alterations of the microbiota have been observed in numerous pathologic conditions [6–11].

Accordingly, there is considerable interest in approaches aimed at altering microbial composition and functions counteracting disease-driving factors and promoting health-beneficial properties. Various approaches including dietary and non-dietary interventions have been described and probiotic and prebiotic modalities are most widely used in clinical practice. Following the definition of probiotics, 'live microorganisms which when administered in adequate amounts confer a health benefit' [12], a prebiotic is considered 'a substrate that is selectively utilized by host microorganisms conferring a health benefit' [13]. These features are thought to demarcate a prebiotic from dietary fibers. Accordingly, even if dietary fibers such as pectins [14] and xylans [15] may cause alterations of gut commensal compositions, either the criterion of selective utilization or a health benefit have not yet been sufficiently demonstrated [13].

Partially hydrolyzed guar gum (PHGG) is a soluble dietary fiber with a linear backbone of β-1,4-linked D-mannose residues, with α-D-galactose residues 1,6-linked to every second mannose. This galactomannan completely dissolves in water, does not form a gel and demonstrates prebiotic properties as previously defined by increasing the abundance of Lactobacilli and Bifidobacteria as well as colonic SCFA contents [16,17]. In functional gastrointestinal disease such as irritable bowel syndrome (IBS), PHGG showed efficacy in improving bloating [18] and improving IBS-related symptoms and quality of life [19] compared to placebo. Fermentation of PHGG by the microbiota increases the abundance of short-chain fatty acids (SCFAs) including acetate, propionate and butyrate. SCFAs are an important energy source for colonic epithelial cells and have a variety of regulatory functions on gut physiology, metabolism and immunity [20].

Despite some evidence for its efficacy and its clinical and nutritional use [21], the prebiotic effects of PHGG, in light of the prebiotic definition and methodological progresses that have been made in studying the microbiota in recent years, are inadequately defined. The aim of this study was to decipher and define the overall prebiotic properties of PHGG in healthy volunteers focusing on taxonomic and functional (i.e., metabolites) properties using state-of-the-art methodologies.

2. Materials and Methods

2.1. Study Design and Criteria for Participation

The PAGODA study is a longitudinal trial including 20 healthy volunteers undergoing supplementation with PHGG. PHGG was from one specific lot and kindly provided by Nestlé Austria. The trial was performed with approval from the ethics committee of the Medical University

Innsbruck (Number: AN2016-0244) and informed consent was obtained from all study subjects. The overall duration of this study was nine weeks, split in three periods (see Figure 1A): during the first three weeks, baseline values were obtained; in weeks 4–6, PHGG was administered in increasing doses (5 g, 10 g, and 15 g per day); finally, PHGG supplementation was stopped and the participants were monitored for another three weeks to distinguish transient from persistent changes. At the baseline, a medical history and information on dietary habits were obtained. Participants were advised to maintain their baseline dietary habits throughout this study. Furthermore, laboratory chemistry analyses were performed during screening in order to exclude candidates with abnormal test values (blood count, C-reactive protein, fecal calprotectin). During this study, sampling was performed once a week. The sample set included fecal matter, urine, serum and plasma. Fecal samples were collected in a Sarstedt stool container within 12 h before and kept at 4 °C until the weekly study visit. Samples were immediately aliquoted and stored at −80 °C until further workup. Additionally, clinical data and information on current well-being were collected on a weekly basis using questionnaires. To be eligible for study participation, the following criteria had to be met: no history of antibiotic therapy within 3 months before this study, history of vaginal delivery and having been breast fed for at least 3 months. Participants were excluded from this study in the case of an acute or chronic gastrointestinal disease, history of major abdominal surgery (appendectomy excluded), if they consumed dietary supplements or probiotics, were on an exclusive vegetarian or vegan diet or showed abnormal laboratory test values at baseline.

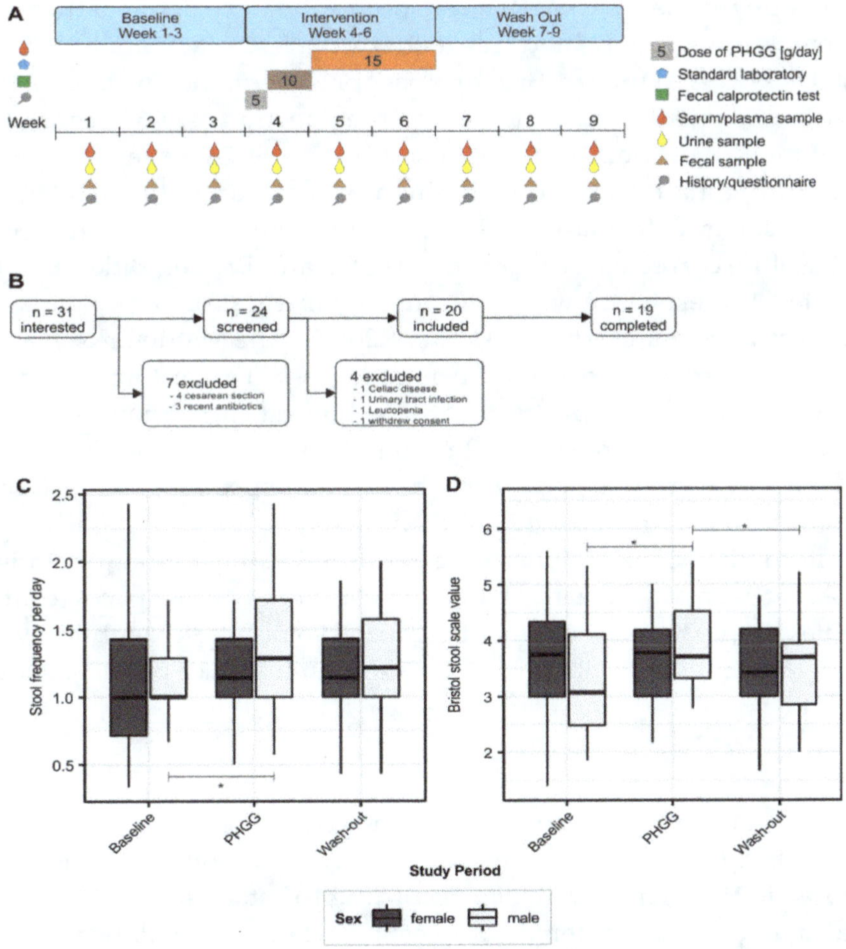

Figure 1. Study design and clinical effects of PHGG supplementation. (**A**) Outline of the design and sampling procedure of the PAGODA study; (**B**) screening process and number of participants included in this study; (**C**) effect of PHGG supplementation on stool frequency; (**D**) effect of PHGG supplementation on stool consistency according to the Bristol stool scale value. PHGG = partially hydrolyzed guar gum; * $p < 0.05$; linear mixed model.

2.2. The 16.S Amplicon-Based Metagenomics

During this study, fecal samples were collected weekly by the participants. Microbial DNA was isolated from these samples using the Qiagen PowerSoil Kit according to the manufacturer's instructions. Isolated DNA was shipped to IMGM (Munich, Germany) for sequencing on the Illumina MISEQ platform using primers targeting the V1–V3 and V3–V4 regions of the bacterial 16S gene [22] (primer sequences detailed in Table S1) aiming for 100,000 reads per region. Generated 16S sequence data are available from the European Nucleotide Archive (accession number ERP120904). All scripts related to our analyses will be provided by the authors upon reasonable request (to SJR). The sequencing results were checked using FASTQC [23] and processed in mothur according to a published protocol (version 1.40.5) [24,25]. Briefly, reads were filtered for a minimum length of 275 nucleotides in prinseq [26]. Filtered fasta files were merged and aligned to the SILVA v128 database [27]. Chimeric reads were removed using vsearch [28]. The SILVA v128 database was also used for taxonomic classification. Finally, operational taxonomic unit (OTU) clustering was performed at a level of 97% identity separately for the V1–V3 and the V3–V4 data. This resulted in 7,509,559 and 7,855,428 high-quality reads clustering into 2,157,950 and 825,683 OTUs in the V1–V3 and the V3–V4 dataset, respectively. After excluding OTUs present only once in the dataset (singleton OTUs), 231,695 (V1–V3) and 177,260 OTUs (V3–V4) were retained.

2.3. NMR Spectroscopy

For nuclear magnetic resonance (NMR) spectroscopy, watery extracts from fecal samples were generated by ultrasonication and repeated freeze–thaw cycles. NMR analysis was performed on a Bruker Avance II 600 MHz. A standard Bruker noesypr1d sequence was used to suppress signals from water molecules. Acquisition parameters for the spectra were 64 scans, a spectral width of 7288 Hz collected into 32K data points, an acquisition time of 2.24 s, and an inter-scan relaxation delay of 5 s. The free induction decay (FID) obtained was multiplied by 0.3 Hz of exponential line broadening before Fourier transformation. The spectra were referenced to TSP (chemical shift 0 ppm), phased, and baseline corrected in Topspin 3.0 software (Bruker, Billerica, MA, USA). Relative quantification of selected 1H resonance was performed by integration of peak areas using Topspin 3.0 (Bruker) [29]. NMR spectra were imported to Matlab R2010b (The Mathworks, Natick, MA, USA), and the misalignments of the spectra were corrected using the icoshift algorithm, based on the correlational shifting of spectral intervals [30]. The spectrum with the highest correlation to the rest of the spectra in the matrix was used as a reference. The 9.5 to 12 ppm region and the region containing residual water resonance (4.8. to 4.7 ppm) were removed from the aligned spectra. The spectra were normalized to unit area and pareto scaled before principal component analysis (PCA) using the PLS Toolbox in MATLAB R2010b. Alternatively, metabolites were identified using automatic statistical identification in complex spectra (ASICS). This approach is based on a library of NMR spectra containing information on 191 pure metabolites [31]. Alternatively, manual attribution of peak identities was performed based on shift values from reference spectra obtained from measurements of pure substances and spike in of pure substances in fecal extracts.

2.4. Statistics

Clinical data were analyzed in R using a linear mixed model (study period, sex, interaction of study period and sex as fixed effect, study week and subject as random effect). Metagenomic data were imported into phyloseq [32] in R and analyzed according to established procedures. Within-sample (α) diversity was calculated from unfiltered samples; for all other calculations, singleton OTUs were removed from the database. Bray–Curtis dissimilarity was calculated on a rarefied dataset and primary coordinate analysis plots were generated. Samples with less than 1000 reads were removed from the database. Vegan [33] was used to perform permutational analysis of variance (PERMANOVA) with study week and subject as predictive variables. Testing for differentially abundant OTUs was performed using DESeq2 using all OTUs, with an absolute abundance of at least three in at least 10% of samples [34,35]. Differential abundance was assumed only if the log2 fold change exceeded 1.7.

NMR spectra were analyzed in a targeted approach integrating intensities of known peaks corresponding to SCFAs, galactose, mannose and PHGG. These peak identities were confirmed by additional NMR measurements of pure substances in the same solvent. Additionally, peak intensities were correlated to microbial abundances in a blinded fashion using SparCC with default parameters [36]. The list of correlations was filtered for interactions with a p value of < 0.05 and a correlation coefficient of >0.2. The peaks included in this filtered correlation matrix were then annotated by hand as described and the network was drawn in Cytoscape v3.7.1 [37].

3. Results

3.1. *Study Cohort and Baseline Nutritional Characteristics*

Thirty-one individuals were interested in participating in this study. After controlling for inclusion/exclusion criteria, 24 underwent screening. Three individuals had to be excluded due to pre-existing medical conditions discovered during screening (celiac disease, urinary tract infection and leucopenia) and one individual declined to participate. Twenty volunteers were included and 19 of them completed this study (8 males, 11 females; Figure 1B). The mean age of study participants was 27.8 years (minimum 20, maximum 46 years) and the mean BMI was 21.7 ± 2.4. Laboratory values and pre-existing medical conditions that did not preclude study participation are listed in Tables S2 and S3. Baseline nutritional habits were characterized in detail using a questionnaire as previously described [38]. Both male and female participants predominantly had three meals a day, with no significance difference in the intake of carbohydrates or dairy products. However, female participants reported higher intake of fruit and fiber, and reduced intake of meat (Figure S1).

3.2. *Effect of PHGG Intake on Intestinal Well-Being and Bowel Function*

First, specific clinical effects of PHGG supplementation on intestinal well-being and bowel function were studied based on the weekly questionnaires. A linear model showed significant changes in the number of bowel movements per day ($p < 0.01$), which was particularly attributable to the male subpopulation ($p < 0.05$). PHGG intake was associated with a significant increase in the number of daily stools (1.13 ± 0.46 vs. 1.27 ± 0.47, $p < 0.01$). This effect did not persist after the end of the intervention period (washout period: 1.22 ± 0.41). These differences were gender dependent: While there was an increase in stool frequency and consistency (BSS value) in male participants, female participants did not experience such effects upon PHGG supplementation (Figure 1C,D). Table S3 summarizes results of the intestinal well-being and symptoms questionnaire during the 9 week study period.

3.3. *PHGG-Associated Changes of Microbial Community Structures*

Samples from all three study periods were compared regarding α-diversity (Figure 2A and Figure S2A). While the number of observed species remained unchanged during PHGG supplementation (species richness, the Chao1 index), species evenness (the Shannon and inverse Simpson indices) decreased significantly ($p < 0.05$; Kruskal–Wallis test). All measures of α-diversity returned to baseline values during the washout period. These effects reached statistical significance in both sexes in the V3–V4 dataset (Figure 2A), but only in the V1–V3 region in males (Figure S2A). No differences between male and female participants were found for each study period ($p > 0.05$, Bonferroni corrected pairwise Wilcoxon tests). Bray–Curtis dissimilarity was used to calculate β-diversity (Figure 2B and Figure S2B). PHGG supplementation significantly affected microbial community composition ($R^2 = 0.023$ and 0.020 respectively; $p < 0.01$; permutational analysis of variance). This resulted in a significant difference of pairwise Bray–Curtis dissimilarities over time between the baseline and the final week of the intervention period (week 6; $p < 0.05$, Wilcoxon test). After stopping PHGG intervention, paired Bray–Curtis dissimilarities quickly returned to individuals' baseline variability measured between weeks 1 and 3. At a personalized level, the reconfiguration of the microbial composition was highly individual (Figures S3 and S4). Inter-individual differences in microbial community composition accounted for most of the variance (factor subject; R2 = 0.67 and 0.68, respectively; $p < 0.01$, permutational analysis of variance).

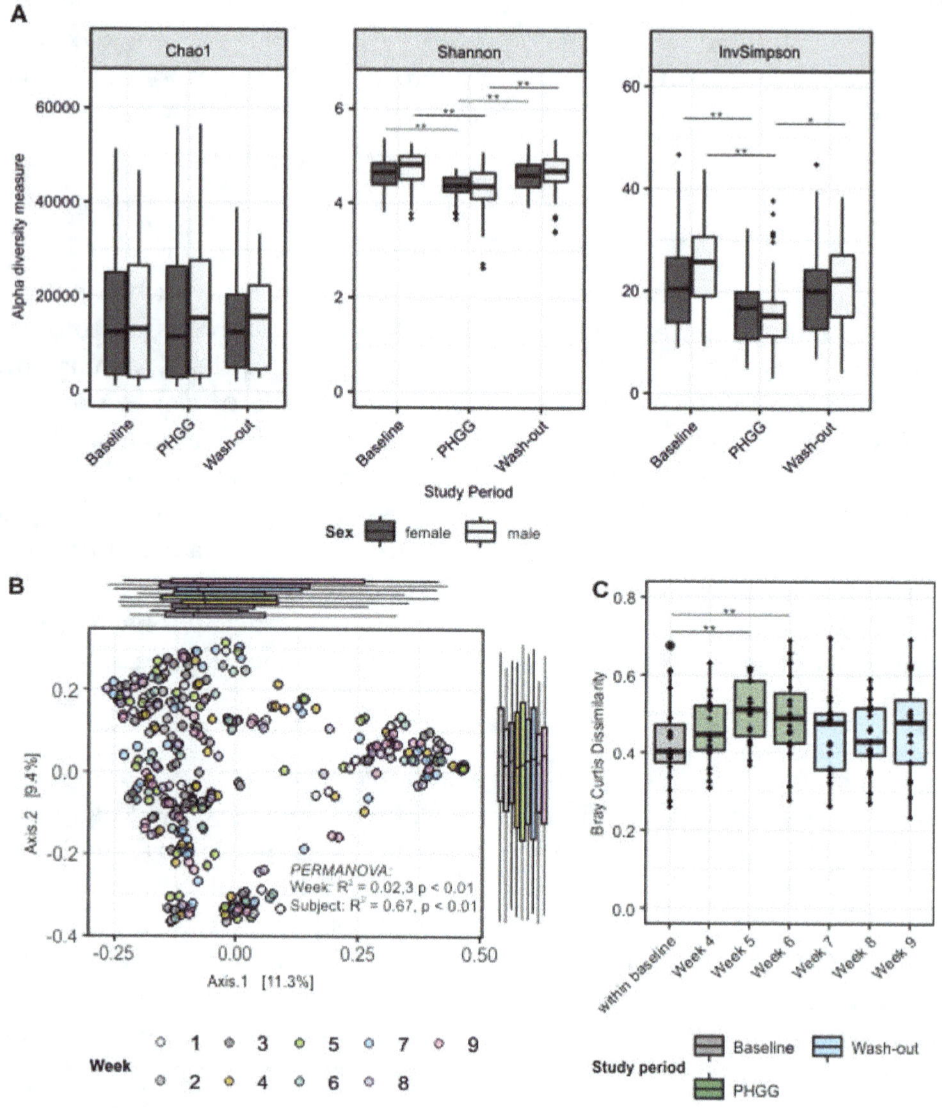

Figure 2. Impact of PHGG supplementation on intestinal microbiota composition. (**A**) α-diversity decreases during intervention in both sexes and returns to baseline during the washout period (pairwise Wilcoxon Test). (**B**) Principal component analysis of microbial compositions over time; study week (i.e., PHGG supplementation status) as determinant was significant (PERMANOVA permutational analysis of variance). (**C**) Pairwise analyses of Bray–Curtis dissimilarities over time (Wilcoxon test). PHGG = partially hydrolyzed guar gum; * $p < 0.05$, ** $p < 0.01$.

To identify potential causes underlying the observed changes in diversity measures, we proceeded to test for differentially abundant bacterial taxa between study periods, accounting for subject as an additional factor (false discovery rate-adjusted $p < 0.01$, negative binomial Wald's test). Using the V3–V4 dataset (Figure 3), 28 taxa predominantly from the Firmicutes phylum were detected. In most of these taxa, an observed change during the intervention period was not sustained during the washout period, (i.e., taxon abundance quickly reverted to baseline values). PHGG had suppressing as well as enhancing effects on the abundance of specific OTUs. Notably, a few OTUs exhibited persistent changes. These belonged to the *Ruminococcus*, *Faecalibacterium* and *Bacteroides* genus. In comparison, in the V1–V3 dataset (Figure S5) 14 OTUs were significantly differentially abundant. Again, most of these OTUs were only transiently affected but one OTU corresponding to Faecalibacterium remained increased during the washout period. These findings widely overlapped between both sequenced 16S regions. OTUs whose abundance was negatively associated with PHGG supplementation mapped to the genera *Roseburia*, *Lachnospiracea* and *Blautia*, while those that bloomed during the intervention period belonged to *Ruminococcus*, *Fusicatenibacter*, *Faecalibacterium* and *Bacteroides* (Figure 3 and Figure S5).

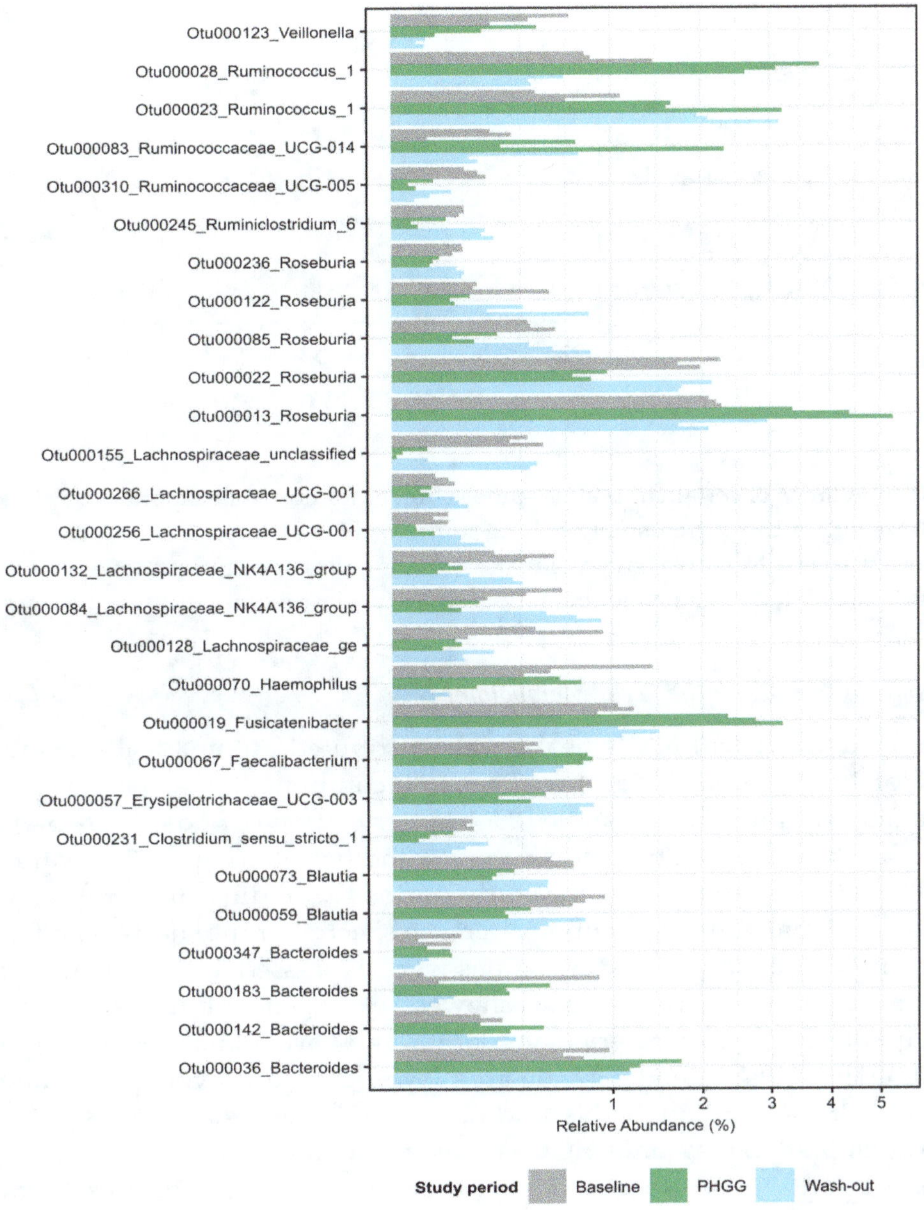

Figure 3. Significantly differentially abundant OTUs and their mapping on the genus level in the V3–V4 dataset. Testing was carried out using a negative binomial model implemented in DESeq2 and a cutoff of 0.01 for the adjusted *p*-value. OTU = operational taxonomic unit; UCG = unknown classification group; PHGG = partially hydrolyzed guar gum.

3.4. Abundance of Specific Taxa in the Steady State Correlates with Clinical Response to PHGG

As there is considerable interest in factors underlying the efficacy of a prebiotic treatment in a given individual, we aimed to identify characteristics of the microbiota during the steady state that would correlate with clinical response to PHGG. Using data from the clinical symptoms questionnaires, responders to PHGG were defined by an increase in stool frequency per day higher than the mean increase observed in the overall study population. Accordingly, future responders to PHGG intervention exhibited a higher baseline abundance of certain members of the Clostridiales order such as *Faecalibacterium*, *Fusicatenibacter* and *Roseburia* ($p < 0.05$; Figure 4).

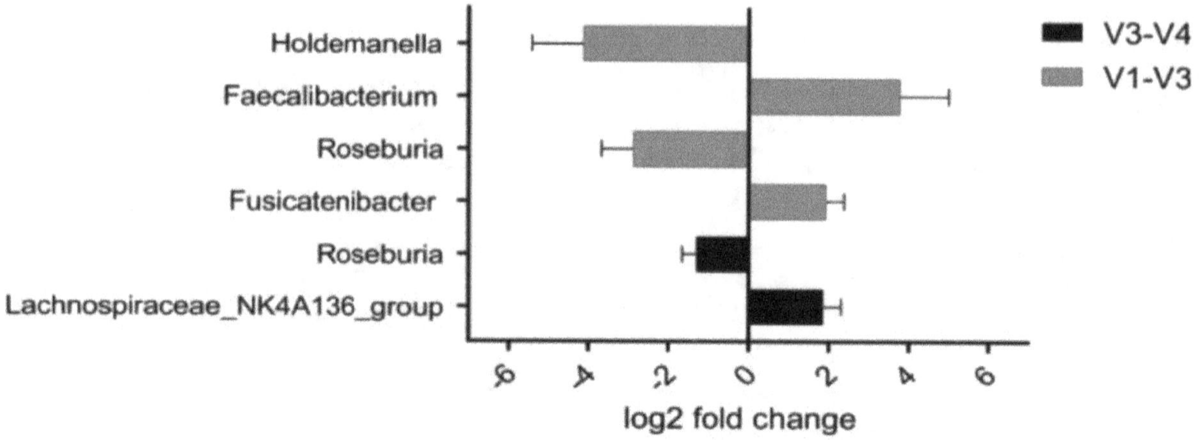

Figure 4. The abundance of certain taxa at baseline is higher in those that experience a clinical response to PHGG. These taxa almost exclusively belong to the order of Clostridiales. Notably, *Roseburia* is detected in both datasets. Negative binomial Wald-test comparing two groups defined by an increase in stool frequency per day larger or smaller than the median increase in this study population; all, $p < 0.05$.

3.5. PHGG-Associated Changes in the Fecal Metabolome

In an untargeted approach, NMR peaks were attributed automatically using ASICS and its reference library of 191 pure NMR spectra. Principle component analysis revealed a slight shift, mainly along the first component during the PHGG intervention period (Figure 5A) and mostly due to differences in the short-chain fatty acids butyrate and acetate (Figure 5B). Various amino acids also contributed to differences between the study periods. Building upon these findings, we next annotated NMR spectra manually based upon reference spectra for the short-chain fatty acids (SCFAs) acetate, butyrate and propionate. Peak intensities were expressed as fold change compared to the individual participant's baseline. This analysis showed sex-dependent differences in SCFA dynamics, with male participants in general experiencing larger and earlier changes during the intervention period (Figure 5C). There was a tendency towards lower butyrate levels at baseline in prospective male responders to PHGG, although this finding did not reach statistical significance (data not shown). We also attempted to measure PHGG and its metabolites galactose and mannose in the feces by comparing participants' NMR spectra during the intervention period to spectra obtained from PHGG, galactose and mannose alone. No increase in the PHGG signal could be detected during supplementation indicating complete metabolization of the soluble fiber. Fittingly, we observed a trend towards increased fecal concentrations of galactose and mannose, the cleavage products of PHGG (Figure S6).

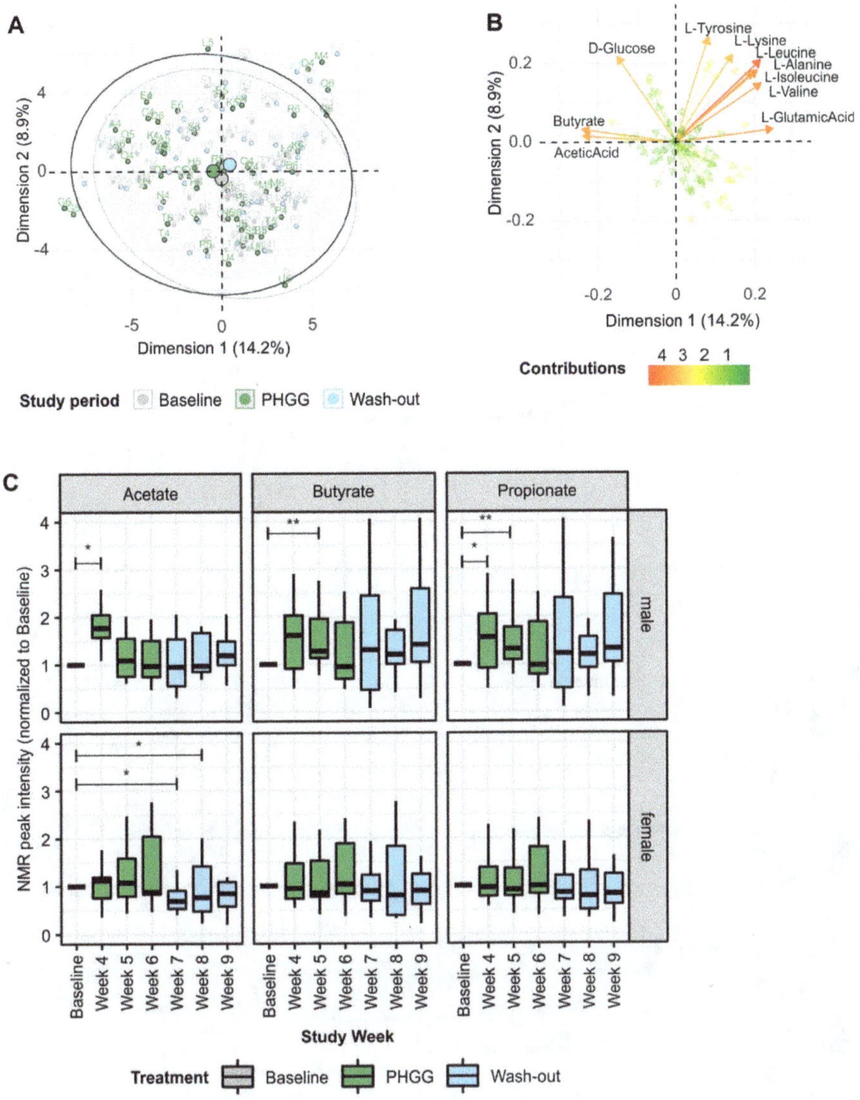

Figure 5. NMR spectroscopy of fecal samples: Peaks were annotated automatically (**A**,**B**) or manually using reference spectra (**C**). (**A**) Principle component analysis of metabolite profiles by study period indicates a small shift during the PHGG intervention. (**B**) Butyrate and acetate contribute most to the changes seen in **A**. (**C**) Targeted analysis of SCFA levels in fecal samples reveals sex-dependent changes over time, with most significant effects at the beginning of the intervention period. Pairwise Wilcoxon tests with Bonferroni correction.

3.6. Correlation Network

Fecal metabolites reflect the biochemical activity of the intestinal microbiota. Hence, we statistically assessed co-occurrence and co-exclusion of bacterial genera of the microbiota and peaks of NMR spectra, resulting in an interaction network centered on butyrate. There were strong links to other SCFAs (acetate, propionate) and certain bacterial genera. These bacteria in part overlapped with those identified by DESeq2 analysis. Bacteria of the Firmicutes phylum, e.g., certain groups of Ruminococcaceae and Lachnospiraceae as well as *Akkermansia* were positively correlated with butyrate abundance. There was a negative interaction of butyrate and *Barnesiella*, and strong negative interactions between *Bacteroides*, *Prevotella* and *Roseburia*, respectively. Importantly, the findings from the V3–V4 and V1–V3 datasets were highly comparable (Figure 6).

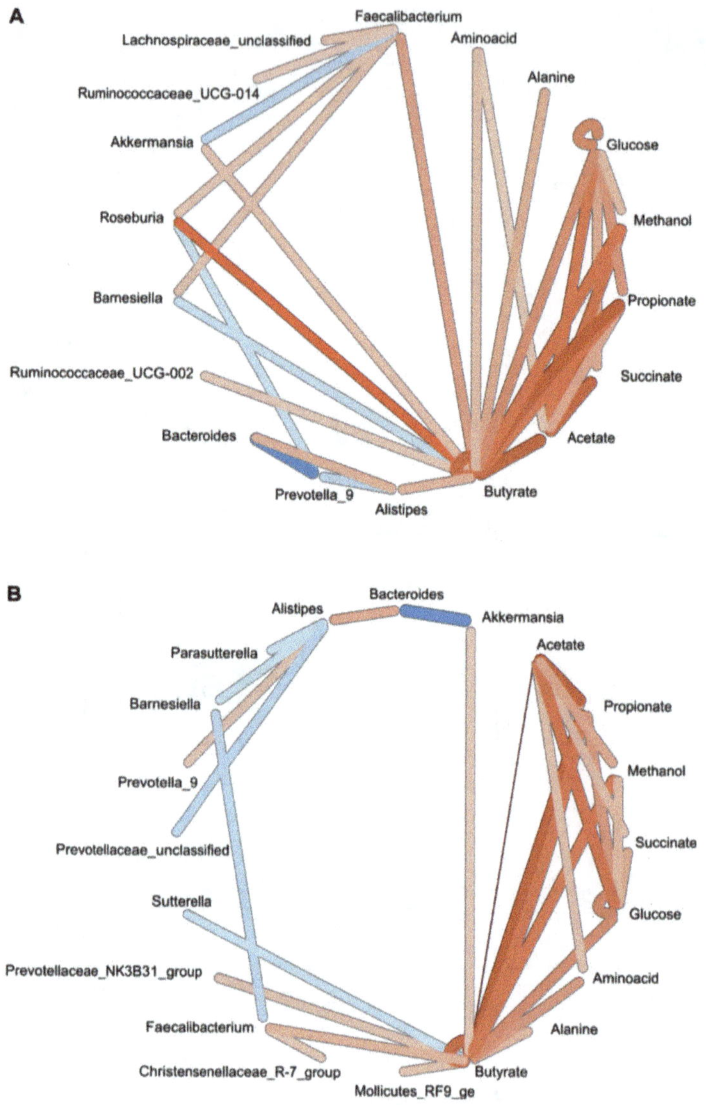

Figure 6. Correlation network of taxa and metabolites. Correlations between taxon abundance and peak intensities were calculated using SparCC and taxonomic abundance data (**A**) for the V3–V4 and (**B**) the V1–V3 region. Both regions reveal an interaction network centered on butyrate, with strong links between the SCFA as well as to certain taxa. In both datasets, Faecalibacterium was positively correlated with butyrate. Edge color = direction of interaction: red = positive; blue = negative; Edge weight = strength of interaction, i.e., correlation coefficient; only interactions with a two-sided p-value of >0.05 were included.

4. Discussion

Microbiota research provides us with fascinating insights into how an altered microbiota may be linked to human disease [39]. Prebiotics look back upon a long tradition in clinical nutrition and their microbiota-modulating properties along with their favorable safety fertilize a growing prebiotic market [40]. This prompted the International Scientific Association for Probiotics and Prebiotics (ISAPP) to revitalize the definition of a prebiotic as 'a substrate that is selectively utilized by host micro-organisms conferring a health benefit' [13]. Herein, we sought to verify and re-define prebiotic effects of the widely used soluble fiber, partially hydrolyzed guar gum (PHGG), applying state-of-the-art methodology in a controlled cohort trial named PAGODA.

In day-to-day clinical practice, prebiotics have been shown to exert beneficial effects in different clinical contexts such as gastrointestinal, cardiometabolic, mental health and bone diseases [40].

Accordingly, PHGG clinical studies have also demonstrated beneficial effects particularly in functional gastrointestinal disorders such as irritable bowel syndrome or constipation [41,42]. The specific study design of the PAGODA trial, involving three serial study periods, allowed measuring specific clinical effects in a time- and exposure-resolved manner. Confirmatory of previously published data [17,18], in our study, PHGG exposure was associated with an increase in stool frequency and a reduction in stool consistency according to the BSS score.

The prebiotic definition by the ISAPP group refers to the feature of 'selective utilization', which translates into utilization of the compound by specific members of the microbiota [13,43], thus conferring a fitness advantage with a respective impact on microbiota composition and function. Due technical limitations in earlier days, this was often equated with an expansion of Bifidobacteria and Lactobacilli and an increase in the abundance of SCFAs [13]. These prebiotic characteristics have also been demonstrated for PHGG [44]. In order to consider this definition, we have chosen a study design in which each study participant can serve his or her own control allowing to compensate for effects driven by the individual microbiota. To minimize the risk of a selection bias determined by the choice of the 16S chemistry, all samples were amplified and sequenced using both V1–V3 and V3–V4 primer pairs. To obtain functional insights we performed untargeted NMR spectroscopy in order to identify PHGG-induced metabolic pathways and to control for PHGG intake and its breakdown products.

Indeed, we identified PHGG-induced alterations of microbial communities with changes in the indices of species evenness and with an increase in pairwise intra-individual Bray–Curtis dissimilarities. Notably, the observed changes were largely reproducible between the two studied regions of the bacterial 16S gene. The nuanced differences between the findings from the two regions reflect their varying sensitivity for detection of certain bacterial groups. In accordance with the suggestions by Bindels et al. [45], we demonstrated that PHGG exerts broader effects on microbial ecology affecting 28 different taxa. In line with Bindels et al., our data provide further evidence that 'selective utilization' may be less dependent on specific taxa but on shared metabolic traits. Such metabolic traits may then provide secondary product that affect other groups microbes by cross-feeding highlighting the complexity of microbial ecology. Interestingly, the majority of these effects were transient and reversed during the washout period. As clinical effects and benefits along the prebiotic–microbiota–host axis are mechanistically linked by bacterial molecules arising from an altered microbial metabolic activity [39], we sought to identify changes in bacterial metabolites induced by PHGG. As expected and in line with previous research [16], induction of SCFAs was the most prominent effect, although additional functional changes in amino acid metabolism were identified. NMR spectroscopy made it possible to quantify fecal concentrations of the prebiotic PHGG itself along with its breakdown products. Interestingly, a daily intake of 15 g PHGG was fully metabolized by microbial metabolism and PHGG remained undetectable in the feces, whereas its cleavage products galactose and mannose were enriched. To link compositional data from 16S metagenomics with the functional metabolomic results, we employed interaction network analysis, which showed associations between OTU abundance and metabolites, particularly SCFAs, hinting at an accumulation of enzymatic functions of these bacterial species.

Another particularly interesting finding of this study was a strong inter-individual difference in response to PHGG between study participants. These differences were very pronounced with regard to clinical effects and generally stronger in male than in female participants. Nutritional data analyses revealed that women had a significantly higher baseline fiber intake, which could be a possible explanation for this discrepancy. However, differences in clinical responsiveness were not paralleled on the metagenomic level. This is consistent with findings reported by De Palma et al., who performed gnotobiotic models in animals that were conventionalized with either IBS or control stool. The authors did not find differences in the taxonomic composition between IBS- and control-conventionalized animals [46]. Nevertheless, IBS-D but not control feces induced typical IBS alterations in gut function and behavior, underscoring the importance of bacterial metabolites mechanistically linking the microbiota with human disease [46]. Strikingly, in our study, these gender-specific differences were reproducible on the metabolomic level, suggesting a mechanistic link between microbial function and clinical phenotype in our study. The absence of a gender difference in the effects of PHGG on a metagenomic level most likely reflects the functional convergence of individua, microbiotas, i.e., analogous biochemical functions are performed by different bacterial taxa within individual hosts.

Taken together, the highly individual responses to PHGG in our study further indicate the need for parameters enabling personalized prebiotic interventions. The complex relationships between the host, its commensal microbiota and their response to a specific prebiotic are influenced by multiple variables and makes a one-fits-all prebiotic becoming available unlikely [47]. Using our dataset, we were able to identify a steady state microbial configuration in combination with a low butyrate concentration to predict clinical response, i.e., an above-average increase in stool frequency and reduction in stool consistency, to PHGG.

Author Contributions: Conceptualization, S.J.R. and A.R.M.; data curation, S.J.R.; formal analysis, S.J.R., S.M., L.T.-G., S.T., L.P. and S.S.; funding acquisition, H.T., H.S. and A.R.M.; investigation, S.J.R., J.T. and N.P.; methodology, S.J.R., S.M., H.S. and T.R.; project administration, S.J.R., J.T. and A.R.M.; resources, S.S., H.T., H.S., T.R. and A.R.M.; software, T.R.; supervision, S.S., H.S., T.R. and A.R.M.; validation, T.R.; visualization, S.J.R.; writing—original draft, S.J.R.; writing—review and editing, S.M., S.S., H.T., H.S., T.R. and A.R.M. All authors have read and agreed to the published version of the manuscript.

Acknowledgments: We are indebted to Alexander Morgner (Nestlé Austria) for providing PHGG for this study. Furthermore, we thank Michael Bonin from IMGM (Munich, Germany) for excellent support with the technical implementations of this study.

References

1. Tilg, H.; Moschen, A.R. Food, immunity, and the microbiome. *Gastroenterology* **2015**, *148*, 1107–1119. [CrossRef] [PubMed]
2. Almeida, A.; Mitchell, A.L.; Boland, M.; Forster, S.C.; Gloor, G.B.; Tarkowska, A.; Lawley, T.D.; Finn, R.D. A new genomic blueprint of the human gut microbiota. *Nature* **2019**, *568*, 499–504. [CrossRef] [PubMed]
3. Lozupone, C.; Faust, K.; Raes, J.; Faith, J.J.; Frank, D.N.; Zaneveld, J.; Gordon, J.I.; Knight, R. Identifying genomic and metabolic features that can underlie early successional and opportunistic lifestyles of human gut symbionts. *Genome Res.* **2012**, *22*, 1974–1984. [CrossRef] [PubMed]
4. Qin, J.; Li, R.; Raes, J.; Arumugam, M.; Burgdorf, K.S.; Manichanh, C.; Nielsen, T.; Pons, N.; Levenez, F.; Yamada, T.; et al. A human gut microbial gene catalogue established by metagenomic sequencing. *Nature* **2010**, *464*, 59–65. [CrossRef]
5. Human Microbiome Project Consortium. Structure, function and diversity of the healthy human microbiome. *Nature* **2012**, *486*, 207–214. [CrossRef]
6. Lozupone, C.A.; Stombaugh, J.I.; Gordon, J.I.; Jansson, J.K.; Knight, R. Diversity, stability and resilience of the human gut microbiota. *Nature* **2012**, *489*, 220–230. [CrossRef]
7. Turnbaugh, P.J.; Ley, R.E.; Mahowald, M.A.; Magrini, V.; Mardis, E.R.; Gordon, J.I. An obesity-associated gut microbiome with increased capacity for energy harvest. *Nature* **2006**, *444*, 1027. [CrossRef]
8. Abdel-Gadir, A.; Stephen-Victor, E.; Gerber, G.K.; Noval Rivas, M.; Wang, S.; Harb, H.; Wang, L.; Li, N.; Crestani, E.; Spielman, S.; et al. Microbiota therapy acts via a regulatory T cell MyD88/RORγt pathway to suppress food allergy. *Nat. Med.* **2019**, *25*, 1164–1174. [CrossRef]
9. Claesson, M.J.; Jeffery, I.B.; Conde, S.; Power, S.E.; O'Connor, E.M.; Cusack, S.; Harris, H.M.; Coakley, M.; Lakshminarayanan, B.; O'Sullivan, O.; et al. Gut microbiota composition correlates with diet and health in the elderly. *Nature* **2012**, *488*, 178–184. [CrossRef]
10. Zhu, W.; Gregory, J.C.; Org, E.; Buffa, J.A.; Gupta, N.; Wang, Z.; Li, L.; Fu, X.; Wu, Y.; Mehrabian, M.; et al. Gut Microbial Metabolite TMAO Enhances Platelet Hyperreactivity and Thrombosis Risk. *Cell* **2016**, *165*, 111–124. [CrossRef]
11. Tang, W.H.W.; Wang, Z.; Levison, B.S.; Koeth, R.A.; Britt, E.B.; Fu, X.; Wu, Y.; Hazen, S.L. Intestinal Microbial Metabolism of Phosphatidylcholine and Cardiovascular Risk. *N. Engl. J. Med.* **2013**, *368*, 1575–1584. [CrossRef] [PubMed]

12. Hill, C.; Guarner, F.; Reid, G.; Gibson, G.R.; Merenstein, D.J.; Pot, B.; Morelli, L.; Canani, R.B.; Flint, H.J.; Salminen, S.; et al. Expert consensus document: The International Scientific Association for Probiotics and Prebiotics consensus statement on the scope and appropriate use of the term probiotic. *Nat. Rev. Gastroenterol. Hepatol.* **2014**, *11*, 506–514. [CrossRef] [PubMed]
13. Gibson, G.R.; Hutkins, R.; Sanders, M.E.; Prescott, S.L.; Reimer, R.A.; Salminen, S.J.; Scott, K.; Stanton, C.; Swanson, K.S.; Cani, P.D.; et al. Expert consensus document: The International Scientific Association for Probiotics and Prebiotics (ISAPP) consensus statement on the definition and scope of prebiotics. *Nat. Rev. Gastroenterol. Hepatol.* **2017**, *14*, 491–502. [CrossRef] [PubMed]
14. Chung, W.S.F.; Meijerink, M.; Zeuner, B.; Holck, J.; Louis, P.; Meyer, A.S.; Wells, J.M.; Flint, H.J.; Duncan, S.H. Prebiotic potential of pectin and pectic oligosaccharides to promote anti-inflammatory commensal bacteria in the human colon. *FEMS Microbiol. Ecol.* **2017**, *93*. [CrossRef] [PubMed]
15. Poeker, S.A.; Geirnaert, A.; Berchtold, L.; Greppi, A.; Krych, L.; Steinert, R.E.; De Wouters, T.; Lacroix, C. Understanding the prebiotic potential of different dietary fibers using an in vitro continuous adult fermentation model (PolyFermS). *Sci. Rep.* **2018**, *8*, 4318. [CrossRef]
16. Ohashi, Y.; Sumitani, K.; Tokunaga, M.; Ishihara, N.; Okubo, T.; Fujisawa, T. Consumption of partially hydrolysed guar gum stimulates Bifidobacteria and butyrate-producing bacteria in the human large intestine. *Benef. Microbes* **2015**, *6*, 451–455. [CrossRef]
17. Yasukawa, Z.; Inoue, R.; Ozeki, M.; Okubo, T.; Takagi, T.; Honda, A.; Naito, Y. Effect of Repeated Consumption of Partially Hydrolyzed Guar Gum on Fecal Characteristics and Gut Microbiota: A Randomized, Double-Blind, Placebo-Controlled, and Parallel-Group Clinical Trial. *Nutrients* **2019**, *11*, 2170. [CrossRef]
18. Niv, E.; Halak, A.; Tiommny, E.; Yanai, H.; Strul, H.; Naftali, T.; Vaisman, N. Randomized clinical study: Partially hydrolyzed guar gum (PHGG) versus placebo in the treatment of patients with irritable bowel syndrome. *Nutr. Metab.* **2016**, *13*, 10. [CrossRef]
19. Parisi, G.C.; Zilli, M.; Miani, M.P.; Carrara, M.; Bottona, E.; Verdianelli, G.; Battaglia, G.; Desideri, S.; Faedo, A.; Marzolino, C.; et al. High-fiber diet supplementation in patients with irritable bowel syndrome (IBS): A multicenter, randomized, open trial comparison between wheat bran diet and partially hydrolyzed guar gum (PHGG). *Dig. Dis. Sci.* **2002**, *47*, 1697–1704. [CrossRef]
20. Koh, A.; De Vadder, F.; Kovatcheva-Datchary, P.; Backhed, F. From Dietary Fiber to Host Physiology: Short-Chain Fatty Acids as Key Bacterial Metabolites. *Cell* **2016**, *165*, 1332–1345. [CrossRef]
21. Kapoor, M.P.; Sugita, M.; Fukuzawa, Y.; Okubo, T. Impact of partially hydrolyzed guar gum (PHGG) on constipation prevention: A systematic review and meta-analysis. *J. Funct. Foods* **2017**, *33*, 52–66. [CrossRef]
22. Klindworth, A.; Pruesse, E.; Schweer, T.; Peplies, J.; Quast, C.; Horn, M.; Glockner, F.O. Evaluation of general 16S ribosomal RNA gene PCR primers for classical and next-generation sequencing-based diversity studies. *Nucleic Acids Res.* **2013**, *41*, e1. [CrossRef] [PubMed]
23. Andrews, S. FastQC: A Quality Control Tool for High throughput Sequence Data; 2010 [M1]. Available online: http://www.bioinformatics.babraham.ac.uk/projects/fastqc (accessed on 1 April 2020).
24. Schloss, P.D.; Westcott, S.L.; Ryabin, T.; Hall, J.R.; Hartmann, M.; Hollister, E.B.; Lesniewski, R.A.; Oakley, B.B.; Parks, D.H.; Robinson, C.J.; et al. Introducing mothur: Open-source, platform-independent, community-supported software for describing and comparing microbial communities. *Appl. Environ. Microbiol.* **2009**, *75*, 7537–7541. [CrossRef] [PubMed]
25. Kozich, J.J.; Westcott, S.L.; Baxter, N.T.; Highlander, S.K.; Schloss, P.D. Development of a dual-index sequencing strategy and curation pipeline for analyzing amplicon sequence data on the MiSeq Illumina sequencing platform. *Appl. Environ. Microbiol.* **2013**, *79*, 5112–5120. [CrossRef]
26. Schmieder, R.; Edwards, R. Quality control and preprocessing of metagenomic datasets. *Bioinformatics* **2011**, *27*, 863–864. [CrossRef]
27. Quast, C.; Pruesse, E.; Yilmaz, P.; Gerken, J.; Schweer, T.; Yarza, P.; Peplies, J.; Glockner, F.O. The SILVA ribosomal RNA gene database project: Improved data processing and web-based tools. *Nucleic Acids Res.* **2013**, *41*, D590–D596. [CrossRef]
28. Rognes, T.; Flouri, T.; Nichols, B.; Quince, C.; Mahe, F. VSEARCH: A versatile open source tool for metagenomics. *PeerJ* **2016**, *4*, e2584. [CrossRef]
29. Moosmang, S.; Pitscheider, M.; Sturm, S.; Seger, C.; Tilg, H.; Halabalaki, M.; Stuppner, H. Metabolomic analysis-Addressing NMR and LC-MS related problems in human feces sample preparation. *Clin. Chim. Acta* **2019**, *489*, 169–176. [CrossRef]

30. Savorani, F.; Tomasi, G.; Engelsen, S.B. icoshift: A versatile tool for the rapid alignment of 1D NMR spectra. *J. Magn. Reson.* **2010**, *202*, 190–202. [CrossRef]
31. Tardivel, P.J.C.; Canlet, C.; Lefort, G.; Tremblay-Franco, M.; Debrauwer, L.; Concordet, D.; Servien, R. ASICS: An automatic method for identification and quantification of metabolites in complex 1D 1H NMR spectra. *Metabolomics* **2017**, *13*, 109. [CrossRef]
32. McMurdie, P.J.; Holmes, S. phyloseq: An R package for reproducible interactive analysis and graphics of microbiome census data. *PLoS ONE* **2013**, *8*, e61217. [CrossRef] [PubMed]
33. Oksanen, J.; Blanchet, F.G.; Friendly, M.; Kindt, R.; Legendre, P.; McGlinn, D.; Minchin, P.R.; O'Hara, R.B.; Simpson, G.L.; Solymos, P.; et al. Vegan: Community Ecology Package; R Package Version 2.4-6; 2018 [M2]. Available online: https://CRAN.R-project.org/package=vegan (accessed on 1 April 2020).
34. Love, M.I.; Huber, W.; Anders, S. Moderated estimation of fold change and dispersion for RNA-seq data with DESeq2. *Genome Biol.* **2014**, *15*, 550. [CrossRef] [PubMed]
35. McMurdie, P.J.; Holmes, S. Waste not, want not: Why rarefying microbiome data is inadmissible. *PLoS Comput. Biol.* **2014**, *10*, e1003531. [CrossRef] [PubMed]
36. Friedman, J.; Alm, E.J. Inferring Correlation Networks from Genomic Survey Data. *PLoS Comput. Biol.* **2012**, *8*, e1002687. [CrossRef]
37. Shannon, P.; Markiel, A.; Ozier, O.; Baliga, N.S.; Wang, J.T.; Ramage, D.; Amin, N.; Schwikowski, B.; Ideker, T. Cytoscape: A software environment for integrated models of biomolecular interaction networks. *Genome Res.* **2003**, *13*, 2498–2504. [CrossRef]
38. Willeit, J.; Kiechl, S.; Oberhollenzer, F.; Rungger, G.; Egger, G.; Bonora, E.; Mitterer, M.; Muggeo, M. Distinct risk profiles of early and advanced atherosclerosis: Prospective results from the Bruneck Study. *Arterioscler. Thromb. Vasc. Biol.* **2000**, *20*, 529–537. [CrossRef]
39. Fischbach, M.A.; Segre, J.A. Signaling in Host-Associated Microbial Communities. *Cell* **2016**, *164*, 1288–1300. [CrossRef]
40. Scott, K.P.; Grimaldi, R.; Cunningham, M.; Sarbini, S.R.; Wijeyesekera, A.; Tang, M.L.K.; Lee, J.C.; Yau, Y.F.; Ansell, J.; Theis, S.; et al. Developments in understanding and applying prebiotics in research and practice-an ISAPP conference paper. *J. Appl. Microbiol.* **2019**. [CrossRef]
41. Giannini, E.G.; Mansi, C.; Dulbecco, P.; Savarino, V. Role of partially hydrolyzed guar gum in the treatment of irritable bowel syndrome. *Nutrition* **2006**, *22*, 334–342. [CrossRef]
42. Polymeros, D.; Beintaris, I.; Gaglia, A.; Karamanolis, G.; Papanikolaou, I.S.; Dimitriadis, G.; Triantafyllou, K. Partially hydrolyzed guar gum accelerates colonic transit time and improves symptoms in adults with chronic constipation. *Dig. Dis. Sci.* **2014**, *59*, 2207–2214. [CrossRef]
43. Gibson, G.R.; Roberfroid, M.B. Dietary modulation of the human colonic microbiota: Introducing the concept of prebiotics. *J. Nutr.* **1995**, *125*, 1401–1412. [CrossRef] [PubMed]
44. Noack, J.; Timm, D.; Hospattankar, A.; Slavin, J. Fermentation profiles of wheat dextrin, inulin and partially hydrolyzed guar gum using an in vitro digestion pretreatment and in vitro batch fermentation system model. *Nutrients* **2013**, *5*, 1500–1510. [CrossRef] [PubMed]
45. Bindels, L.B.; Delzenne, N.M.; Cani, P.D.; Walter, J. Towards a more comprehensive concept for prebiotics. *Nat. Rev. Gastroenterol. Hepatol.* **2015**, *12*, 303–310. [CrossRef] [PubMed]
46. De Palma, G.; Lynch, M.D.; Lu, J.; Dang, V.T.; Deng, Y.; Jury, J.; Umeh, G.; Miranda, P.M.; Pigrau Pastor, M.; Sidani, S.; et al. Transplantation of fecal microbiota from patients with irritable bowel syndrome alters gut function and behavior in recipient mice. *Sci. Transl. Med.* **2017**, *9*. [CrossRef]
47. Zmora, N.; Suez, J.; Elinav, E. You are what you eat: Diet, health and the gut microbiota. *Nat. Rev. Gastroenterol. Hepatol.* **2019**, *16*, 35–56. [CrossRef]

5

Short- and Long-Term Effects of Wholegrain Oat Intake on Weight Management and Glucolipid Metabolism in Overweight Type-2 Diabetics

Xue Li [1,2], Xiaxia Cai [1,3], Xiaotao Ma [1,4], Lulu Jing [1], Jiaojiao Gu [1], Lei Bao [1,5], Jun Li [6], Meihong Xu [1], Zhaofeng Zhang [1] and Yong Li [1,*]

1 Department of Nutrition and Food Hygiene, School of Public Health, Peking University, Beijing 100191, China; xue.li@ed.ac.uk (X.L.); shuiruoran8886@126.com (X.C.); maxt2008@sina.com (X.M.); jingll_wit@bjmu.edu.cn (L.J.); jiaojiaogu442@gmail.com (J.G.); baolei6230@163.com (L.B.); xumeihong@bjmu.edu.cn (M.X.); zzfeng1104@bjmu.edu.cn (Z.Z.)
2 Centre for Population Health Sciences, University of Edinburgh, Edinburgh EH8 9AG, UK
3 Department of Nutrition and Food Hygiene, School of Public Health, Capital Medical University, Beijing 100191, China
4 Department of Clinical Nutrition, China-Japan Friendship Hospital, Peking University, Beijing 100191, China
5 Department of Clinical Nutrition, International Hospital, Peking University, Beijing 100191, China
6 The 153 Hospital of People's Liberation Army, Zhengzhou 450001, China; pla153ywc@163.com
* Correspondence: liyongbmu@163.com;

Abstract: Glycemic control and weight reduction are primary goals for the management of overweight and obese type 2 diabetes mellitus (T2DM). Effective management cannot be achieved without an appropriate diet. Our study aimed to evaluate the short- and long-term effects of oat intake and develop a reasonable dietary plan for overweight T2DM patients. A randomized control trial, registered under ClinicalTrials.gov (Identification code: NCT01495052), was carried out among adult T2DM patients. A subgroup of 298 overweight subjects was selected and received a 30-day centralized intervention and 1-year free-living follow-up. Participants were randomly allocated to one of the following four groups. The usual care group ($n = 60$) received no intervention; the healthy diet group ($n = 79$) received a low-fat and high-fiber diet ("healthy diet"); the 50 g-oats group ($n = 80$) and 100 g-oats group ($n = 79$) received the "healthy diet" with the same amount of cereals replaced by 50 g and 100 g oats respectively. Anthropometric, blood glycemic and lipid variables were measured. For the 30-day intervention, significant differences in the changes of FPG (fasting plasma glucose), PPG (postprandial plasma glucose), HbA1c (glycosylated hemoglobin), HOMA-IR (homeostasis model assessment of insulin resistance), TC (total cholesterol), TG (total triglycerides), and LDL-c (low-density lipoprotein cholesterol) were observed among the four groups. Compared to the healthy diet group, the 50 g-oats group had a bigger reduction in PPG (mean difference (MD): −1.04 mmol/L; 95% CI: −2.03, −0.05) and TC (MD: −0.24 mmol/L; 95% CI: −0.47, −0.01); the 100 g-oats group had a bigger reduction in PPG (MD: −1.48 mmol/L; 95% CI: −2.57, −0.39), HOMA-IR (MD: −1.77 mU·mol/L^2; 95% CI: −3.49, −0.05), TC (MD: −0.33 mmol/L; 95% CI: −0.56, −0.10) and LDL-c (MD: −0.22 mmol/L; 95% CI: −0.41, −0.03). In the 1-year follow-up, greater effects in reducing weight (MD: −0.89 kg; 95% CI: −1.56, −0.22), HbA1c (MD: −0.64%; 95% CI: −1.19, −0.09) and TG (MD: −0.70 mmol/L; 95% CI: −1.11, −0.29) were observed in the 100 g-oats group. In conclusion, short- and long-term oat intake had significant effects on controlling hyperglycemia, lowering blood lipid and reducing weight. Our study provided some supportive evidence for recommending oat as a good whole grain selection for overweight diabetics.

Keywords: type 2 diabetes; obesity; whole grain; oats; fiber

---

1. Introduction

Type 2 diabetes (T2DM) and obesity are both major global health problems, which have been linked with an increased risk of life-threatening comorbidities and enormous economic burdens [1,2]. Epidemiological studies report that most of the patients with T2DM are overweight or obese and, similarly, a significant number of obese individuals have diabetes [3]. This parallel prevalence indicates a strong association between T2DM and obesity. It has been further estimated that every 1 kilogram increase in body weight is associated with a 9% relative increase in diabetes prevalence [4]. Identification of this association has changed the primary goal of diabetes management in obese and overweight T2DM patients, and now controlling the blood glucose and reducing weight are both promoted [5].

Effective management of diabetes cannot be achieved without an appropriate diet, especially for type 2 diabetics who are overweight or obese. The recommended diet for controlling diabetes should be rich in dietary fiber, preferably provided by nature and less processed whole grains [6]. A Harvard study of health professionals found that high intake of whole grains was associated with lower incidence of T2DM [7] and therefore its benefit could be an important part of a diet which can help to improve diabetic control.

Wholegrain foods can be found in a variety of cereals, but the content and solubility of fiber can vary significantly [8]. People with diabetes are often advised to select a good source of whole grains. Oat, with the advantage of having a high concentration of β-glucan, can be used for the management of diabetes [9]. The effects of oat intake have been investigated in several aspects [10–12]. Soluble fiber from oats has been found to be effective in lowering total cholesterol and low-density lipoprotein (5%–10% reduction with 3 g β-glucan intake per day), and thus oat and oat-products have already been recommended to patients with hyperlipidemia [13]. Besides, it has been suggested that oat intake can improve insulin response and decrease postprandial hyperglycemia [11,14]. Although these effects have been supported in many studies, others failed to replicate these. In particular, the effects of oat intake on fasting glucose concentration and weight control remain conflicting [11,14]. Therefore, further work is needed to determine whether oat intake has the reported benefits and whether these benefits could be observed similarly in specific populations, particularly in overweight T2DM patients.

To develop a reasonable dietary plan, which includes wholegrain oats, a randomized control trail was conducted among adults with T2DM in Baotou, Inner Mongolia, China. This study aimed to compare the short- and long-term integrative effects of oat intake with a low-fat and high-fiber diet ("healthy diet") on weight management, blood glucose control and lipid-profile improvement in overweight T2DM patients.

2. Methods

2.1. Participants

A subgroup of 298 subjects, meeting the Chinese criteria of overweight (body mass index $\geq$ 24 kg/m^2), was selected from 445 adult patients with T2DM, who had participated in the 30-day centralized management of a dietary program and the 1-year free-living follow-up in Baotou, China. The sample size of the original study was calculated based on an estimated standard deviation (SD) of 2.7 mmol/L in HbA1c. A total of 420 participants were required to detect a difference of 0.80 SD of HbA1c with 90% power and allowing for 10% missing data. Individuals who were heavy smokers (smoking more than or equal to 25 cigarettes per day) or heavy drinkers (drinking more than 25 mL alcohol per day), or had recent changes (less than 3 months) in diet and physical activities, or had severe cardiovascular, renal or hepatic complications, mental illness or other serious diseases, or recently accepted glucocorticoid treatment, or had already been eating oats or oat products as part of their diet, were excluded. At the end of recruitment, a total of 445 individuals were included and randomized, of which 298 overweight participants were selected for this subgroup analysis.

Eleven patients dropped out during the 1-year follow-up due to personal reasons with no difference in drop-out rates among the four groups ($p = 0.774$) (Figure 1).

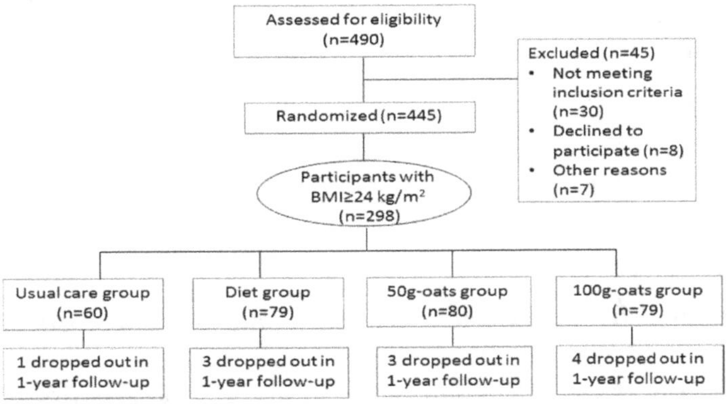

Figure 1. Flow chart for subject enrollment, allocation, intervention and follow-up.

2.2. Ethics

This study was approved by the ethic review board of China-Japan Friendship Hospital of Health Ministry China in December 2011 and registered under ClinicalTrials.gov (Identification code: NCT01495052 available at https://clinicaltrials.gov/). Written and oral information of the study protocol was given prior to the study initiation. Informed consent was signed by every participant.

2.3. Study Design

During the 30-day centralized intervention, all participants were arranged to live in a hotel and have meals together under the supervision of 12 qualified dietitians and 18 well trained investigators. Food intake and compliance of participants were recorded every day by the investigators. Physical activities were assessed and categorized using the recommendations of the international physical activity questionnaire (IPAQ). Participants were required to record uncomfortable symptoms and maintain their normal physical activities and medications. After a one-week run-in period, participants were randomly allocated to one of the following four groups by computer-generated random numbers. The usual care group ($n = 60$) served as the control group and received no dietry intervention. They took meals depending on their own eating habits. The healthy diet group ($n = 79$) received a low-fat and high-fiber diet ("healthy diet"). A 7-day cyclical menu (Supplementary Materials Table S1) was designed according to the China Food Composition [15], the Dietary Guidelines for Chinese Resident [16] and the China Medical Nutrition Therapy Guideline for Diabetes [17] to provide a low-fat and high-fiber diet. Each participant was provided with three meals a day, which contained 2275 kcal for men and 1890 kcal for women (60% from carbohydrate, 22% from fat, 18% from protein) and 30 g of dietary fiber. In addition, a maximum of an extra 10% of daily kcal intake was allowed according to the individual need of participants. For the 50 g and 100 g-oats groups, participants received the "healthy diet" with the same amount of cereals replaced by 50 g and 100 g of wholegrain oats respectively. The daily intake of energy and macronutrients for each group is shown in Table 1. Apart from the dietary intervention, the study dieticians gave nutritional education and training to the three intervention groups six times per week to encourage the participants to have a general healthy diet in daily life.

After the centralized management, all participants returned home and were asked to continue with their intervention and record their daily diet, uncomfortable symptoms and medication changes. Wholegrain oats were continuously provided for the 50 g and 100 g-oats groups. Investigators continued to give diet recommendations and supervise the daily life of participants by monthly group interviews through network-chat, telephone or face-to-face interviews. Scheduled clinical checks were performed every three months. The follow-up lasted for one year.

Table 1. The daily intake of energy and macronutrients (one day's intake).

Dietary Components	Usual Care Group	Treatment Diet		
		Healthy Diet Group	50 g-oats Group	100 g-oats Group
Energy (kcal) *	2441 (478)	2279 (196)	2281 (185)	2233 (204)
Carbohydrate (% of total energy)	50	60	59	58
Fat (% of total energy)	31	22	23	23
Protein (% of total energy)	19	18	18	19
Total fiber (g) *	22.1 (4.0)	33.0 (5.8)	36.1 (4.2)	39.0 (4.8)
Oat β-glucan (g)	0	0	2.65	5.30

* Variables are presented as mean with (SD (standard deviation)).

2.4. Wholegrain Oats

The wholegrain oats used in this study were provided by Inner Mongolia Sanzhuliang Natural Oats Industry Corporation (IMSNOIC) (Hohhot, Inner Mongolia, China). The oats were grown in northwest China and were processed by a peeling technology which retained the necessary ingredients and beneficial nutrients of the whole grain [18]. The nutrient composition of this product was analyzed by the laboratory of the School of Life Sciences, Sun Yat-sen University, according to a standard procedure (GB/T 5009). Each 100 g of wholegrain oats contained 63.5 g carbohydrate, 7.6 g fat, 13.7 g protein, and 8.7 g fiber, of which approximately 5.3 g was β-glucan.

2.5. Outcome Measurement

Physical examinations were performed at baseline, at the end of the 30-day intervention and at the end of the 1-year follow-up. Anthropometric measurements were carried out for weight, height, waist and hip circumference, and blood pressure. Body fat percent and visceral fat index (VFI) were measured using bioelectrical impedance scales (Tanita BF-622W, Tanita Corporation of the United State). Venus blood samples were collected after an overnight fast for testing fasting plasma glucose (FPG), 2-h postprandial plasma glucose (PPG), glycosylated hemoglobin (HbA1c), fasting plasma insulin, 2-h postprandial plasma insulin, total triglycerides (TG), total cholesterol (TC), low-density lipoprotein cholesterol (LDL-c), and high-density lipoprotein cholesterol (HDL-c). Insulin resistance was calculated by the formula: HOMA-IR = fasting serum insulin (μU/mL) × FPG (mmol/L)/22.5. All measurements were conducted with standard procedures by the same clinical staff in the third hospital of Inner Mongolia medical college, who were blinded to the group allocation.

2.6. Statistical Analyses

Categorical and continuous variables were analyzed by either Chi-squared test or sample *t*-test. Responses to interventions were assessed by the changes in anthropometric and metabolic variables, determined at baseline and at the end of the intervention. A generalized linear model (GLM) was applied to estimate the changes after adjusting for potential confounding factors including sex, age, drinking, smoking, physical activity level, education level, family history of diabetes, diabetic medications and the duration of diabetes. The mean differences (MD) of changes among groups were calculated to compare the effects of different interventions. We performed multiple imputations to account for missing data (SAS Institute, Inc., Cary, NC, USA). Results are presented as means with standard deviation (SD) or 95% confidence intervals (95% CI). All tests were two-sided and $p < 0.05$ was considered to be statistically significant. Analyses were conducted with the IBM SPSS Statistics 22 (IBM Corp., Armonk, NY, USA, 2013), unless otherwise stated.

3. Results

The main characteristics of the participants in each group are shown in Table 2. Among the four groups, there were no significant differences in the baseline characteristics of sex, age, drinking, smoking, physical activity, education level, the duration of diabetes, family history of diabetes, diabetic medications and blood pressure.

Table 2. The baseline characteristics of the study participants *.

Variables	Usual Care Group (n = 60)	Healthy Diet Group (n = 79)	50 g-oats Group (n = 80)	100 g-oats Group (n = 79)	p-Value
Male/female	39/21	42/37	41/39	33/46	0.059
Age (years)	59.00 (3.94)	59.73 (6.53)	59.72 (6.10)	59.44 (6.78)	0.886
Mild drinking	15 (25.0%)	20 (25.3%)	17 (21.3%)	16 (20.3%)	0.838
Mild smoking	14 (23.3%)	16 (20.3%)	14 (17.5%)	11 (13.9%)	0.523
Physical activity level	-	-	-	-	0.541
Low	13 (21.7%)	18 (22.8%)	17 (21.2%)	22 (27.8%)	-
Moderate	30 (50.0%)	42 (53.1%)	45 (56.3%)	46 (58.2%)	-
High	17 (28.3%)	19 (24.1%)	18 (22.5%)	11 (13.9%)	-
Education level	-	-	-	-	0.473
Less than primary school	9 (15.0%)	9 (11.4%)	15 (18.8%)	8 (10.1%)	-
Middle and high school	39 (65.0%)	56 (70.9%)	47 (58.8%)	49 (62.0%)	-
College or more	12 (20.0%)	14 (17.7%)	18 (22.5%)	22 (27.8%)	-
Duration of diabetes (month)	79.00 (36.52)	74.87 (61.92)	100.08 (75.73)	94.71 (76.63)	0.060
Family history of diabetes	19 (31.7%)	24 (30.4%)	36 (45.0%)	38 (48.1%)	0.051
Diabetic medications	-	-	-	-	0.999
No diabetic medication	5 (8.3%)	7 (8.9%)	6 (7.5%)	6 (7.6%)	-
Oral diabetic medication	32 (53.3%)	45 (57.0%)	43 (53.8%)	47 (59.5%)	-
Insulin injection	12 (20.0%)	14 (17.7%)	16 (20.0%)	12 (15.2%)	-
Combined treatment	11 (18.3%)	13 (16.4%)	15 (18.7%)	14(17.7%)	-
Systolic blood pressure (mmHg)	143.71 (15.83)	147.23 (21.31)	144.90 (19.18)	147.19 (17.68)	0.613
Diastolic blood pressure (mmHg)	84.43 (16.05)	84.63 (11.78)	82.93 (9.39)	83.10 (10.20)	0.737

* Continuous variables are presented as mean with (SD) and categorical variables are presented as a number (with percentage).

Changes in variables, and the mean differences of changes among the four groups after the 30-day intervention, are presented in Table 3. When compared to the baseline values of the anthropometric variables, the three intervention groups had a significant reduction in weight, BMI and waist circumference, while significant reduction in visceral fat index (VFI) was only observed in the 50 g oats group (adjusted change: −0.48; 95% CI: −0.69, −0.27) and the 100 g oats group (adjusted change: −0.44; 95% CI: −0.78, −0.10). When comparing the mean differences between groups, there were no statistically significant differences in the changes of anthropometric variables between the healthy diet group and the oats groups.

For the glycemic variables, a significant reduction in FPG, PPG and HbA1c from baseline was observed in the three intervention groups, while a significant decrease in HOMA-IR was observed in 50 g oats group (adjusted change: −1.80 mU·mol/L^2; 95% CI: −3.48, −0.12) and 100 g oats group (adjusted change: −2.65 mU·mol/L^2; 95% CI: −4.72, −0.58). When comparing the changes between groups (the healthy diet group was the reference), the 50 g oats group showed a bigger reduction in PPG (MD: −1.04 mmol/L; 95% CI: −2.03, −0.05), and the 100 g oats group showed a bigger reduction in PPG (MD: −1.48 mmol/L; 95% CI: −2.57, −0.39) and HOMA-IR (MD: −1.77 mU·mol/L^2; 95% CI: −3.49, −0.05).

Compared to the baseline values of the lipid variables, the three intervention groups had a significant reduction in TC and LDL-c. When comparing between groups, the 50 g oats group had a bigger reduction in TC (MD: −0.24 mmol/L; 95% CI: −0.47, −0.01) and the 100 g oats group had a bigger reduction in TC (MD: −0.33 mmol/L; 95% CI: −0.56, −0.10) and LDL-c (MD: −0.22 mmol/L; 95% CI: −0.41, −0.03) than the healthy diet group. For TG, no statistically significant difference in the reduction was observed in the two oats groups when compared to the healthy diet group.

The changes and mean differences of changes in variables between the baseline and the end of the 1-year intervention are shown in Table 4. Compared with the baseline values, the three intervention groups had significant reduction in FPG, PPG, HbA1c, TC, and LDL-c, while the significant decrease in weight, BMI and TG was only observed in the 50 g and 100 g oats groups. Comparing the oats groups to the healthy diet group, the 50 g oats group had a bigger reduction in TG (MD: −0.42 mmol/L; 95% CI: −0.83, −0.01) and LDL-c (MD: −0.27 mmol/L; 95% CI: −0.49, −0.05), and the 100 g oats group had a bigger reduction in weight (MD: −0.89 kg; 95% CI: −1.56, −0.22), PPG (MD: −1.17 mmol/L; 95% CI: −2.27, −0.07), HbA1c (MD: −0.64%; 95% CI: −1.19, −0.09), TC (MD: −0.30 mmol/L; 95% CI: −0.57, −0.03), TG (MD: −0.70 mmol/L; 95% CI: −1.11, −0.29), and LDL-c (MD: −0.37 mmol/L; 95% CI: −0.59, −0.15).

Table 3. Changes in variables and mean differences (MD) in changes among groups after 30-day intervention *.

Variables	Usual Care Group (n = 60)	Healthy Diet Group (n = 79)	50 g-oats Group (n = 80)	100 g-oats Group (n = 79)	p-Value
Weight (kg)					
Baseline	71.54 (5.82)	73.77 (8.58)	72.60 (8.67)	74.44 (7.63)	0.141
30-day intervention	71.45 (6.00)	72.59 (7.94)	71.74 (8.50)	72.70 (7.21)	-
Adjusted changes	−0.18 (−1.39, 1.02)	−1.20 (−2.22, −0.19)	−1.67(−2.69, −0.65)	−1.74 (−2.76, −0.71)	0.178
MD (vs. usual care group)	-	−1.02 (−2.56, 0.52)	−1.49 (−3.03, 0.05)	−1.56 (−3.14, 0.02)	-
MD (vs. diet group)	-	-	−0.47 (−1.89, 0.96)	−0.54 (−1.97, 0.89)	-
BMI (kg/m^2)					
Baseline	25.17 (0.89)	27.19 (2.82)	26.91 (2.69)	27.39 (2.42)	0.000
30-day intervention	25.14 (0.94)	26.77 (2.66)	26.28 (3.86)	26.77 (2.33)	-
Adjusted changes	−0.08 (−0.49, 0.33)	−0.43 (−0.78, −0.08)	−0.60(−0.95, −0.25)	−0.63 (−0.98, −0.28)	0.160
MD (vs. usual care group)	-	−0.35 (−0.88, 0.18)	−0.52 (−1.05, 0.01)	−0.55 (−1.10, 0.00)	-
MD (vs. diet group)	-	-	−0.17 (−0.66, 0.32)	−0.20 (−0.69, 0.29)	-
Waist circumference (cm)					
Baseline	92.69 (7.94)	94.81 (7.01)	93.38 (6.79)	94.86 (7.65)	0.210
30-day intervention	91.92 (8.22)	92.02 (8.63)	91.08 (3.98)	92.07 (7.27)	-
Adjusted changes	−0.78 (−2.92, 1.36)	−2.79 (−3.85, −1.73)	−2.32 (−3.37, −1.27)	−2.77 (−3.83, −1.70)	0.028
MD (vs. usual care group)	-	−2.01 (−3.54, −0.48)	−1.54 (−3.08, 0.00)	−1.99 (−3.48, −0.50)	-
MD (vs. diet group)	-	-	0.47 (−1.01, 1.95)	0.02 (−1.47, 1.50)	-
Waist-to-hip ratio(WHR)					
Baseline	0.91 (0.05)	0.92 (0.05)	0.91 (0.05)	0.92 (0.05)	0.398
30-day intervention	0.90 (0.05)	0.91(0.07)	0.90 (0.05)	0.90 (0.05)	-
Adjusted changes	−0.01(−0.02, 0.01)	−0.01 (−0.02, 0.01)	−0.01 (−0.02, 0.01)	−0.02 (−0.03, −0.01)	0.259
MD (vs. usual care group)	-	0.00 (−0.02, 0.02)	0.00 (−0.02, 0.02)	−0.01 (−0.03, 0.01)	-
MD (vs. diet group)	-	-	0.00 (−0.02, 0.02)	0.00 (−0.02, 0.02)	-
Body fat percent (%)					
Baseline	32.46 (5.49)	31.58 (6.11)	31.54 (5.87)	33.31 (5.12)	0.162
30-day intervention	32.21 (5.88)	31.05 (6.23)	31.37 (5.75)	32.78 (5.34)	-
Adjusted changes	−0.25 (−1.09, 0.59)	−0.59 (−1.20, 0.02)	−0.52 (−1.12, 0.08)	−0.52 (−1.13, 0.08)	0.878
MD (vs. usual care group)	-	−0.34 (−1.06, 0.36)	−0.27 (−0.85, 0.31)	−0.27 (−0.81, 0.26)	-
MD (vs. diet group)	-	-	0.07 (−0.51, 0.65)	0.07 (−0.51, 0.65)	-
Visceral fat index (VFI)					
Baseline	12.37 (3.64)	12.38 (3.86)	12.53 (4.14)	12.33 (3.59)	0.988
30-day intervention	12.13 (3.77)	12.13 (3.53)	12.06 (4.42)	11.87 (3.47)	-
Adjusted changes	−0.25 (−0.55, 0.05)	−0.27 (−0.62, 0.07)	−0.48 (−0.69, −0.27)	−0.44 (−0.78, −0.10)	0.380

Table 3. *Cont.*

Variables	Usual Care Group (n = 60)	Healthy Diet Group (n = 79)	50 g-oats Group (n = 80)	100 g-oats Group (n = 79)	p-Value
MD (vs. usual care group)	-	−0.02 (−0.44, 0.40)	−0.24 (−0.74, 0.26)	−0.19 (−0.73, 0.35)	-
MD (vs. diet group)	-	-	−0.22 (−0.70, 0.27)	−0.17 (−0.64, 0.31)	-
Fasting plasma glucose (mmol/L)					
Baseline	9.38 (2.81)	9.52 (2.87)	9.87 (2.83)	9.70 (3.30)	0.719
30-day intervention	9.40 (0.75)	8.16 (2.53)	8.67 (2.49)	8.03 (2.56)	-
Adjusted changes	−0.20 (−0.91, 0.52)	−1.27 (−1.88, −0.67)	−1.23 (−1.84, −0.62)	−1.70 (−2.31, −1.10)	0.002
MD (vs. usual care group)	-	−1.07 (−1.99, −0.15)	−1.03 (−1.94, −0.11)	−1.50 (−2.42, −0.58)	-
MD (vs. diet group)	-	-	0.04 (−0.81, 0.89)	−0.43 (−1.28, 0.42)	-
2-h postprandial plasma glucose (mmol/L)					
Baseline	19.10 (3.22)	17.58 (4.87)	18.23 (4.84)	17.89 (5.45)	0.284
30-day intervention	18.66 (3.07)	15.42 (4.31)	14.97 (4.10)	14.08 (4.62)	-
Adjusted changes	−0.53 (−1.45, 0.39)	−2.14 (−2.92, −1.36)	−3.18 (−3.95, −2.41)	−3.62 (−4.39., −2.84)	0.001
MD (vs. usual care group)	-	−1.61 (−2.79, −0.43)	−2.65 (−3.82, −1.47)	−3.09 (−4.27, −1.91)	-
MD (vs. diet group)	-	-	−1.04 (−2.03, −0.05)	−1.48 (−2.57, −0.39)	-
HbA1c (%)					
Baseline	8.05 (1.52)	8.10 (1.77)	8.37 (1.44)	8.28 (1.35)	0.463
30-day intervention	8.07 (1.52)	7.88 (1.82)	7.71 (1.94)	7.65 (1.93)	-
Adjusted changes	0.10 (−0.34, 0.54)	−0.61 (−0.98, −0.24)	−0.76 (−1.13, −0.39)	−0.71 (−1.09, −0.34)	0.001
MD (vs. usual care group)	-	−0.71 (−1.29, −0.13)	−0.86 (−1.43, −0.29)	−0.81 (−1.37, −0.24)	-
MD (vs. diet group)	-	-	−0.14 (−0.67, 0.39)	−0.10 (−0.63, 0.43)	-
HOMA-IR (mU·mol/L^2)					
Baseline	5.49 (4.99)	5.48 (5.40)	4.68 (3.78)	6.20 (5.78)	0.312
30-day intervention	5.31 (3.16)	4.50 (4.89)	3.41 (3.23)	3.76 (4.75)	-
Adjusted changes	−0.25 (−2.66, 2.16)	−0.89 (−3.52, 1.74)	−1.80 (−3.48, −0.12)	−2.65 (−4.72, −0.58)	0.010
MD (vs. usual care group)	-	−0.64 (−2.40, 1.12)	−1.55 (−3.30, 0.20)	−2.41 (−4.59, −0.23)	-
MD (vs. diet group)	-	-	−0.91 (−1.93, 0.11)	−1.77 (−3.49, −0.05)	-
TC (total cholesterol) (mmol/L)					
Baseline	5.84 (1.83)	4.98 (0.86)	5.04 (0.98)	5.24 (1.03)	0.000
30-day intervention	5.82 (1.88)	4.81 (0.87)	4.66 (0.87)	4.72 (0.85)	-
Adjusted changes	−0.07 (−0.26, 0.12)	−0.18 (−0.34, −0.02)	−0.42 (−0.59, −0.26)	−0.51 (−0.67, −0.35)	0.000
MD (vs. usual care group)	-	−0.11 (−0.35, 0.14)	−0.35 (−0.60, −0.10)	−0.44 (−0.69, −0.19)	
MD (vs. diet group)	-	-	−0.24 (−0.47, −0.01)	−0.33 (−0.56, −0.10)	-

Table 3. *Cont.*

Variables	Usual Care Group (n = 60)	Healthy Diet Group (n = 79)	50 g-oats Group (n = 80)	100 g-oats Group (n = 79)	p-Value
TG (total triglycerides) (mmol/L)					
Baseline	1.92 (0.94)	1.83 (0.88)	2.06 (1.06)	1.98 (1.00)	0.510
30-day intervention	1.95 (1.02)	1.57 (0.84)	1.98 (1.65)	1.56 (0.77)	-
Adjusted changes	0.01 (−0.25, 0.27)	−0.25 (−0.47, −0.03)	−0.09 (−0.31, 0.13)	−0.43 (−0.65, −0.21)	0.003
MD (vs. usual care group)	-	−0.26 (−0.60, 0.08)	−0.10 (−0.43, 0.23)	−0.44 (−0.78, −0.10)	-
MD (vs. diet group)	-	-	0.16 (−0.26, 0.58)	−0.17 (−0.59, 0.26)	-
LDL-c (low-density lipoprotein cholesterol) (mmol/L)					
Baseline	3.20 (1.05)	2.96 (0.71)	2.90 (0.77)	3.15 (0.85)	0.128
30-day intervention	3.18 (1.05)	2.85 (0.74)	2.70 (0.70)	2.79 (0.63)	-
Adjusted changes	−0.06 (−0.21, 0.10)	−0.12 (−0.25, 0.01)	−0.23 (−0.36, −0.10)	−0.34 (−0.47, −0.21)	0.001
MD (vs. usual care group)	-	−0.06 (−0.26, 0.14)	−0.17 (−0.37, 0.02)	−0.28 (−0.48, −0.08)	-
MD (vs. diet group)	-	-	−0.10 (−0.28, 0.08)	−0.22 (−0.41, −0.03)	-
HDL-c (high-density lipoprotein cholesterol) (mmol/L)					
Baseline	1.41 (0.45)	1.30 (0.24)	1.25 (0.21)	1.36 (0.36)	0.022
30-day intervention	1.39 (0.42)	1.22 (0.24)	1.20 (0.22)	1.28 (0.26)	-
Adjusted changes	−0.02 (−0.07, 0.04)	−0.08 (−0.19, 0.03)	−0.07 (−0.11, −0.02)	−0.08 (−0.13, −0.03)	0.635
MD (vs. usual care group)	-	−0.06 (−0.14, 0.01)	−0.05 (−0.12, 0.02)	−0.06 (−0.14, 0.02)	-
MD (vs. diet group)	-	-	0.01 (−0.05, 0.07)	0.00 (−0.07, 0.07)	-

* All values were presented as means (SD) or means (95% CI). Changes from the baseline were adjusted for potential confounding variables (sex, age, drinking, smoking, physical activity level, education level, family history of diabetes, diabetic medications and duration of diabetes) in the analysis of covariance model.

Table 4. Changes in variables and mean differences (MD) in changes among groups after 1-year follow-up *.

Variables	Usual Care Group (n = 59)	Healthy Diet Group (n = 76)	50 g-oats Group (n = 77)	100 g-oats Group (n = 75)	p-Value
Weight (kg)					
Baseline	71.54 (5.82)	73.77 (8.58)	72.60 (8.67)	74.44 (7.63)	0.141
1-year follow-up	71.47 (7.35)	72.76 (8.70)	71.39 (8.68)	72.43 (7.58)	-
Adjusted changes	−0.11 (−0.68, 0.46)	−1.08 (−2.31, 0.16)	−1.44 (−2.74, −0.15)	−1.97 (−3.06, −0.88)	0.012
MD (vs. usual care group)	-	−0.97 (−2.23, 0.29)	−1.33 (−2.69, 0.03)	−1.86 (−3.25, −0.47)	-
MD (vs. diet group)	-	-	−0.36 (−1.10, 0.38)	−0.89 (−1.56, −0.22)	-
BMI (kg/m^2)					
Baseline	25.17 (0.89)	27.19 (2.82)	26.91 (2.69)	27.39 (2.42)	0.000
1-year follow-up	25.13 (1.25)	26.80 (2.91)	26.48 (2.33)	26.64 (2.74)	-
Adjusted changes	−0.05 (−0.39, 0.29)	−0.37 (−0.74, 0.00)	−0.50 (−0.91, −0.09)	−0.73 (−1.08, −0.39)	0.128
MD (vs. usual care group)	-	−0.33 (−1.05, 0.39)	−0.45 (−1.19, 0.29)	−0.68 (−1.43, 0.07)	-
MD (vs. diet group)	-	-	−0.12 (−0.64, 0.40)	−0.33 (−0.83, 0.17)	-
Fasting plasma glucose (mmol/L)					
Baseline	9.38 (2.81)	9.52 (2.87)	9.87 (2.83)	9.70 (3.30)	0.719
1-year follow-up	9.52 (1.44)	7.94 (2.14)	8.19 (2.01)	7.74 (2.43)	-
Adjusted changes	0.08 (−0.63, 0.46)	−1.65 (−2.21, −1.10)	−1.62 (−2.17, −1.07)	−1.87 (−2.44, −1.31)	0.000
MD (vs. usual care group)	-	−1.57 (−2.36, −0.78)	−1.54 (−2.33, −0.75)	−1.79 (−2.58, −1.00)	-
MD (vs. diet group)	-	-	0.03 (−0.76, 0.82)	−0.22 (−1.02, 0.58)	-
2-h postprandial plasma glucose (mmol/L)					
Baseline	19.10 (3.22)	17.58 (4.87)	18.23 (4.84)	17.89 (5.45)	0.284
1-year follow-up	19.69 (3.27)	15.01 (3.63)	14.98 (3.02)	14.22 (3.78)	-
Adjusted changes	0.63 (−0.36, 1.63)	−2.41 (−3.40, −1.42)	−3.16 (−4.16, −2.16)	−3.58 (−4.63, −2.53)	0.000
MD (vs. usual care group)	-	−3.04 (−4.48, −1.60)	−3.79 (−5.22, −2.36)	−4.21 (−5.67, −2.75)	-
MD (vs. diet group)	-	-	−0.75 (−1.91, 0.41)	−1.17 (−2.27, −0.07)	-
HbA1c (%)					
Baseline	8.05 (1.52)	8.10 (1.77)	8.37 (1.44)	8.28 (1.35)	0.463
1-year follow-up	8.47 (1.86)	7.63 (1.89)	7.41 (1.18)	7.27 (1.72)	-
Adjusted changes	0.35 (−0.01, 0.71)	−0.42 (−0.79, −0.06)	−0.90 (−1.27, −0.54)	−1.06 (−1.44, −0.69)	0.000
MD (vs. usual care group)	-	−0.77 (−1.31, −0.23)	−1.25 (−1.79, −0.71)	−1.41 (−1.95, −0.87)	-
MD (vs. diet group)		-	−0.48 (−1.02, 0.06)	−0.64 (−1.19, −0.09)	-
TC (mmol/L)					
Baseline	5.84 (1.83)	4.98 (0.86)	5.04 (0.98)	5.24 (1.03)	0.000
1-year follow-up	6.01 (1.87)	4.8 (1.04)	4.69 (0.95)	4.76 (0.97)	-
Adjusted changes	0.12 (0.07, 0.31)	−0.19 (−0.38, −0.01)	−0.37 (−0.56, −0.18)	−0.49 (−0.68, −0.29)	0.000

Table 4. *Cont.*

Variables	Usual Care Group (n = 59)	Healthy Diet Group (n = 76)	50 g-oats Group (n = 77)	100 g-oats Group (n = 75)	p-Value
MD (vs. usual care group)	-	−0.31 (−0.62, 0.00)	−0.49 (−0.75, −0.23)	−0.61 (−0.88, −0.34)	-
MD (vs. diet group)	-	-	−0.18 (−0.45, 0.09)	−0.30 (−0.57, −0.03)	-
TG (mmol/L)					
Baseline	1.92 (0.94)	1.83 (0.88)	2.06 (1.06)	1.98 (1.00)	0.510
1-year follow-up	2.13 (1.41)	2.00 (1.91)	1.83 (1.19)	1.55 (0.97)	-
Adjusted changes	0.21 (−0.08, 0.50)	0.17 (−0.12, 0.46)	−0.27 (−0.56, 0.02)	−0.45 (−0.75, −0.16)	0.005
MD (vs. usual care group)	-	−0.04 (−0.45, 0.38)	−0.46 (−0.87, −0.05)	−0.66 (−1.07, −0.25)	-
MD (vs. diet group)	-	-	−0.42 (−0.83, −0.01)	−0.70 (−1.11, −0.29)	-
LDL-c (mmol/L)					
Baseline	3.20 (1.05)	2.96 (0.71)	2.90 (0.77)	3.15 (0.85)	0.128
1-year follow-up	3.35 (0.99)	2.84 (0.88)	2.50 (0.79)	2.64 (0.75)	-
Adjusted changes	0.16 (−0.01, 0.33)	−0.14 (−0.30, 0.01)	−0.41 (−0.56, −0.26)	−0.51 (−0.67, −0.35)	0.000
MD (vs. usual care group)	-	−0.30 (−0.51, −0.09)	−0.57 (−0.78, −0.36)	−0.67 (−0.89, −0.45)	-
MD (vs. diet group)	-	-	−0.27 (−0.49, −0.05)	−0.37 (−0.59, −0.15)	-
HDL-c (mmol/L)					
Baseline	1.41 (0.45)	1.30 (0.24)	1.25 (0.21)	1.36 (0.36)	0.022
1-year follow-up	1.39 (0.34)	1.34 (0.57)	1.29 (0.40)	1.39 (0.41)	-
Adjusted changes	−0.02 (−0.11, 0.07)	0.06 (−0.15, 0.03)	0.06 (−0.03, 0.15)	0.01 (−0.09, 0.10)	0.636
MD (vs. usual care group)	-	0.08 (−0.09, 0.26)	0.09 (−0.08, 0.26)	0.03 (−0.15, 0.21)	-
MD (vs. diet group)	-	-	0.00 (−0.17, 0.18)	−0.05 (−0.23, 0.12)	-

* All values were presented as means (SD) or means (95% CI). Changes from the baseline were adjusted for potential confounding variables (sex, age, drinking/smoking, physical activity level, education level, family history, medications and duration of diabetes) in the analysis of covariance model.

4. Discussion

The present study showed that a low-fat and high-fiber diet ("healthy diet") had beneficial effects on glucolipid metabolism in overweight T2DM patients, and these effects were more evident when combined with oat intake. In particular, the combination of short-term (30 days) oat intake with the "healthy diet" had greater effects on lowering the PPG, HOMA-IR, TC and LDL-c than that of merely having a low-fat and high-fiber diet. The 1-year follow-up showed that the reduction of PPG, HOMA-IR, TC and LDL-c can be maintained for long time, and significantly greater effects in decreasing weight, HbA1c and TG were observed.

The primary finding of this study was the significant effect of oat intake on hyperglycemia control. A growing number of studies have suggested that oats and oat-enriched products can significantly decrease the postprandial hyperglycemia [11,14]. Consistently, our study provided supportive evidence for the PPG lowering effect of oat intake in overweight T2DM patients. Although the mechanism of lowering PPG has not been fully understood, at least parts of the contribution could be attributed to the property of oat β-glucan. Oat β-glucan can increase the viscosity in the intestine, slow the absorption of carbohydrates, and thus reduce the PPG [19,20]. Research findings on the FPG lowering effects of oat intake are less consistent. A few human trials and diabetic mice laboratory studies have found that oat intake can significantly decrease the FPG concertation [14,21,22], but this finding was not supported by the majority of randomized control trials (RCTs) [11]. Although a subgroup analysis of high quality RCTs in a meta-analysis indicated that oat intake can slightly lower FPG concentration in the long-term intervention [11], our study did not find any FPG lowering effect that could be attributed to either short-term or long-term oat intake. The long-term oat intake had a significant effect in reducing HbA1c, but short-term oat intake did not. This finding is not totally unexpected. Considering that HbA1c levels usually reflect the blood glucose levels for the period of 8–12 weeks, the duration of a 30-day intervention may not be long enough to have significant changes in HbA1c, whereas a significant reduction in HbA1c could be shown in the longer 1-year follow-up. So far, a few studies have evaluated the effect of oat intake on HOMA-IR. A meta-analysis of three RCTs reported that oat intake had no effect on the improvement of HOMA-IR [11]. In contrast, our study suggested a significant effect on decreasing HOMA-IR. Our finding was consistent with a recent published RCT, which suggested oats consumption can significantly decrease the HOMA-IR index [23]. These varying results may be partly due to the different characteristics of study populations, probably because overweight and obese T2DM patients are likely to result in more severe insulin resistance, and insulin resistance is more likely to be modifiable in this population [24].

Furthermore, this study confirmed the serum lipid lowering effect of oat intake in overweight T2DM patients. The effect of oat intake on lowering TC and LDL-c has been supported in most published studies [10,13]. The main controversy is the magnitude of the effect. In some studies, the reduction of TC and LDL-c could be more than 10% [25,26], while in others, the reduction was less than 5% [27,28]. In our study, the decrease of TC and LDL-c was around 10%. However, the effect size in this study was not comparable with others, considering the study population, the dose of oats and oat processing were different from other studies. Comparing the duration of the intervention, the long-term oat intake had a significant effect on the reduction of TG. The mechanism of serum lipid-lowering effect also seems to be related to the increased viscosity attributed to the oat β-glucan, which can lead to the reduction in cholesterol absorption [20].

Another finding which is important for overweight T2DM patients is the weight loss effect of long-term oat intake. During the 30-day intervention, the three intervention groups had a significant decrease in body weight and the weight reduction was similar among the three diet groups. However, during the 1-year follow-up, the 100 g oats group had a significantly greater decrease in weight than the healthy diet group. Considering that oat intake was combined with the "healthy diet", it is possible that the moderate weight-reducing effect of a short-term (30 days) oat intake was covered up by the weight reduction due to the low-fat and high-fiber diet; or the duration of a 30-day oat intake was too short to have changes on weight. The bigger weight reduction observed in the 1-year oat intake was unlikely to be caused by the poorly controlled blood glucose level, since a significant reduction in FPG, PPG and HbA1c was also observed. The weight reduction effect is probably related to the oat β-glucan, which may enhance the viscosity of meals, decrease the starch digestion and reduce the food intake by increasing satiety [29]. In addition to our studies, a few other studies also indicated a weigh-reducing effect of oats in certain populations [23,29,30], but these findings were not consistently in agreement, as some studies found no decrease in weight [12,25,31]. Further research is needed to verify the weight-reducing effect of oat intake.

The predominant effect of oats on diabetic management is most likely to be attributed to the bioactivity of β-glucan. Although, compared to other cereals, wholegrain oats have distinct bioactive composition in lipids and phenolics, the most significant difference is in the high content of β-glucan, especially when considering that the effective dose of the other two components is not likely to be achieved through 50 g or 100 g wholegrain oats consumption [30,31]. As mentioned above, β-glucan has been reported to increase the intestinal viscosity, decrease the absorption of carbohydrates and lipids, and reduce food intake to control hyperglycemia, lower lipid and reduce weight. In addition, another important role of β-glucan involves the impact on gut microbiota. Specifically, the bacterial metabolism of β-glucan can increase the production of short-chain fatty acids and drive the release of bioactive compounds, which may interact with host biology to affect the risk of obesity and associated disorders [32,33]. Oat β-glucan has been shown to decrease the protein fermentation and thus reduce the detrimental metabolites produced [34]. Furthermore, the fermentation of β-glucan has also been reported to increase the diversity of gut microbiota, which is a potential benefit, considering that the reduced microbiota diversity is associated with obesity [35,36]. Studies exploring the mechanisms behind the health benefits of β-glucan and gut microbiota may provide more evidence to encourage an increase in oat intake and to maximize the health benefits derived from oats.

Strengths and limitations of the study design should be noted. In the first phase, a 30-day centralized management of intervention was designed to improve the compliance of participants. Potential dietary confounding factors for assessing the effects of oat intake were homogenized among groups by providing a general "healthy diet" to the intervention groups of oat intake and using a healthy diet group as the reference group. To estimate the beneficial effects due to the "healthy diet", a usual care group, with no dietry intervention, was established as a control group. To provide information for recommending a proper dose of daily oat intake (or oat β-glucan), we designed two intervention groups with different doses (50 g and 100 g) of oat intake. Considering that the duration of a 30-day intervention is probably too short for some variables, such as HbAc1 and weight, to have significant changes, a 1-year follow-up was designed to investigate the long-term changes of the variables and to determine if the significant changes observed in the 30-day intervention could be maintained for a long time. However, in this subgroup analysis, we only reported that the anthropometric and blood biochemical variables, cardiovascular events and other diabetic complications were not presented, which led us to consider that the duration of a 1-year intervention was relatively short for evaluating the diabetic complications. Another limitation was that the subjects were not fully blinded because of the different taste of oats and other cereals. Furthermore, the benefits of oat intake were assessed in comparison to an already healthy diet, and as discussed above, it is possible that the moderate beneficial effects of oat intake were covered up or magnified by the healthy reference diet. However, in either case, it should be emphasized that the whole grain oat intake should be recommended with a healthy diet.

5. Conclusions

In conclusion, our study provided some supportive evidence that oats can be a good selection of whole grains for overweight diabetics, but further larger scale studies are needed to evaluate these findings further.

Acknowledgments: The authors would like to thank the Beijing Nutrition Society for the consistent support in the field study and data collection herein. The authors would also like to thank the Third Hospital of Inner Mongolia Medical College for helping with the clinical examinations.

Author Contributions: Y.L. conceived the idea for the study. X.L. performed the statistical analysis and drafted the manuscript. All authors participated in the design of the study, study supervision, data collection and interpretation, revised and approved the final version of the manuscript.

References

1. Series, W.T. Obesity: Preventing and managing the global epidemic. Report of a WHO consultation. *World Health Organ. Tech. Rep. Ser.* **2000**, *894*, 1–253.
2. NCD Risk Factor Collaboration. Effects of diabetes definition on global surveillance of diabetes prevalence and diagnosis: A pooled analysis of 96 population-based studies with 331,288 participants. *Lancet Diabetes Endocrinol.* **2015**, *3*, 624–637.
3. Yaturu, S. Obesity and type 2 diabetes. *J. Diabetes Mellit.* **2011**, *1*, 79–95. [CrossRef]
4. Mokdad, A.H.; Ford, E.S.; Bowman, B.A.; Nelson, D.E.; Engelgau, M.M.; Vinicor, F.; Marks, J.S. Diabetes trends in the U.S.: 1990–1998. *Diabetes Care* **2000**, *23*, 1278–1283. [CrossRef] [PubMed]
5. American Diabetes Association. Standards of medical care in diabetes-2015 abridged for primary care providers. *Clin. Diabetes* **2015**, *33*, 97–111.
6. American Diabetes Association. Evidence-based nutrition principles and recommendations for the treatment and prevention of diabetes and related complications. *Diabetes Care* **2002**, *25*, 202–212.
7. Fung, T.T.; Hu, F.B.; Pereira, M.A.; Liu, S.; Stampfer, M.J.; Colditz, G.A.; Willett, W.C. Whole-grain intake and the risk of type 2 diabetes: A prospective study in men. *Am. J. Clin. Nutr.* **2002**, *76*, 535–540. [PubMed]
8. Brennan, C.S.; Cleary, L.J. The potential use of cereal (1→3,1→4)-β-D-glucans as functional food ingredients. *J. Cereal Sci.* **2005**, *42*, 1–13. [CrossRef]
9. Clemens, R.; van Klinken, B.J. Oats, more than just a whole grain: An introduction. *Br. J. Nutr.* **2014**, *112* (Suppl. S2), S1–S3. [CrossRef] [PubMed]
10. Whitehead, A.; Beck, E.J.; Tosh, S.; Wolever, T.M. Cholesterol-lowering effects of oat beta-glucan: A meta-analysis of randomized controlled trials. *Am. J. Clin. Nutr.* **2014**, *100*, 1413–1421. [CrossRef] [PubMed]
11. Bao, L.; Cai, X.; Xu, M.; Li, Y. Effect of oat intake on glycaemic control and insulin sensitivity: A meta-analysis of randomised controlled trials. *Br. J. Nutr.* **2014**, *112*, 457–466. [CrossRef] [PubMed]
12. Saltzman, E.; Das, S.K.; Lichtenstein, A.H.; Dallal, G.E.; Corrales, A.; Schaefer, E.J.; Greenberg, A.S.; Roberts, S.B. An oat-containing hypocaloric diet reduces systolic blood pressure and improves lipid profile beyond effects of weight loss in men and women. *J. Nutr.* **2001**, *131*, 1465–1470. [PubMed]
13. Othman, R.A.; Moghadasian, M.H.; Jones, P.J. Cholesterol-lowering effects of oat beta-glucan. *Nutr. Rev.* **2011**, *69*, 299–309. [CrossRef] [PubMed]
14. Shen, X.L.; Zhao, T.; Zhou, Y.; Shi, X.; Zou, Y.; Zhao, G. Effect of oat beta-glucan intake on glycaemic control and insulin sensitivity of diabetic patients: A meta-analysis of randomized controlled trials. *Nutrients* **2016**, *8*, 39. [CrossRef] [PubMed]
15. Institute of Nutrition and Food Safety. *China CDC 2005 China Food Composition*; Peking University Medical Press: Beijing, China, 2005.
16. Chinese Nutrition Society. *Dietary Guidelines for Chinese Residents*; Tibet People's Publishing House: Lhasa, China, 2010.
17. Chinese Diabetes Society. China Medical Nutrition Therapy Guideline for Diabetes. Available online: http://www.cdschina.org/news_show.jsp?id=509.html (accessed on 16 October 2012).
18. Sun, Z. Process for Dehulling Oats without Removing Plumules. CN101264459 17 September 2008.
19. Hlebowicz, J. Postprandial blood glucose response in relation to gastric emptying and satiety in healthy subjects. *Appetite* **2009**, *53*, 249–252. [CrossRef] [PubMed]
20. Wang, Q.; Ellis, P.R. Oat beta-glucan: Physico-chemical characteristics in relation to its blood-glucose and cholesterol-lowering properties. *Br. J. Nutr.* **2014**, *112* (Suppl. S2), S4–S13. [CrossRef] [PubMed]
21. Pick, M.E.; Hawrysh, Z.J.; Gee, M.I.; Toth, E.; Garg, M.L.; Hardin, R.T. Oat bran concentrate bread products improve long-term control of diabetes: A pilot study. *J. Am. Diet. Assoc.* **1996**, *96*, 1254–1261. [CrossRef]

22. Shen, R.L.; Cai, F.L.; Dong, J.L.; Hu, X.Z. Hypoglycemic effects and biochemical mechanisms of oat products on streptozotocin-induced diabetic mice. *J. Agric. Food Chem.* **2011**, *59*, 8895–8900. [CrossRef] [PubMed]
23. Schuster, J.; Beninca, G.; Vitorazzi, R.; Morelo Dal Bosco, S. Effects of oats on lipid profile, insulin resistance and weight loss. *Nutr. Hosp.* **2015**, *32*, 2111–2116. [PubMed]
24. Qatanani, M.; Lazar, M.A. Mechanisms of obesity-associated insulin resistance: Many choices on the menu. *Genes Dev.* **2007**, *21*, 1443–1455. [CrossRef] [PubMed]
25. Charlton, K.E.; Tapsell, L.C.; Batterham, M.J.; O'Shea, J.; Thorne, R.; Beck, E.; Tosh, S.M. Effect of 6 weeks' consumption of beta-glucan-rich oat products on cholesterol levels in mildly hypercholesterolaemic overweight adults. *Br. J. Nutr.* **2012**, *107*, 1037–1047. [CrossRef] [PubMed]
26. Ma, X.; Gu, J.; Zhang, Z.; Jing, L.; Xu, M.; Dai, X.; Jiang, Y.; Li, Y.; Bao, L.; Cai, X.; et al. Effects of avena nuda l. On metabolic control and cardiovascular disease risk among Chinese patients with diabetes and meeting metabolic syndrome criteria: Secondary analysis of a randomized clinical trial. *Eur. J. Clin. Nutr.* **2013**, *67*, 1291–1297. [CrossRef] [PubMed]
27. Torronen, R.; Kansanen, L.; Uusitupa, M.; Hanninen, O.; Myllymaki, O.; Harkonen, H.; Malkki, Y. Effects of an oat bran concentrate on serum lipids in free-living men with mild to moderate hypercholesterolaemia. *Eur. J. Clin. Nutr.* **1992**, *46*, 621–627. [PubMed]
28. Kerckhoffs, D.A.; Hornstra, G.; Mensink, R.P. Cholesterol-lowering effect of beta-glucan from oat bran in mildly hypercholesterolemic subjects may decrease when beta-glucan is incorporated into bread and cookies. *Am. J. Clin. Nutr.* **2003**, *78*, 221–227. [PubMed]
29. Lyly, M.; Liukkonen, K.H.; Salmenkallio-Marttila, M.; Karhunen, L.; Poutanen, K.; Lahteenmaki, L. Fibre in beverages can enhance perceived satiety. *Eur. J. Nutr.* **2009**, *48*, 251–258. [CrossRef] [PubMed]
30. Rose, D.J. Impact of whole grains on the gut microbiota: The next frontier for oats? *Br. J. Nutr.* **2014**, *112* (Suppl. S2), S44–S49. [CrossRef] [PubMed]
31. Viscidi, K.A.; Dougherty, M.P.; Briggs, J.; Camire, M.E. Complex phenolic compounds reduce lipid oxidation in extruded oat cereals. *Food Sci. Technol.* **2004**, *37*, 789–796. [CrossRef]
32. El Khoury, D.; Cuda, C.; Luhovyy, B.L.; Anderson, G.H. Beta glucan: Health benefits in obesity and metabolic syndrome. *J. Nutr. Metab.* **2012**, *2012*, 851362. [CrossRef] [PubMed]
33. Den Besten, G.; van Eunen, K.; Groen, A.K.; Venema, K.; Reijngoud, D.J.; Bakker, B.M. The role of short-chain fatty acids in the interplay between diet, gut microbiota, and host energy metabolism. *J. Lipid Res.* **2013**, *54*, 2325–2340. [CrossRef] [PubMed]
34. Ross, A.B.; Pere-Trepat, E.; Montoliu, I.; Martin, F.P.; Collino, S.; Moco, S.; Godin, J.P.; Cleroux, M.; Guy, P.A.; Breton, I.; et al. A whole-grain-rich diet reduces urinary excretion of markers of protein catabolism and gut microbiota metabolism in healthy men after one week. *J. Nutr.* **2013**, *143*, 766–773. [CrossRef] [PubMed]
35. Martinez, I.; Lattimer, J.M.; Hubach, K.L.; Case, J.A.; Yang, J.; Weber, C.G.; Louk, J.A.; Rose, D.J.; Kyureghian, G.; Peterson, D.A.; et al. Gut microbiome composition is linked to whole grain-induced immunological improvements. *ISME J.* **2013**, *7*, 269–280. [CrossRef] [PubMed]
36. De Vos, W.M.; de Vos, E.A. Role of the intestinal microbiome in health and disease: From correlation to causation. *Nutr. Rev.* **2012**, *70* (Suppl. S1), S45–S56. [CrossRef] [PubMed]

6

The Effects of Early Post-Operative Soluble Dietary Fiber Enteral Nutrition for Colon Cancer

Rui Xu, Zhi Ding, Ping Zhao, Lingchao Tang, Xiaoli Tang and Shuomeng Xiao *

Department of Gastrointestinal Surgery, Sichuan Cancer Hospital, Chengdu 610041, China; xrscu2012@163.com (R.X.); dzscch@sina.com (Z.D.); zpscch@sina.com (P.Z.); scch2015@163.com (L.T.); txlscch@sina.com (X.T.)

* Correspondence: ambition123@foxmail.com;

Abstract: We examined colon cancer patients who received soluble dietary fiber enteral nutrition (SDFEN) to evaluate the feasibility and potential benefit of early SDFEN compared to EN. Sixty patients who were confirmed as having colon cancer with histologically and accepted radical resection of colon cancer were randomized into an SDFEN group and an EN group. The postoperative complications, length of hospital stay (LOH), days for first fecal passage, and the difference in nutritional status, immune function and inflammatory reaction between pre-operation and post-operation were all recorded. The statistical analyses were performed using the t-test and the chi square test. Statistical significance was defined as $p < 0.05$. After the nutrition support, differences in the levels of albumin, prealbumin and transferrin in each group were not statistically significant ($p > 0.05$); the levels of CD4+, IgA and IgM in the SDFEN group were higher than that of the EN group at seven days ($p < 0.05$); the levels of TNF-α and IL-6 in the SDFEN group were lower than that of the EN group at seven days ($p < 0.05$); and patients in the SDFEN group had a significantly shorter first flatus time than the EN group ($p < 0.05$). Early post-operative SDFEN used in colon cancer patients was feasible and beneficial in immune function and reducing inflammatory reaction, gastrointestinal function and speeding up the recovery.

Keywords: colon cancer; dietary fiber; early enteral nutrition

1. Introduction

In the 21st century, cancer incidence and mortality has not reduced; moreover, it has even increased year by year. The total number of patients with colorectal cancer increased to 1.23 million globally in 2008; it is ranked third in cancer incidence and fourth in mortality [1]. However, the incidence and mortality of colorectal cancer were ranked third and fifth, respectively [2] in China. Many studies showed that the incidence of malnutrition in patients with a malignant tumor was as high as 31%–97% [3,4], especially for gastrointestinal cancer, so choosing a proper nutrition therapy for colorectal cancer patients with malnutrition is necessary. Early enteral nutrition support is promoted after gastrointestinal surgery, and there are many kinds of nutrient elements, such as probiotics, ω-3PUFA, Gln and fiber. We know that dietary fiber is a kind of nutrient, which is divided into soluble dietary fiber and insoluble dietary fiber and can protect the intestinal barrier, modulate immune function, induce inflammatory response and postoperative complications [5,6]. SCFA is the main source of energy for intestinal epithelial cells and plays a key role in maintaining colonic health and moderating cell growth and differentiation. This depends on the fermentation of dietary fiber. Soluble dietary fiber is fermented, but insoluble dietary fiber is difficult to ferment. The relationship between dietary fiber and colon cancer prevention was studied widely, but there is little study about the early postoperative application of soluble dietary fiber in colon cancer [7–9]. Thus, we decide to add soluble dietary fiber to verify the feasibility and potential benefit of SDFEN for colon cancer for the postoperative course.

2. Patients and Methods

2.1. Patient Selection

We recruited 60 subjects from the department of gastrointestinal surgery of the Sichuan cancer Hospital between June 2014 and June 2015. All patients who confirmed colon cancer with histologically and accepted radical resection of colon cancer were randomized into an SDFEN group (30 cases) and EN group (30 cases). Informed consents were obtained according to the Declaration of Helsinki. Patients suffering from diabetes or underlying cardiopulmonary diseases were excluded. Moreover, the patients whose tumor staging was Stage IV (the cancer had spread to other parts of the body) were also excluded.

2.2. Methods

No patients had a decompression tube before the operation, and all were given sequential nutrition support for 7 days consecutively after the operation. The total daily calories for all the patients should reach 125.52 kJ (30 kcal)/kg. All enteral nutrition was ingested through mouth, and if energy was insufficient, we would obtain residual energy by infusing the Fat Emulsion, Amino Acids (17) and Glucose (1%) Injection (1440 mL/bag) made by Sino-Swed Pharmaceutical Corp. (Wuxi, China). Intervention in detail is in the following Table 1.

Table 1. Intervention of the cases and control.

Time	Nutrients	SDFEN	EN
Day 1	5% GNS	500 mL	500 mL
	dietary fiber	25 g	-
	Probiotics	4g	4 g
Day 2–3	Enteral Nutrition	500 mL	500 mL
	dietary fiber	25 g	-
	Probiotics	4 g	4 g
Day 4–7	Enteral Nutrition	1000 mL	1000 mL
	dietary fiber	25 g	-
	Probiotics	4 g	4 g
Total energy	125.52 kJ (30 kcal)/kg		
Insufficient energy	Amino Acids (17) and Glucose (1%) Injection (1440 mL/bag)		

SDFEN: soluble dietary fiber enteral nutrition. EN: enteral nutrition. Dietary fiber: Soluble dietary fiber from fruit and vegetables made by Beijing yikang Biotechnology Corp. (Beijing, China); Enteral Nutrition: Enteral Nutritional Emulsion (TP-HE) (500 mL/bag, 750 kcal) made by Sino-Swed Pharmaceutical Corp; Probiotics: Live Combined Bifidobacterium and Lactobacillus Tablets made by Inner Mongolia shuangqi Pharmaceutical Corp. (Huhhot, China).

2.3. Clinical Assessment

Clinical factors included age, gender, smoking, drinking habits, and tumor stage according to the tumor-node-metastasis classification of the International Union against Cancer (7th edition) [10]. Peripheral blood was collected on the pre-operative day, and post-operative second and seventh day. Nutritional status was expressed by the levels of albumin, prealbumin and transferring; and immune function was shown by the levels of CD3+, CD4+, CD8+, CD4+/CD8+, IgA, IgM and IgG; The levels of TNF-α, IL-6 and PCT reflected the immune function. Length of hospital stay (LOH), and bowel movement recovery were expressed as days and the first fecal passage was recorded. Postoperative complications including pneumonia, anastomotic fistula and severe abdominal distension were also recorded.

2.4. Statistical Analysis

All analyses were carried out with the SPSS 19.0 software package (IBM, New York, NY, USA), and measurement data were indicated with the mean ± standard deviation. The *t*-test was used to examine measurement data, the chi-square test was used to categorize data. p value < 0.05 was considered significant for statistical analysis.

3. Results

3.1. Demography

Among 30 colon cancer cases, there were 16 males and 14 females, and the mean age was 52.20 ± 14.20 years; among the 30 control cases, there were 19 males and 11 females, and the mean age was 53.20 ± 13.10 years. The characteristics of the cases and controls are summarized in Table 2. There was no significant difference between the distributions of the age, gender, smoking, drinking habits and TNM stage of the two groups.

Table 2. Characteristics of the cases and control.

Variable	SDFEN (n = 30)	EN (n = 30)	p
Gender (%)			
Male	16 (53.3)	19 (63.3)	0.735
Female	14 (46.7)	11 (36.7)	0.690
Age mean (SD) year	52.2 ± 14.2	53.2 ± 13.1	0.750
Smoking status (%)			
Smokers	12 (40)	9 (30)	0.664
Nonsmokers	18 (60)	21 (70)	0.749
Drinking (%)			
Drinkers	10 (33)	13 (43.3)	0.678
Nondrinkers	20 (67)	17 (56.7)	0.868
TNM stage (%)			
I, II	13 (43.3)	11 (36.7)	0.839
III	17 (56.7)	19 (63.3)	0.868

SDFEN: soluble dietary fiber enteral nutrition; EN: enteral nutrition; SD: standard deviation.

3.2. Pre-Operative and Post-Operative Nutritional Index

After the nutrition support, differences of the levels of albumin, prealbumin and transferrin in each group were not statistically significant ($p > 0.05$) (Table 3).

Table 3. Comparison of the two groups' nutrition index.

	Pre Op	POD 2	POD 7
ALB (g/L)			
SDFEN	40.15 ± 2.45	32.64 ± 2.32	35.45 ± 2.21
EN	39.39 ± 2.87	31.81 ± 1.72	34.30 ± 1.86
p	0.22	0.09	0.05
PAB (mg/L)			
SDFEN	194.78 ± 31.74	177.32 ± 22.82	192.67 ± 21.30
EN	191.47 ± 30.61	178.09 ± 28.24	189.97 ± 25.32
p	0.62	0.88	0.58
TRF (g/L)			
SDFEN	2.58 ± 0.50	2.05 ± 0.39	2.29 ± 0.33
EN	2.55 ± 0.39	2.09 ± 0.20	2.23 ± 0.28
p	0.75	0.57	0.30

Pre Op: pre-operation; POD: postoperative day; SDFEN: soluble dietary fiber enteral nutrition; EN: enteral nutrition; ALB; albumin; PAB; prealbumin; TRF; transferring.

3.3. Pre-Operative and Post-Operative Immune Index

Differences of CD3+, CD8+, CD4+/CD8+ and IgG in each group were not statistically significant at two and seven days. The levels of CD4+, IgA and IgM in SDFEN group were higher than the EN group at seven days ($p < 0.05$) (Table 4).

Table 4. Comparison of the two groups' immune index.

	Pre Op	POD 2	POD 7
CD3+ (%)			
SDFEN	62.77 ± 6.46	54.32 ± 6.95	61.34 ± 4.32
EN	60.99 ± 7.00	53.59 ± 6.42	59.80 ± 6.23
p	0.321	0.669	0.285
CD4+ (%)			
SDFEN	34.28 ± 4.83	28.40 ± 3.32	35.90 ± 2.24
EN	33.70 ± 5.31	29.76 ± 3.32	34.41 ± 2.64
p	0.61	0.155	0.024
CD8+ (%)			
SDFEN	23.20 ± 4.83	21.58 ± 3.91	21.30 ± 3.03
EN	22.03 ± 3.83	21.11 ± 2.72	21.35 ± 1.94
p	0.377	0.659	0.949
CD4+/CD8+			
SDFEN	1.55 ±0.43	1.36 ± 0.31	1.72 ± 0.29
EN	1.58 ±0.41	1.44 ± 0.27	1.62 ± 0.20
p	0.766	0.387	0.190
IgA (g/L)			
SDFEN	2.13 ± 0.95	1.81 ± 0.94	2.25 ± 0.79
EN	2.03 ± 0.56	1.69 ± 0.59	1.88 ± 0.54
p	0.622	0.567	0.045
IgM (g/L)			
SDFEN	1.26 ± 0.64	0.94 ± 0.20	1.30 ± 0.33
EN	1.12 ± 0.19	0.96 ± 0.13	1.11 ± 0.15
p	0.241	0.693	0.002
IgG (g/L)			
SDFEN	11.22 ± 1.54	9.57 ± 1.59	11.55 ± 1.44
EN	11.12 ± 1.73	9.74 ± 0.87	11.41 ± 1.32
p	0.799	0.618	0.590

Pre Op: pre-operation; POD: postoperative day; SDFEN: soluble dietary fiber enteral nutrition; EN: enteral nutrition.

3.4. Pre-Operative and Post-Operative Inflammatory Index

The levels of TNF-α and IL-6 in the SDFEN group were lower than the EN group at seven days ($p < 0.05$) (Table 5).

Table 5. Comparison of the two groups' immune index.

	Pre Op	POD 2	POD 7
TNF-α (pg/mL)			
SDFEN	12.88 ± 5.62	20.32 ± 6.35	13.02 ± 2.85
EN	13.91 ± 6.47	22.14 ± 6.81	14.73 ± 4.07
p	0.524	0.333	0.045
IL-6(pg/mL)			
SDFEN	47.54 ± 34.30	110.72 ± 46.86	58.75 ± 24.82
EN	45.83 ± 42.14	115.57 ± 56.93	70.83 ± 35.65
p	0.850	0.682	0.044
PCT (ng/mL)			
SDFEN	0.11 ± 0.11	0.26 ± 0.18	0.15 ± 0.07
EN	0.15 ± 0.15	0.28 ± 0.18	0.16 ± 0.08
p	0.086	0.489	0.539

Pre Op: pre-operation; POD: postoperative day; SDFEN: soluble dietary fiber enteral nutrition; EN: enteral nutrition.

3.5. Post-Operative Recovery

Patients in the SDFEN group had a significantly shorter first flatus time than the EN group ($p < 0.05$). However, abdominal distension, pneumonia, Anastomotic fistula and total postoperative hospitalization time were similar between the two groups (Table 6).

Table 6. Post-operative recovery.

	SDFEN	EN	*p*
First flatus time (h)	58.93 ± 6.5	63.03 ± 4.8	0.015
Abdominal distension	1	2	-
Pneumonia	1	2	-
Anastomotic fistula	0	1	-
Length of hospital stay (day)	7.4 ± 0.72	7.63 ± 0.61	0.257

SDFEN: soluble dietary fiber enteral nutrition; EN: enteral nutrition.

4. Discussion

Colon cancer is a common gastrointestinal malignancy, the incidence of which has increased year by year. Seventy percent of patients with GI cancer may be suffering from malnutrition and 39.3% of patients with colon cancer had different degrees of malnutrition [11,12]. Surgery is still the first choice for treatment, but surgical trauma and anesthesia can cause body metabolic disorder and aggravated malnutrition. Widespread attention has been given on how to further improve the postoperative nutritional status and the prognosis.

Early enteral nutrition began at 24 h after surgery in our study. ASPEN [13] suggested that ideal enteral nutrition should begin within 24 to 48 h after surgery. Actually, intestine had recovered its absorption function and EMG activity within 4 to 8 h after surgery [14]. The gastrointestinal tract can not only absorb nutrients, but also plays an important role in immunity because it is a central organ after surgical stress [15] and it is also the motor of the MODS. Intestine mucosal atrophy and abnormal intestinal permeability can occur after not eating for several days. Early enteral nutrition is more close to the human physiological needs. The application of enteral nutrition can reverse the loss of gut mucosal integrity resulting from surgical trauma [16], and early enteral nutrition support is associated with a decreased infection risk, a reduced hospital stay, and a clear trend of a reduction in anastomotic breakdown [17,18]. Therefore, it could be the first choice for patients who have had an operation.

Some studies proposed that early application of soluble dietary fiber enteral nutrition could increase nutritional indicators, make patients' weight decline slowly and reduce the incidence of digestive tract complications [19,20]. However, there was no obvious difference in post-operative nutrition status and complication between the SDFEN group and EN group in our study. Fortunately, there was a trend of an increased post-operative nutrition status and declined incidence of complications. Dietary fiber are not a static collection of indigestible plant materials that pass through the human GI tract without any function; instead, they bind potential nutrients, result in new metabolites, and modulate nutrient absorption/metabolism, and they can promote the growth of the small intestinal villus to increase the absorption of nutrients to improve nutrition status. Dietary fiber is divided into soluble dietary fiber and insoluble dietary fiber. In general, soluble dietary fiber is fermented, but insoluble dietary fiber is difficult to ferment. Studies found that dietary fiber could be fermented into SCFAs in colon and unoxidized SCFA through the portal system into the liver. They can thus be converted to glutamine, and then glutamine enters into the circulation of blood to nourish the small intestine [21]. Therefore, statistical differences in post-operative nutrition status and complication will exist between the SDFEN group and EN group, if observation time is enough.

A large amount of research has reported that soluble dietary fiber had health benefits with immunomodulatory and anti-inflammatory effects [8,22]. In our study, there were significant differences in the indicators of immune conditions including deviations in CD4+, IgA and IgG at seven days between the SDFEN group and EN group (35.90% ± 2.24% vs. 34.41% ± 2.64%, 2.25% ± 0.79 g/L vs. 1.88 ± 0.54 g/L, and 11.55 ± 1.44 g/L vs. 11.41 ± 1.32 g/L, respectively, $p < 0.05$), and the levels of TNF-α and IL-6 in the SDFEN group was lower than those in the EN group (13.02 ± 2.85 pg/mL vs. 14.73 ± 4.07 pg/mL, and 58.75 ± 24.82 pg/mL vs. 70.83 ± 35.65 pg/mL, respectively, $p < 0.05$). These health benefits can be attributed to the fermentation of soluble dietary fiber into SCFAs in the colon. The three major colonic SCFAs are acetate, propionate and butyrate, which is the main source of energy for intestinal epithelial cells and plays a key role in maintaining colonic health and moderating cell growth and differentiation [23]. Acetate plays a role in the host immune system through interacting with the G protein-coupled receptor (GPCR43, 41) in immune cells [24]. Butyrate exhibits strong anti-inflammatory properties, and this effect is likely mediated by inhibition of TNF-α production, NF-κB activation, and IL-8, IL-10, and IL-12 expression in immune and colonic epithelial cells [25,26]. Leukocytes are recruited and migrate from the bloodstream to the inflamed tissue through a multistep process that involves expression and activation of several proteins such as adhesion molecules and chemokines, and SCFAs modify this leukocyte recruitment [27,28] by modulating the amount or type of adhesion molecules and chemokines. SCFAs may alter the recruitment of leukocytes to reduce the chronic GI tract inflammatory response. Therefore, intakes of dietary fiber can reduce inflammatory reaction and improve the postoperative immune function.

Under the stimulation of mixed dietary fiber food, the gastrointestinal hormone is increased, such as gastrin and cholecystokinin, which can promote recovery of intestinal movement. Furthermore, SCFAs also have the same function; Kamath et al. [29] found that the movement of the free small bowel was increased after being stimulated with SCFAs. In our study, patients in the SDFEN group had a significantly shorter first flatus time than the EN group (58.93 ± 6.5 h vs. 63.03 ± 4.8 h, $p < 0.05$), so that SDFEN can promote recovery of intestinal movement.

5. Conclusions

Early post-operative soluble dietary fiber enteral nutrition used in colon cancer patients was feasible and has advantages in improving immune function, reducing inflammatory response and promoting early recovery of intestinal movement.

Acknowledgments: Thanks to the support of gastrointestinal surgery centre, department of pathology and nutrition in Sichuan cancer hospital.

Author Contributions: R.X. and S.X. designed the study; R.X. and S.X. collected the data; X.T. and S.X. entered the data; R.X. and S.X. drafted the manuscript; and Z.D., L.T. and P.Z. undertook the statistical analysis. All authors read and approved the final manuscript.

References

1. Ferlay, J.; Shin, H.R.; Bray, F.; Forman, D.; Mathers, C.; Parkin, D.M. Estimates of worldwide burden of cancer in 2008: GLOBOCAN 2008. *Int. J. Cancer* **2010**, *127*, 2893–2917. [CrossRef] [PubMed]
2. Chen, W.Q.; Zhang, S.W.; Zheng, R.S.; Zhao, P.; Li, G.; Wu, L.; He, J. Report of cancer incidence and mortality in China, 2009. *Chin. J. Cancer Res.* **2013**, *22*, 1–12.
3. Huhmann, M.B.; Cunningham, R.S. Importance of nutritional screening in treatment of cancer related weight loss. *Lancet Oncol.* **2005**, *6*, 334–343. [CrossRef]
4. Segura, A.; Pardo, J.; Jara, C.; Zugazabeitia, L.; Carulla, J.; de Las Peñas, R.; García-Cabrera, E.; Luz Azuara, M.; Casadó, J.; Gómez-Candela, C. An epidemiological evaluation of the prevalence of malnutrition in Spanish patients with locally advanced or metastatic cancer. *Clin. Nutr.* **2005**, *24*, 801–814. [CrossRef] [PubMed]
5. Zeng, H.W.; Lazarova, D.L.; Bordonaro, M. Mechanisms linking dietary fiber, gut microbiota and colon cancer prevention. *World J. Gastrointest. Oncol.* **2014**, *6*, 41–51. [CrossRef] [PubMed]
6. Vieira, A.T.; Galvão, I.; Macia, L.M.; Sernaglia, E.M.; Vinolo, M.A.; Garcia, C.C.; Tavares, L.P.; Amaral, F.A.; Sousa, L.P.; Martins, F.S.; et al. Dietary fiber and the short-chain fatty acid acetate promote resolution of neutrophilic inflammation in a model of gout in mice. *J. Leukoc. Biol.* **2016**. [CrossRef] [PubMed]

7. Kaczmarczyk, M.M.; Miller, M.J.; Freund, G.G. The health benefis of dietary fiber: Beyond the usual suspects of type 2 diabetes mellitus, cardiovascular disease and colon cancer. *Metabolism* **2012**, *61*, 1058–1066. [CrossRef] [PubMed]
8. Peters, U.; Sinha, R.; Chatterjee, N.; Subar, A.F.; Ziegler, R.G.; Kulldorff, M.; Bresalier, R.; Weissfeld, J.L.; Flood, A.; Schatzkin, A.; Hayes, R.B.; et al. Dietary fire and colorectal adenoma in a colorectal cancer early detection programme. *Lancet* **2003**, *361*, 1491–1495. [CrossRef]
9. Nomura, A.M.; Hankin, J.H.; Henderson, B.E.; Wilkens, L.R.; Murphy, S.P.; Pike, M.C.; Le Marchand, L.; Stram, D.O.; Monroe, K.R.; Kolonel, L.N. Dietary fier and colorectal cancer risk: The multiethnic cohort study. *Cancer Causes Control* **2007**, *18*, 753–764. [CrossRef] [PubMed]
10. Sobin, L.H.; Gospodarowicz, M.K.; Wittekind, C. *TNM Classification of Malignant Tumors*, 7th ed.; Wiley: New York, NY, USA, 2010.
11. Yang, Z.H.; Li, G.N. Clinical analysis of perioperative enteral nutrition in patients with gastrointestinal tumor. *Appl. J. Gen. Prac.* **2008**, *6*, 483–484.
12. Schwegler, I.; von Holzen, A.; Gutzwiller, J.P.; Schlumpf, R.; Mühlebach, S.; Stanga, Z. Nutritional risk is a clinical predictor of postoperative mortality and morbidity in surgery for colorectal cancer. *Br. J. Surg.* **2010**, *97*, 92–97. [CrossRef] [PubMed]
13. McClave, S.A.; Martindale, R.G.; Vanek, V.W.; McCarthy, M.; Roberts, P.; Taylor, B.; Ochoa, J.B.; Napolitano, L.; Cresci, G. Guidelines for the provision and assessment of nutritionsupport therapyintheadult critically ill patient: Society of Critical Caremedicine (SCCM) and American Society for Parenteral and Enteral Nutrition (ASPEN). *J. Parenter. Enter. Nutr.* **2009**, *33*, 277–316. [CrossRef] [PubMed]
14. Sakurai, Y.; Kanaya, S.; Komori, Y.; Uyama, I. Is postoperative early enteral nutrition with regular or disease-specific enteral formula really beneficial in patients undergoing esophagectomy? *Esophagus* **2009**, *3*, 149–154. [CrossRef]
15. Wilmore, D.W.; Smith, R.J.; O'Dwyer, S.T.; Jacobs, D.O.; Ziegler, T.R.; Wang, X.D. The gut: A central organ after surgical stress. *Surgery* **1988**, *104*, 917–923. [PubMed]
16. Jiang, X.H.; Li, N.; Li, J.S. Intestinal permeability in patients after surgical trauma and effect of enteral nutrition versus parenteral nutrition. *World J. Gastroenterol.* **2003**, *9*, 1878–1880. [CrossRef] [PubMed]
17. Ochoa, J.B.; Caba, D. Advances in surgical nutrition. *Surg. Clin. N. Am.* **2006**, *86*, 1483–1493. [CrossRef] [PubMed]
18. Fearon, K.C.; Ljungqvist, O.; Von Meyenfeldt, M.; Revhaug, A.; Dejong, C.H.; Lassen, K.; Nygren, J.; Hausel, J.; Soop, M.; Andersen, J.; et al. Enhanced recovery after surgery: A consensus review of clinical care for patients undergoing colonic resection. *Clin. Nutr.* **2005**, *24*, 466–477. [CrossRef] [PubMed]
19. Yan, M.; Li, S.F.; Li, C.; Zhang, J.; Ji, F.; Xu, H.; Cao, W.H. Clinical studies on early post-operative enteral nutrition with dietary fibers for GI tumor. *Parenter. Enter. Nutr.* **2001**, *8*, 15–18.
20. Lu, J.; Zhao, Z.M.; Wang, F.; Ding, Y.P.; Ma, D.N.; Ye, X.L.; Song, X.L. High dietary fiber enteral nutrition improves the nutritional status and tolerance in critically ill patients. *Chin. J. Crit. Care Med.* **2011**, *5*, 300–305.
21. Dosmoulin, F.; Caninoni, P.; Cozzone, P.J. Glutamate-glutamine metabolism in the perfused rat liver. ^{13}C NMR study using ^{13}C-enriched acetate. *FEBS Lett.* **1985**, *185*, 29–32. [CrossRef]
22. Macfarlane, G.T.; Steed, H.; Macfarlane, S. Bacterial metabolism and health-related effects of galacto-oligosaccharides and other prebiotics. *Appl. Microbiol.* **2008**, *104*, 305–344. [CrossRef] [PubMed]
23. Macfarlane, G.T.; Macfarlane, S. Fermentation in the human large intestine: Its physiologic consequences and the potential contribution of prebiotics. *Clin. Gastroenterol.* **2011**, *45*, S120–S127. [CrossRef] [PubMed]
24. Brown, A.J.; Goldsworthy, S.M.; Barnes, A.A.; Eilert, M.M.; Tcheang, L.; Daniels, D.; Muir, A.I.; Wigglesworth, M.J.; Kinghorn, I.; Fraser, N.J.; et al. The orphan G protein-coupled receptors GPR41 and GPR4 are activated by propionate and other short chain carboxylic acids. *J. Biol. Chem.* **2003**, *278*, 11312–11319. [CrossRef] [PubMed]
25. Bailón, E.; Cueto-Sola, M.; Utrilla, P.; Rodríguez-Cabezas, M.E.; Garrido-Mesa, N.; Zarzuelo, A.; Xaus, J.; Gálvez, J.; Comalada, M. Butyrate in vitro immune-modulatory effects might be mediated through a proliferation-related induction of apoptosis. *Immunobiology* **2010**, *215*, 863–873. [CrossRef] [PubMed]
26. Lührs, H.; Gerke, T.; Müller, J.G.; Melcher, R.; Schauber, J.; Box-berge, F.; Scheppach, W.; Menzel, T. Butyrate inhibits NF-kappaB activation in lamina propria macrophages of patients with ulcerative colitis. *Scand. J. Gastroenterol.* **2002**, *37*, 458–466. [CrossRef] [PubMed]

27. Maslowski, K.M.; Vieira, A.T.; Ng, A.; Kranich, J.; Sierro, F.; Yu, D.; Schilter, H.C.; Rolph, M.S.; Mackay, F.; Artis, D.; et al. Regulation of inflmmatory responses by gut microbiota and chemoattractant receptor GPR4. *Nature* **2009**, *461*, 1282–1286. [CrossRef] [PubMed]
28. Vinolo, M.A.; Rodrigues, H.G.; Hatanaka, E.; Hebeda, C.B.; Farsky, S.H.; Curi, R. Short-chain fatty acids stimulate the migration of neutrophils to inflmmatory sites. *Clin. Sci.* **2009**, *117*, 331–338. [CrossRef] [PubMed]
29. Kamath, P.S.; Hoepfner, M.T.; Phillips, S.F. Short-chain fatty acids stimulate ileal motility in humans. *Gastroenterology* **1988**, *95*, 1496–1502. [CrossRef]

7

Effect on Insulin, Glucose and Lipids in Overweight/Obese Australian Adults of 12 Months Consumption of Two Different Fibre Supplements in a Randomised Trial

Sebely Pal [1,*], Suleen Ho [1], Roland J. Gahler [2] and Simon Wood [3]

1 School of Public Health, Curtin University, Perth 6845, Australia; suleen.ho@curtin.edu.au
2 Factors Group Research, Burnaby, BC V3N 4S9, Canada; rgahler@naturalfactors.com
3 Food, Nutrition and Health Program, University of British Columbia, Vancouver, BC V6T 1Z4, Canada; simonwood@shaw.ca
* Correspondence: s.pal@curtin.edu.au;

Abstract: Higher fibre intakes are associated with risk reduction for chronic diseases. This study investigated the effects of supplementation with PolyGlycopleX® (PGX), a complexed polysaccharide, on insulin, glucose and lipids in overweight and obese individuals. In this double-blind 12 months study, participants were randomised into three groups: control (rice flour); PGX or psyllium (PSY). Participants followed their usual lifestyle and diet but consumed 5 g of their supplement before meals. Insulin was significantly lower in the PGX and PSY groups compared to control at 3 and 6 months and in the PSY group compared to control at 12 months. Serum glucose was significantly lower in the PGX group at 3 months compared to control. Total cholesterol was significantly lower in the PGX and PSY groups compared to control at 3 and 6 months. High density lipoprotein (HDL) cholesterol was significantly increased in the PGX group compared to control at 12 months. low density lipoprotein (LDL) cholesterol was significantly lower in the PGX group at 3 and 6 months compared to control and in the PSY group at 3 months compared to control. A simple strategy of fibre supplementation may offer an effective solution to glucose, insulin and lipid management without the need for other nutrient modification.

Keywords: obesity; PGX; psyllium; cholesterol; insulin

---

1. Introduction

Previous studies have consistently shown that higher fibre intakes are correlated with lower body weight, body mass index (BMI), waist circumference [1,2] and improved plasma lipid profiles [3–12], glycaemia and insulinaemia [13], indicating benefits and risk reduction for metabolic syndrome, cardiovascular disease (CVD) and type 2 diabetes.

While the benefits of a high fibre diet are well known, increasing fruit and vegetable intake to meet the recommended intake of fibre is difficult for many [14]. Present estimations of dietary fibre intake in Australian, Canadian, European and American adults is approximately 15–25 g/day [3,15], which is below the current recommendations for adults in Australia, Canada, Europe and the USA of 25–30 g/day [16]. Therefore, fibre supplements can provide a cost effective and easy alternative method for increasing the fibre content of a diet without the need for other major nutrient modifications.

PolyGlycopleX (PGX) has been shown to have lipid lowering effects in healthy subjects [17] as well as in overweight and obese adults [18]. In a clinical trial with healthy subjects, 25 males and 29 females, mean age of 31.6 ± 10.5 years entered the study [17] and consumed 2.5 g of PGX twice a day as part of two main meals (breakfast and/or lunch, and/or dinner) for the first seven days, followed by 5 g PGX for the last 14 days of the study. The control product was a skimmed milk powder. PGX's effects on decreasing total and low density lipoprotein (LDL) cholesterol levels in the study concur with similar reports in the literature [19]. Studies are required to investigate if these benefits are sustainable over a longer duration and also in those who are overweight/obese. Another study with 29 overweight and obese adults, ages 20–65 with a BMI between 25–36 kg/m^2, consuming 5 g of PGX in 500 mL of water 5–10 min before each meal, 2–3 times a day for 14 days showed a significant reduction of total cholesterol (TC) and LDL levels of 19% and 25% respectively, compared to baseline [18]. However, the supplement was combined with advice for healthy eating, weight loss and exercise so it is difficult to evaluate the effect of the fibre alone on lipids. This was not a randomised controlled trial as there was no control group in this study. Recent human studies have shown that the addition of 2.5 to 5 g of PGX with a meal is highly effective in reducing postprandial glycaemia, lowering the glycaemic index of food [20] and modifying satiety hormones in healthy adults [21]. However, these studies have some limitations; they were acute or short term, mostly conducted in healthy, normal weight participants or combined with lifestyle changes.

Psyllium has been evaluated in various human studies for effects on glucose and insulin homeostasis, body weight, body composition and appetite as well as lipids and lipoproteins [22–30 Psyllium was reviewed in 2012 for its effect on metabolic syndrome [31]. The authors concluded that "Collectively, research to date does support the notion that the consumption of psyllium may provide benefits to many components of the metabolic syndrome". Psyllium fibre decreased fat absorption in overweight and obese men, but had no effect on postprandial glucose and insulin concentrations [32]. In another study, simply adding a psyllium fibre supplement to a normal diet (10.2 g/day) was sufficient to see improvements in TC and LDL cholesterol but not fasting glucose or insulin concentrations when compared to the control group [22]. However, a meta-analysis [33 found that in type 2 diabetes patients, psyllium fibre significantly improved fasting blood glucose, proportional to loss of glycaemic control.

Apart from these few studies, limited research is available on the effect of PGX fibre on blood insulin, glucose and lipids. Randomised controlled clinical trials are required to verify whether PGX can be used for improving insulin, glucose and lipids in the long term and whether this fibre type is better than other soluble fibres, such as psyllium. Therefore the aim of this study was to investigate the effect of PGX on insulin, glucose and lipid concentrations. Given the effect of PGX on total and LDL cholesterol in healthy weight participants and its considerably higher viscosity, we hypothesise that PGX will have a greater health outcome than psyllium in overweight and obese individuals.

2. Materials and Methods

2.1. Subjects

Overweight and obese individuals with a body mass index (BMI) between 25–47 kg/m^2 and aged between 19 and 68 years, were recruited from the community in Perth, Australia (via newspaper and radio). Potential participants were screened by telephone or online questionnaire and attended Curtin University to assess suitability for the study, at which time the details of the study were explained. Exclusion criteria included smoking, lipid lowering medication, use of steroids and other agents that may influence lipid metabolism, use of warfarin, diabetes mellitus, hypo- and hyperthyroidism, cardiovascular events within the last 6 months, psychological unsuitability, major systemic diseases, gastrointestinal problems, proteinuria, liver, renal failure, weight fluctuations over the past 6 months, vegetarianism and participation in any other clinical trials within the last 6 months. This study was approved by and conducted in accordance with the ethical standards of Curtin Human Research Ethics Committee. Written consent was obtained from all participants. ANZCTR number: ACTRN12611000415909.

2.2. Study Design

This study is part of a larger trial, which was a randomised, double blind, parallel design study over a 52 week period. Study participants were randomised by the trial sponsors using a Web site (http://www.randomization.com) to one of the three groups (three randomly permuted blocks): the control group who consumed the placebo with their usual diet; the psyllium supplement group (PSY) who consumed a psyllium supplement with their usual diet and a PGX supplement group (PGX) who consumed a PGX supplement with their usual diet. Psyllium is a soluble fibre and PolyGlycopleX (PGX) is a novel, highly viscous functional non-starch polysaccharide complex, with developing viscosity, manufactured from konjac (glucomannan), sodium alginate and xanthan gum by a proprietary process (EnviroSimplex®). The fibre supplementation consisted of either 5 g of psyllium (a proprietary psyllium product with the trade name PgxSyl™) (InovoBiologic, Inc., Calgary, AB, Canada) or 5 g of PGX (InovoBiologic, Inc., Calgary, AB, Canada). Placebo consisted of 5 g rice flour. All supplements were artificially sweetened and flavoured. The rice flour provided an appropriate placebo due to its low energy and fibre content and similarity in texture and appearance to the psyllium and PGX supplement. Participants were instructed to take either 5 g of the fibre supplements or placebo, mixed with a minimum of 250 mL water followed by a further 250 mL water, three times daily, 5–10 min before breakfast, lunch and dinner. Extra water was allowed to be taken *ad libitum* during or after the meal if desired and subjects were encouraged to do this. The supplement packages (control, PGX and psyllium) were from a single batch provided by the manufacturer, and appeared identical so that the research assistants and participants were blinded to the type of supplement being consumed. Packages consisted of 5 g doses of the control, PGX or psyllium and were only marked by the participant ID, with the group allocation only known to the trial sponsors to ensure blinding. Quantities of rice flour and psyllium were determined by input, with the amounts weighed and checked by the dispensing and blending department while PGX was analysed according to USP Monograph FCC9 3rd Sup 2015 [34]. All identifiable information from participants was coded to ensure privacy.

The subjects attended a briefing session on how to consume the supplement, complete food records and comply with the study protocol as previously reported [35]. Briefly, the dietary intake over the course of the trial was monitored through the completion of 3-day food diaries at baseline, 12, 26 and 52 weeks. All participants in the control and the fibre supplement groups were asked to maintain their usual dietary intake for the duration of the study. To monitor compliance, all participants were required to complete a diary to record their supplement consumption and asked to return both the empty and unused sachets of the supplements at their visits.

2.3. Anthropometry and Body Composition

Measures of body weight, height, waist and hip circumference were undertaken at baseline, 3, 6 and 12 months. Body weight (HBF-514, Omron, Kyoto, Japan) was recorded in light clothing without shoes. Height was measured to the nearest 0.1 cm using a stadiometer without shoes. Waist circumference was measured in the standing position at the narrowest area between the lateral lower rib and the iliac crest. Hip measurement was taken at the largest circumference of the lower abdomen.

2.4. Diet and Physical Activity

Participants completed 3-day food and drink diaries at baseline, 3, 6 and 12 months to monitor for changes in food intake. Data were analysed with Foodworks 7 Professional (Xyris Software, Brisbane, Australia), based on data from the AUSNUT database. Participants also completed the International Physical Activity Questionnaire (IPAQ) at the same time points.

2.5. *Measurements of Lipids, Glucose and Insulin Levels*

Participants attended clinical rooms at Curtin University Bentley, after a 10–12 h fast, for baseline measurements. Fasting blood samples (20 mL) were drawn by venipuncture. The collection of fasting blood samples was repeated at 3, 6 and 12 months. Serum tubes were allowed to clot and blood samples were centrifuged at 2500 rpm at 4 °C for 10 min using a Hettich Rottina 48R centrifuge. Serum and plasma were then aliquoted and samples stored at −80 °C and analysed after study completion.

Serum triglyceride and total cholesterol was measured by enzymatic colorimetric kits (TRACE Scientific Ltd., Melbourne, Australia). Serum HDL cholesterol was determined after precipitation of apoB (apolipoprotein B)-containing lipoproteins with phosphotungstic acid and $MgCl_2$ (magnesium chloride); the supernatant containing the HDL cholesterol was determined by enzymatic colorimetry (TRACE Scientific Ltd., Melbourne, Australia). Serum LDL cholesterol was determined by using the Friedewald equation [36]. Non-esterified fatty acid (NEFA) was determined using WAKO NEFA C kit (Osaka, Japan). ApoB was analysed using an ELISA kit obtained from Mabtech AB (Nacka Strand, Stockholm, Sweden).

Plasma glucose concentrations were measured using the Randox glucose GOD-PAP kit (Antrim, UK), according to the manufacturer's instructions. Plasma insulin was measured by an ELISA kit (Alpha Diagnostics International, San Antonio, TX, USA). HOMA2-IR (homeostasis model assessment of insulin resistance) was used to assess insulin resistance from fasting glucose and insulin concentrations using a computer model [37].

2.6. *Statistical Analysis*

A sample size of 24 subjects per group was predicted to provide sufficient power (80%) to detect a 3% difference in weight before and after treatment within a group. We recruited a total of 53 subjects per group to accommodate for 50% dropouts. Calculations were based on an average mean weight of 80 kg and a standard deviation of 5% within a group on all eligible subjects. Statistical analysis was undertaken using SPSS 22 for Windows (SPSS Inc., Chicago, IL, USA). Data were expressed as mean (±SD or SEM) and assessed for normality to ensure that the assumptions of the analysis were met. Baseline differences between groups were analysed with one-way ANOVA. The data were analysed using general linear models with baseline value covariates. If significant between–groups effects were present, post hoc comparisons between the treatment groups was made using the least significant difference (LSD) method. Statistical significance was considered at $p < 0.05$. Intention–to–treat analysis was also carried out with missing data replaced with the last observation carried forward.

3. Results

3.1. *Participants*

The 159 participants (19 to 68 years) who met the eligibility criteria were randomised to one of three groups (Control, PSY, PGX) by assignment of an ID number and the corresponding numbered supplement. Participant flow through the study can be seen in Figure 1. Although the PGX group had the highest attrition rate, it was generally due to factors unrelated to the study. A total of 127 participants (54 male, 73 female) completed at least 3 months of the study and were included in the analysis (45 in Control (24 male), 43 in PSY (15 male) and 39 in PGX (15 male)). Thirty-two participants withdrew before 3 months and were excluded from analysis due to non-compliance, unrelated health issues, minor adverse effects and personal reasons. A total of 108 participants at 6 months (38 in Control, 39 in PSY and 31 in PGX) and 93 participants at 12 months (32 in Control, 36 in PSY and 25 in PGX) were analysed. Results for intention–to–treat analysis for the primary outcome variables can be found in supplementary files.

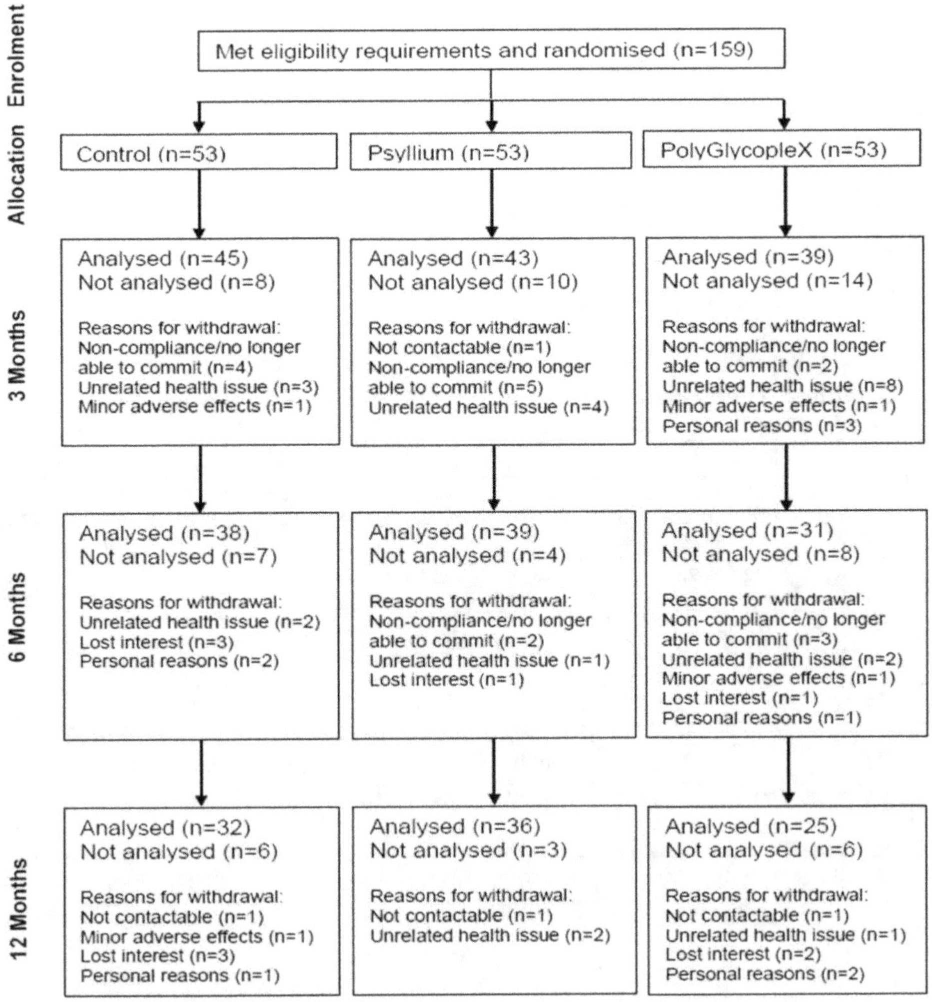

Figure 1. Participant flow diagram.

3.2. Baseline Characteristics

There were no significant differences at baseline between groups for major characteristics, energy intake, fibre intake, lipids, insulin or glucose (Table 1).

Table 1. Baseline characteristics.

	Control (n = 45)	PSY (n = 43)	PGX (n = 39)	p
Gender (Male/Female)	24/21	15/28	15/24	
Age (year)	49.82 ± 11.75	49.93 ± 11.04	47.87 ± 12.08	
Height (cm)	171.68 ± 10.04	169.16 ± 10.52	169.76 ± 10.51	
Weight (kg)	94.69 ± 17.05	91.17 ± 14.74	96.24 ± 18.02	0.365
BMI (kg/m^2)	32.01 ± 4.2	31.74 ± 3.22	33.25 ± 4.3	0.189
Waist (cm)	103.12 ± 11.02	101.17 ± 9.76	105.97 ± 12.72	0.154
Hip (cm)	112.87 ± 9.04	114.63 ± 8.63	115.71 ± 9.37	0.414
Waist Hip Ratio	0.91 ± 0.08	0.88 ± 0.08	0.92 ± 0.1	0.158
TC (mmol/L)	5 ± 0.85	4.93 ± 1.06	5.02 ± 0.85	0.904
HDL (mmol/L)	1.33 ± 0.37	1.36 ± 0.38	1.28 ± 0.26	0.563
LDL (mmol/L)	3.02 ± 0.87	3.04 ± 0.96	3.2 ± 0.77	0.592
TG (mmol/L)	1.44 ± 1.12	1.18 ± 0.67	1.2 ± 0.56	0.269
Insulin (μIU/mL)	6.11 ± 1.43	5.87 ± 1.64	6.56 ± 1.94	0.172
Glucose (mmol/L)	4.94 ± 0.73	4.79 ± 0.52	4.99 ± 0.56	0.302

Values are mean ± SD. PSY (Psyllium), PGX (PolyGlycopleX), TC (Total Cholesterol), TG (Triglyceride). p values are differences between groups.

3.3. Diet

The dietary analysis can be seen in Table 2. When examining differences between groups, energy intake was significantly lower compared to control at 3 months and 6 months in the PGX and PSY groups and at 12 months only the PGX group demonstrated significantly lower energy intake compared to the control. Carbohydrate intake was significantly lower at 3 months and 6 months in the PGX and PSY groups compared to control. Fat intake and protein intake were significantly lower compared to control at 3 months in the PGX and PSY groups and at 6 months in the PGX group compared to control.

Table 2. Dietary intake during 12 months of fibre supplementation.

Variable		3 Months	*n*	P	6 Months	*n*	P	12 Months	*n*	*p*
Energy (kJ/day)	CTR	9013.1 ± 223.6 [a]	39	0.641	8803.3 ± 282.9 [a]	34	0.928	8218 ± 295.4 [a]	31	0.111
	PSY	7272.3 ± 218 [b]	41	<0.001	7539.2 ± 278.8 [b]	35	<0.001	7657.1 ± 277.9 [a,b]	35	0.001
	PGX	7556.3 ± 243.1 [b]	33	0.001	7453.7 ± 323.5 [b]	26	0.009	7315.3 ± 342.4 [b]	23	0.012
CHO (g/day)	CTR	212.6 ± 7.7 [a]	39	0.827	213.4 ± 10 [a]	34	0.787	200.5 ± 8.4	31	0.212
	PSY	181 ± 7.5 [b]	41	0.002	164.7 ± 9.8 [b]	35	0.002	183.9 ± 7.9	35	0.015
	PGX	175.3 ± 8.4 [b]	33	0.003	177.2 ± 11.4 [b]	26	0.032	176.3 ± 9.7	23	0.012
Fat (g/day)	CTR	83.8 ± 3.2 [a]	39	0.907	82.3 ± 4.3 [a]	34	0.887	73 ± 4	31	0.066
	PSY	66.9 ± 3.1 [b]	41	<0.001	72.9 ± 4.2 [a,b]	35	0.147	73 ± 3.8	35	0.070
	PGX	72.2 ± 3.4 [b]	33	0.055	69.1 ± 4.9 [b]	26	0.047	66 ± 4.7	23	0.020
Total Fibre (g/day)	CTR	24.2 ±1.2 [a]	39	0.599	22.1 ± 1 [a]	34	0.790	21.6 ± 1.3 [a]	31	0.613
	PSY	36.4 ± 1.2 [b]	41	<0.001	35.1 ± 0.9 [b]	35	<0.001	36.6 ± 1.3 [b]	35	<0.001
	PGX	36.6 ± 1.3 [b]	33	<0.001	34.1 ± 1.1 [b]	26	<0.001	36.1 ± 1.6 [b]	23	<0.001

Values are mean ± SEM with baseline as a covariate. Different letters in superscript represent significant differences between groups $p < 0.05$. p Values are within group differences compared to baseline. CHO (carbohydrate), CTR (control), PGX (PolyGlycopleX), PSY (psyllium).

3.4. Physical Activity

Physical activity levels did not significantly change from baseline within any groups and there were no significant differences between groups at any time point (Table 3).

Table 3. Physical activity during 12 months of fibre supplementation.

	3 Months	Mean Change	*n*	P	6 Months	Mean Change	*n*	P	12 Months	Mean Change	*n*	*p*
CTR	2802.4 ± 449.3	−130.5	29	0.837	2868.2 ± 454.7	−141.2	32	0.823	3294.5 ± 525.6	415.4	30	0.569
PSY	2933 ± 443.6	620.8	30	0.345	3009.3 ± 433.2	187	35	0.876	2879.1 ± 497.8	609.6	33	0.526
PGX	2181.7 ± 470.6	751.3	27	0.254	2681.1 ± 495.5	328.2	27	0.711	2684.9 ± 619.1	194.3	22	0.886

Values are mean kJ/day ± SEM with baseline as a covariate. Mean change from baseline. p Values are within group differences compared to baseline.

3.5. Lipids

Total cholesterol was significantly lower in the PGX group at 3 months (−8%, $p < 0.001$) and 6 months (−5.1%, $p = 0.048$) compared to baseline, as shown in Figure 2A. Total cholesterol was significantly lower in the PSY group at 3 months (−6.5%, $p < 0.001$) and 6 months (−4.8%, $p = 0.006$) compared to baseline. Total cholesterol was significantly lower at 3 months in the PGX (−8.2%, $p < 0.001$) and PSY (−7%, $p = 0.001$) groups and at 6 months in the PGX (−5.5%, $p = 0.047$) and PSY (−5.3%, $p = 0.042$) groups compared to control. There were no significant differences in total cholesterol between PSY and PGX groups at 3, 6 or 12 months.

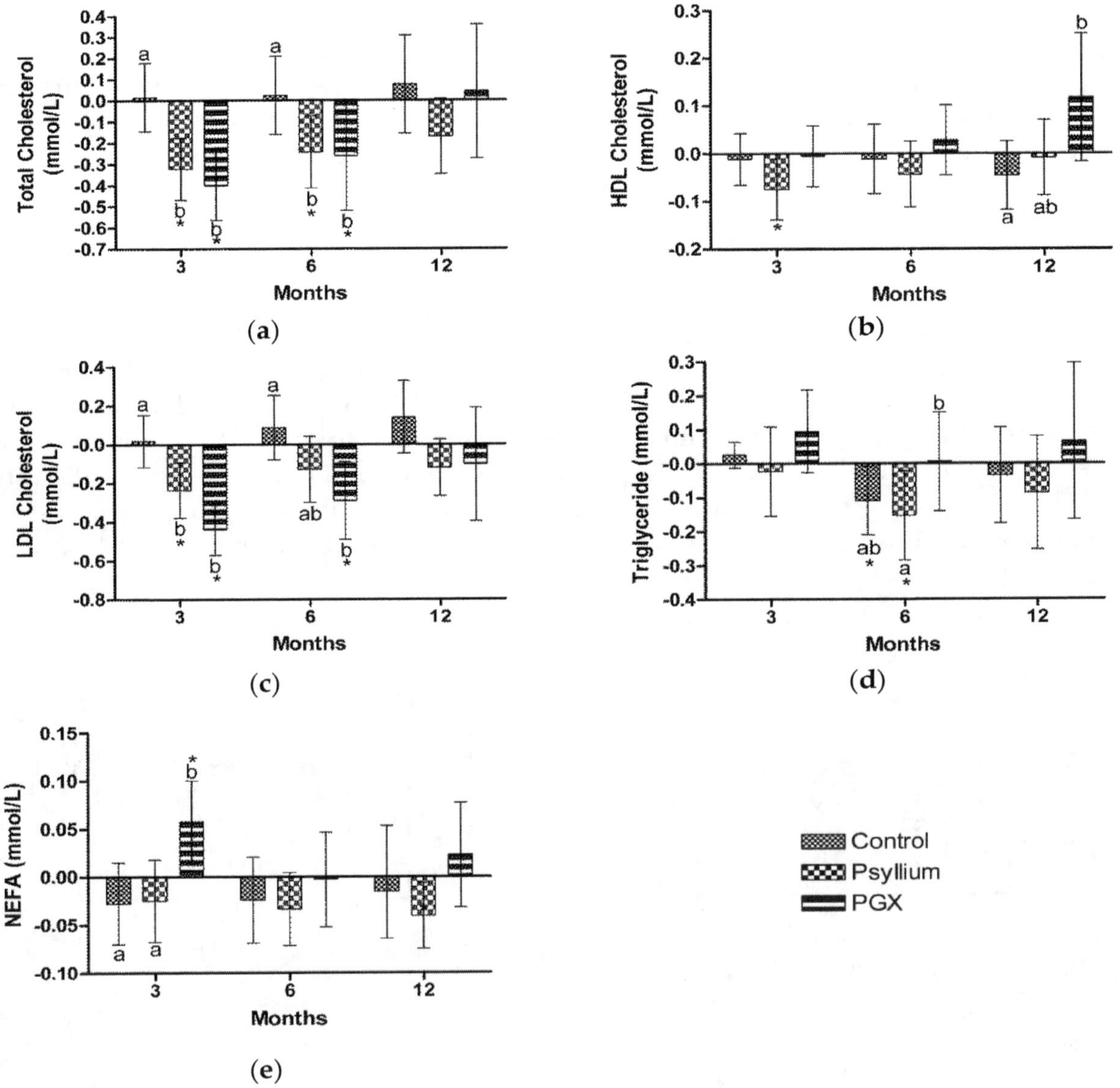

Figure 2. Changes in fasting blood lipids during 12 months of fibre supplementation (**a**) Total Cholesterol; (**b**) high density lipoprotein (HDL); (**c**) low density lipoprotein (LDL); (**d**) Triglyceride; (**e**) NEFA (non-esterified fatty acid). Values are mean ± 95% CI with baseline as a covariate. * indicates within group differences compared to baseline. Different letters represent significant differences between groups $p < 0.05$.

High density lipoprotein (HDL) cholesterol was significantly lower in the PSY group at 3 months (−5.5%, $p = 0.022$) compared to baseline, as shown in Figure 2B. HDL was significantly higher at 12 months in the PGX group (11.5%, $p = 0.019$) compared to control. There were no significant differences in HDL between control and PSY or between PSY and PGX groups at 3, 6 or 12 months.

LDL was significantly lower in the PGX group at 3 months (−13.7%, $p < 0.001$) and 6 months (−9.1%, $p = 0.006$) compared to baseline, shown in Figure 2C. LDL cholesterol was significantly lower in the PSY group at 3 months (−7.8%, $p = 0.002$) compared to baseline. LDL was significantly lower compared to control at 3 months in the PGX (−13.9%, $p < 0.001$) and PSY (−8.1%, $p = 0.007$) groups and at 6 months in the PGX (−11%, $p = 0.006$) group compared to control. There were no significant differences in LDL between PSY and PGX groups at 3, 6 or 12 months.

Triglyceride was significantly lower in the control group at 6 months (−7.6%, $p = 0.033$) compared to baseline (Figure 2D). TG was significantly lower in the PSY group at 6 months (−12.7%, $p = 0.023$) compared to baseline.

Non-esterified fatty acid (NEFA) was significantly lower in the PSY group at 12 months (−9.5%, $p = 0.021$) compared to baseline, as shown in Figure 2E. NEFA was significantly higher in the PGX group at 3 months (15.7%, $p = 0.009$) compared to baseline. NEFA was significantly higher in the PGX group compared to control (16.9%, $p = 0.027$) and PSY (18.2%, $p = 0.017$) at 3 months. There were no significant differences in NEFA between control and PSY at 3, 6 or 12 months.

ApoB did not significantly change within any of the study groups. There were no significant differences in apoB between control, PSY or PGX groups at 3, 6 or 12 months (data not shown).

3.6. Insulin

Insulin was significantly lower in the PGX group at 3 months (−7.6%, $p < 0.001$) compared to baseline (Figure 3A). Insulin was significantly lower in the PSY group at 3 months (−5.5%, $p = 0.032$) compared to baseline. Insulin was significantly lower compared to control at 3 months in the PGX (−9%, $p = 0.008$) and PSY (−9.4%, $p = 0.004$) groups, at 6 months in PGX (−9.8%, $p = 0.038$) and PSY (−9.1%, $p = 0.040$) groups compared to control and at 12 months in the PSY group (−9.4%, $p = 0.029$) compared to control. There were no significant differences in insulin between PSY and PGX groups at 3, 6 or 12 months.

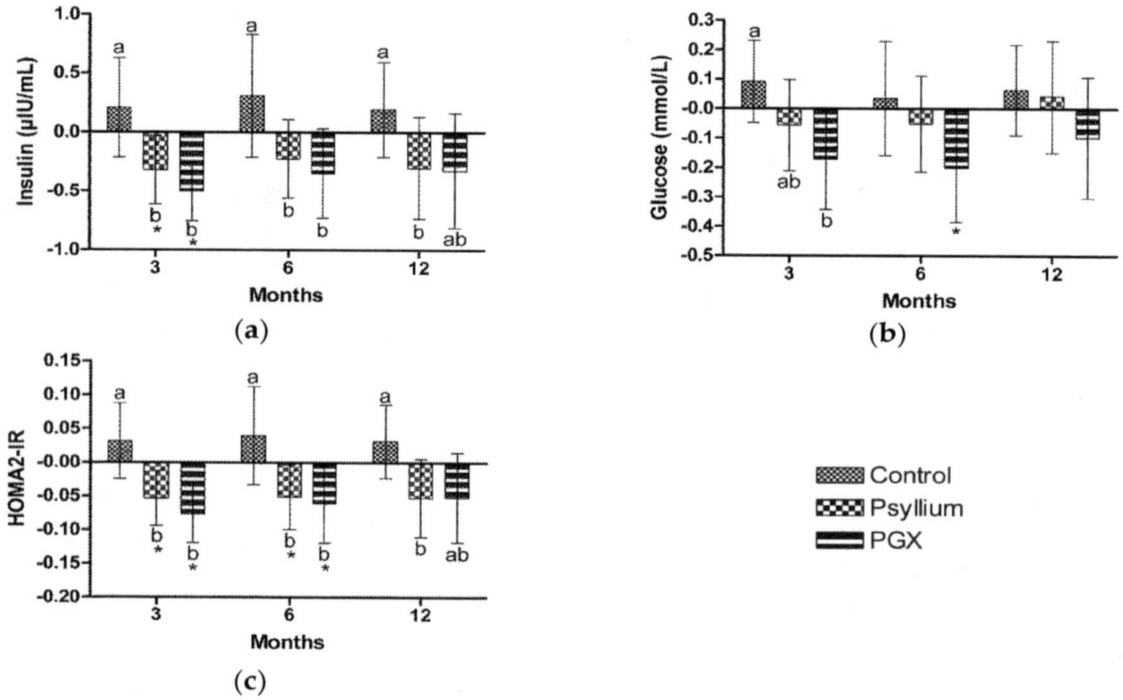

Figure 3. Changes in fasting blood parameters during 12 months of fibre supplementation (**a**) Insulin, (**b**) Glucose; (**c**) HOMA2-IR. Values are mean ± 95% CI with baseline as a covariate. * indicates within group differences compared to baseline. Different letters represent significant differences between groups $p < 0.05$.

3.7. Glucose

Glucose was significantly lower in the PGX group at 6 months (−3.9%, $p = 0.033$) compared to baseline, while the decrease at 3 months did not reach significance (−3.4%, $p = 0.053$) (Figure 3B). Glucose was significantly lower compared to control at 3 months in the PGX (−4.8%, $p = 0.019$) group. There were no significant differences in glucose between control and PSY or between PSY and PGX groups at 3, 6 or 12 months.

3.8. Homeostasis Model Assessment of Insulin Resistance

The HOMA2-IR score was significantly lower in the PGX group at 3 months (−9%, $p = 0.001$) and 6 months (−7.3%, $p = 0.039$) compared to baseline (Figure 3C). HOMA2-IR was significantly lower in the PSY group at 3 months (−7%, $p = 0.011$) and 6 months (−6.7%, $p = 0.037$) compared to baseline. HOMA2-IR was significantly lower compared to control at 3 months in the PGX (−10.8%, $p = 0.005$) and PSY (−10.8%, $p = 0.001$) groups, at 6 months in PGX (−11.9%, $p = 0.033$) and PSY (−11.9%, $p = 0.018$) groups compared to control and at 12 months in the PSY group (−11%, $p = 0.011$) compared to control. There was a trend for HOMA2-IR to be lower in the PGX group compared to control at 12 months but this was not significant (−8.5%, $p = 0.068$). There were no significant differences in HOMA2-IR score between PSY and PGX groups at 3, 6 or 12 months.

3.9. Adverse Events

Minor adverse events were gastrointestinal related (e.g., flatulence, diarrhoea) with four withdrawing from the study, two in the PGX group and two in the control group. The PSY supplement was better tolerated and participants did not report any adverse effects.

4. Discussion

Previous epidemiological and cohort studies have consistently revealed that higher fibre intakes are correlated with lower body weight, BMI, waist circumference [1,2], and improved plasma lipid profiles [3–12], glycaemia and insulinaemia [13], indicating the benefits and risk reduction for the metabolic syndrome, CVD and type 2 diabetes. Given that individuals find it difficult to eat the required amounts of fibre by increasing fruit and vegetable intake, it was hypothesised that fibre supplements can provide similar health benefits compared with increased dietary fibre intake. Therefore, this study investigated the effects of 15 g of PGX or psyllium compared to control (rice flour) supplementation for one year on lipids, insulin and glucose. Specifically, both the PGX and PSY groups demonstrated significant reductions at 3 months in fasting concentrations of total cholesterol by 8.2% and 7% respectively, LDL cholesterol by 13.9% and 8.1% respectively, insulin by 9% and 9.4% respectively and HOMA2-IR score by 11.9%, compared to control group. Only the PGX intervention improved fasting glucose and HDL cholesterol during the study.

Our results herein are supported by recent human and animal studies which suggest that psyllium fibre supplementation may provide cardiovascular benefits [22,31]. The effect of PGX on decreasing total and LDL cholesterol levels in this study concurs with similar reports in the literature describing the effects of viscous dietary fibre on lowering serum cholesterol levels. Carabin et al. [17] conducted a clinical trial with healthy subjects, 25 males and 29 females, mean age of 31.6 ± 10.5 years who consumed 2.5 g of PGX packaged with cereal and yoghurt twice a day as part of two main meals (breakfast and/or lunch, and/or dinner), for the first seven days, followed by 5 g PGX twice a day for the last 14 days of the study. The control product was a skimmed milk powder. Investigators observed significantly lower total and LDL cholesterol in the test group compared to the control group at day 8 (9.4% vs. 3.3% for total and 10.4% vs. 2.5% for LDL cholesterol, respectively) and at day 22 (14.1% vs. 8.3% for total and 16.6% vs. 8.2% for LDL cholesterol, respectively). The differences between groups was similar to the magnitude observed in our study. Reimer et al. [38] observed the effects of 14 weeks of short-term PGX supplementation in adults with abdominal obesity and also observed significant reductions in total and LDL cholesterol. In a pre-post study by Lyon & Reichert [18], 29 overweight and obese adults with a BMI between 25–36 kg/m^2, consumed 5 g of PGX in 500 mL of water 5–10 min before each meal, 2–3 times a day for 14 days and showed a significant reduction of total cholesterol and LDL cholesterol levels of 19% and 25% respectively, compared to baseline. As the supplement intervention in this latter study was combined with lifestyle changes, the decreases in cholesterol levels were greater than those observed in our current study. Although neither of the studies described above reported changes in HDL after PGX supplementation, we only observed this effect at 12 months, indicating a possible long term effect that has not been demonstrated previously. When looking at the effect of psyllium, another study [22] also found that simply adding a psyllium fibre supplement to a normal diet (10.2 g/day) was sufficient to see improvements in total cholesterol (−21%) and LDL cholesterol (−22%) at 12 weeks compared to control. Similar findings for psyllium have also been reported in various meta-analyses [39].

Animal studies have demonstrated a beneficial effect of PGX supplementation on glucose control and fasting insulin [40]. While many human studies have examined the short-term postprandial glucose response to PGX supplementation [20,41,42], few have looked at the long term effects. Lyon & Reichert [18] assessed changes to fasting insulin and glucose in their study. The PGX and lifestyle intervention caused a 6.96% reduction in fasting glucose and a 27.26% reduction in fasting insulin which is in agreement with our PGX intervention findings. Psyllium has been previously shown to improve glucose and insulin response [31,33]. In a study by Ziai et al. [23], psyllium was taken in combination with medication and a significant reduction in fasting glucose was observed. Gibb et al. [33] reported that psyllium improved glycaemic control proportional to loss of glycaemic control, which may explain why our non-diabetic psyllium group did not demonstrate any significant improvements to fasting blood glucose concentrations.

Due to its high viscosity, PGX swells in the stomach and increases feelings of fullness [23,42–45]. Psyllium has also been shown to increase fullness [29] but has a far lower viscosity than PGX [18]. This characteristic may have caused participants to decrease their food intake, which then lead to significant weight loss [46]. The changes to blood lipids and insulin observed are likely due to the changes in dietary intake and weight loss observed as well as the possible effect of PGX slowing gastric emptying and absorption of nutrients in the small intestine [47].

When comparing the PGX and PSY groups in the current study, there were no significant differences between them except for a lower concentration of TG at 3 months in the PSY group compared to the PGX group. However, when examining differences compared to control, HDL cholesterol was significantly higher in the PGX group at 12 months but not in the PSY group. LDL cholesterol was significantly lower in the PGX group at 3 and 6 months compared to control whereas LDL cholesterol was only significantly lower in the PSY group at 3 months compared to control. Glucose was significantly lower in the PGX group at 3 months but not in the PSY group. Intent-to-treat analysis was carried out but the outcome results were no different from the results presented. In this regard, the PGX group performed better overall than the PSY group and elicited more health benefits over the 12 months intervention period.

One of the strengths of this study was the duration, with a 12 months intervention period. Comparable studies have only been conducted for 14 weeks. This allowed us to investigate the long term effects of the fibre supplements, especially weight maintenance. This was a double-blinded study and supplements were packed in identical foil sachets. Investigators were not aware which participants were taking which supplement; however, due to the different characteristics of the supplements, participants may have been able to guess if they were taking a fibre supplement or the control, which is a limitation. The intervention was not combined with any other lifestyle modification advice, thus it would be simple for consumers to incorporate into their lifestyle or there could be added benefits if the supplements were combined with healthy lifestyle advice. Other study limitations include the use of a generally healthy population. We did not specifically recruit participants with elevated lipid, insulin or glucose concentrations which would have limited our ability to detect significant improvements. The majority of participants were women and hormonal changes over the 12 months may have impacted on lipids levels.

5. Conclusions

It is thought the high viscosity of PGX caused participants to decrease their food intake, which then lead to significant weight loss, lipid, insulin, and glucose reductions. Taking a fibre supplement before meals was a relatively easy task for people to incorporate into their daily routine and would be a simple intervention to implement. We observed similar results between PGX and PSY supplements when compared to the control group, however the PGX supplement was superior in terms of increased HDL cholesterol and decreased fasting blood glucose. Therefore, regular consumption of a PolyGlycopleX or a psyllium supplement is a simple and effective method to improve blood lipids, insulin and glucose control in overweight or obese people and may lead to risk reduction for metabolic syndrome, CVD and type 2 diabetes.

Acknowledgments: PGX®, PolyGlycopleX® and EnviroSimplex® are registered trademarks of InovoBiologic Inc., Calgary, AB, Canada. The proprietary Psyllium product (PgxSyl™) (PSY) was formulated by InovoBiologic Inc. We thank Michael Lyon, MD for helping with the design of this study. We thank all the participants for their time and contributions to this study.

Author Contributions: S.P., S.W. and R.J.G. designed research; S.H. (and Jenny McKay) conducted research; S.H. analysed data; S.P., S.H., S.W. and R.J.G. wrote the paper; S.P. and S.H. had primary responsibility for final content. All authors read and approved the final manuscript.

References

1. Du, H.; van der, A.D.L.; Boshuizen, H.C.; Forouhi, N.G.; Wareham, N.J.; Halkjaer, J.; Tjonneland, A.; Overvad, K.; Jakobsen, M.U.; Boeing, H.; et al. Dietary fiber and subsequent changes in body weight and waist circumference in European men and women. *Am. J. Clin. Nutr.* **2010**, *91*, 329–336. [CrossRef] [PubMed]
2. Newby, P.K.; Maras, J.; Bakun, P.; Muller, D.; Ferrucci, L.; Tucker, K.L. Intake of whole grains, refined grains, and cereal fiber measured with 7-D diet records and associations with risk factors for chronic disease. *Am. J. Clin. Nutr.* **2007**, *86*, 1745–1753. [PubMed]
3. National Health and Medical Research Council. *Australian Dietary Guidelines*; National Health and Medical Research Council: Canberra, Australia, 2013.
4. Wu, H.; Dwyer, K.M.; Fan, Z.; Shircore, A.; Fan, J.; Dwyer, J.H. Dietary fiber and progression of atherosclerosis: The Los Angeles Atherosclerosis Study. *Am. J. Clin. Nutr.* **2003**, *78*, 1085–1091. [PubMed]
5. Lairon, D. Macronutrient intake and modulation on chylomicron production and clearance. *Atheroscler. Suppl.* **2008**, *9*, 45–48. [CrossRef] [PubMed]
6. Kan, H.; Stevens, J.; Heiss, G.; Klein, R.; Rose, K.M.; London, S.J. Dietary fiber intake and retinal vascular caliber in the atherosclerosis risk in communities study. *Am. J. Clin. Nutr.* **2007**, *86*, 1626–1632. [PubMed]
7. Lairon, D.; Arnault, N.; Bertrais, S.; Planells, R.; Clero, E.; Hercberg, S.; Boutron-Ruault, M.C. Dietary fiber intake and risk factors for cardiovascular disease in French adults. *Am. J. Clin. Nutr.* **2005**, *82*, 1185–1194. [PubMed]
8. Venn, B.J.; Mann, J.I. Cereal grains, legumes and diabetes. *Eur. J. Clin. Nutr.* **2004**, *58*, 1443–1461. [CrossRef] [PubMed]
9. Weickert, M.O.; Pfeiffer, A.F. Metabolic effects of dietary fiber consumption and prevention of diabetes. *J. Nutr.* **2008**, *138*, 439–442. [PubMed]
10. McKeown, N.M.; Meigs, J.B.; Liu, S.; Wilson, P.W.; Jacques, P.F. Whole-grain intake is favorably associated with metabolic risk factors for type 2 diabetes and cardiovascular disease in the Framingham Offspring Study. *Am. J. Clin. Nutr.* **2002**, *76*, 390–398. [PubMed]
11. Pittler, M.H.; Ernst, E. Guar gum for body weight reduction: Meta-analysis of randomized trials. *Am. J. Med.* **2001**, *110*, 724–730. [CrossRef]
12. Brown, L.; Rosner, B.; Willett, W.W.; Sacks, F.M. Cholesterol-lowering effects of dietary fiber: A meta-analysis. *Am. J. Clin. Nutr.* **1999**, *69*, 30–42. [PubMed]
13. Ludwig, D.S.; Pereira, M.A.; Kroenke, C.H.; Hilner, J.E.; Van Horn, L.; Slattery, M.L.; Jacobs, D.R., Jr. Dietary fiber, weight gain, and cardiovascular disease risk factors in young adults. *JAMA* **1999**, *282*, 1539–1546. [CrossRef] [PubMed]
14. Clemens, R.; Kranz, S.; Mobley, A.; Nicklas, R.; Raimondi, M.; Rodriguez, J.; Slavin, J.; Jacobs, D.J. Filling America's Fiber Intake Gap: Summary of a Roundtable to Probe Realistic Solutions with a Focus on Grain-Based Foods. *J. Nutr.* **2012**, *142*, 1390S–1401S. [CrossRef] [PubMed]

15. US Department of Agriculture; US Department of Health and Human Services. *Dietary Guidelines for Americans*; US Government Printing Office: Washington, DC, USA, 2005.
16. Marlett, J.A.; McBurney, M.I.; Slavin, J.L. Position of the American Dietetic Association: Health implications of dietary fiber. *J. Am. Diet. Assoc.* **2002**, *102*, 993–1000. [CrossRef]
17. Carabin, I.G.; Lyon, M.R.; Wood, S.; Pelletier, X.; Donazzolo, Y.; Burdock, G.A. Supplementation of the diet with the functional fiber PolyGlycoplex is well tolerated by healthy subjects in a clinical trial. *Nutr. J.* **2009**, *8*, 9. [CrossRef] [PubMed]
18. Lyon, M.R.; Reichert, R.G. The effect of a novel viscous polysaccharide along with lifestyle changes on short-term weight loss and associated risk factors in overweight and obese adults: an observational retrospective clinical program analysis. *Altern. Med. Rev.* **2010**, *15*, 68–75. [PubMed]
19. Food and Nutrition Board of the Institute of Medicine of the National Academies. Dietary, functional, and total fiber. In *Dietary Reference Intakes for Energy, Carbohydrate, Fiber, Fat, Fatty Acids, Cholesterol, Protein, and Amino Acids*; Spears, G.E., Ed.; The National Academies Press: Washington, DC, USA, 2005; pp. 339–421.
20. Jenkins, A.L.; Kacinik, V.; Lyon, M.; Wolever, T.M. Effect of adding the novel fiber, PGX®, to commonly consumed foods on glycemic response, glycemic index and GRIP: A simple and effective strategy for reducing post prandial blood glucose levels—A randomized, controlled trial. *Nutr. J.* **2010**, *9*, 58. [CrossRef] [PubMed]
21. Reimer, R.A.; Pelletier, X.; Carabin, I.G.; Lyon, M.; Gahler, R.; Parnell, J.A.; Wood, S. Increased plasma PYY levels following supplementation with the functional fiber PolyGlycopleX in healthy adults. *Eur. J. Clin. Nutr.* **2010**, *64*, 1186–1191. [CrossRef] [PubMed]
22. Pal, S.; Khossousi, A.; Binns, C.; Dhaliwal, S.; Ellis, V. The effect of a fibre supplement compared to a healthy diet on body composition, lipids, glucose, insulin and other metabolic syndrome risk factors in overweight and obese individuals. *Br. J. Nutr.* **2011**, *105*, 90–100. [CrossRef] [PubMed]
23. Ziai, S.; Larijani, B.; Akhoondzadeh, S.; Fakhrzadeh, H.; Dastpak, A.; Bandarian, F.; Rezai, A.; Badi, H.; Emami, T. Psyllium decreased serum glucose and glycosylated hemoglobin significantly in diabetic outpatients. *J. Ethnopharmacol.* **2005**, *102*, 202–207. [CrossRef] [PubMed]
24. Karhunen, L.; Juvonen, K.; Flander, S.; Liukkonen, K.; Lahteenmaki, L.; Siloaho, M.; Laaksonen, D.; Herzig, K.; Uusitupa, M.; Poutanen, K. A psyllium fiber-enriched meal strongly attenuates postprandial gastrointestinal peptide release in healthy young adults. *J. Nutr.* **2010**, *140*, 737–744. [CrossRef] [PubMed]
25. Anderson, J.; Allgood, L.; Lawrence, A.; Altringer, L.; Jerdack, G.; Hengehold, D.; Morel, J. Cholesterol-lowering effects of psyllium intake adjuctive to diet therapy in men and women with hypercholesterolemia: Meta-analysis of 8 controlled trials. *Am. J. Clin. Nutr.* **2000**, *71*, 472–479. [PubMed]
26. Rodriguez-Moran, M.; Guerrero-Romero, F.; Lazcano-Burciaga, G. Lipid- and glucose-lowering efficacy of *Plantago*. Psyllium in type II diabetes. *J. Diabetes Complic.* **1998**, *12*, 273–278. [CrossRef]
27. Vuksan, V.; Jenkins, A.L.; Rogovik, A.L.; Fairgrieve, C.; Jovanovski, E.; Leiter, L. Viscosity rather than quantity of dietary fibre predicts cholesterol-lowering effect in healthy individuals. *Br. J. Nutr.* **2011**, *106*, 1349–1352. [CrossRef] [PubMed]
28. Tai, E.; Fok, A.; Chu, R.; Tan, C. A study to assess the effect of dietary supplementation with soluble fibre (Minolest) on lipid levels in normal subjects with hypercholesterolaemia. *Ann. Acad. Med. Singapore* **1999**, *28*, 209–213. [PubMed]
29. Turnbull, W.; Thomas, H. The effect of a *Plantago ovata* seed containing preparation on appetite variables, nutrient and energy intake. *Int. J. Obes. Relat. Metab. Disord.* **1995**, *19*, 338–342. [PubMed]
30. Delargy, H.; O'Sullivan, K.; Fletcher, R.; Blundell, J. Effects of amount and type of dietary fibre (soluble and insoluble) on short-term control of appetite. *Int. J. Food Sci. Nutr.* **1997**, *48*, 67–77. [CrossRef] [PubMed]
31. Pal, S.; Radavelli-Bagatini, S. Effects of psyllium on metabolic syndrome risk factors. *Obes. Rev.* **2012**, *13*, 1034–1047. [CrossRef] [PubMed]
32. Khossousi, A.; Binns, C.W.; Dhaliwal, S.S.; Pal, S. The acute effects of psyllium on postprandial lipaemia and thermogenesis in overweight and obese men. *Br. J. Nutr.* **2008**, *99*, 1068–1075. [CrossRef] [PubMed]
33. Gibb, R.; McRorie, J.; Russel, D.; Hasselblad, V.; D'Alessio, D. Psyllium fiber improves glycemic control proportional to loss of glycemic control: A meta-analysis of data in euglycemic subjects, patients at risk of type 2 diabetes mellitus, and patients being treated for type 2 diabetes mellitus. *Am. J. Clin. Nutr.* **2015**, *102*, 1604–1614. [CrossRef] [PubMed]

34. US Pharmacopeia. *Food Chemicals Codex (FCC)*, 9th ed.; US Pharmacopeia: Rockville, MD, USA, 2015.
35. Pal, S.; Ellis, V.; Dhaliwal, S. Effects of whey protein isolate on body composition, lipids, insulin and glucose in overweight and obese individuals. *Br. J. Nutr.* **2010**, *104*, 716–723. [CrossRef] [PubMed]
36. Bairaktari, E.; Hatzidimou, K.; Tzallas, C.; Vini, M.; Katsaraki, A.; Tselepis, A.; Elisaf, M.; Tsolas, O. Estimation of LDL cholesterol based on the Friedewald formula and on apo B levels. *Clin. Biochem.* **2000**, *33*, 549–555. [CrossRef]
37. Wallace, T.M.; Levy, J.C.; Matthews, D.R. Use and abuse of HOMA modeling. *Diabetes Care* **2004**, *27*, 1487–1495. [CrossRef] [PubMed]
38. Reimer, R.A.; Yamaguchi, H.; Eller, L.K.; Lyon, M.R.; Gahler, R.J.; Kacinik, V.; Juneja, P.; Wood, S. Changes in visceral adiposity and serum cholesterol with a novel viscous polysaccharide in Japanese adults with abdominal obesity. *Obesity* **2013**, *21*, E379–E387. [PubMed]
39. Bernstein, A.; Titgemeier, B.; Kirkpatrick, K.; Golubic, M.; Roizen, M. Major cereal grain fibers and psyllium in relation to cardiovascular health. *Nutrients* **2013**, *5*, 1471–1487. [CrossRef] [PubMed]
40. Grover, G.J.; Koetzner, L.; Wicks, J.; Gahler, R.J.; Lyon, M.R.; Reimer, R.A.; Wood, S. Effects of the soluble fiber complex PolyGlycopleX® on glucose homeostasis and body weight in young Zucker diabetic rats. *Front. Pharmacol.* **2011**, *2*, 47. [CrossRef] [PubMed]
41. Brand-Miller, J.C.; Atkinson, F.S.; Gahler, R.J.; Kacinik, V.; Lyon, M.R.; Wood, S. Effects of PGX, a novel functional fibre, on acute and delayed postprandial glycaemia. *Eur. J. Clin. Nutr.* **2010**, *64*, 1488–1493. [CrossRef] [PubMed]
42. Solah, V.A.; Brand-Miller, J.C.; Atkinson, F.S.; Gahler, R.J.; Kacinik, V.; Lyon, M.R.; Wood, S. Dose-response effect of a novel functional fibre, PolyGlycopleX®, PGX®, on satiety. *Appetite* **2014**, *77C*, 72–76. [CrossRef] [PubMed]
43. Vuksan, V.; Panahi, S.; Lyon, M.; Rogovik, A.L.; Jenkins, A.L.; Leiter, L.A. Viscosity of fiber preloads affects food intake in adolescents. *Nutr. Metab. Cardiovasc. Dis.* **2009**, *19*, 498–503. [CrossRef] [PubMed]
44. Yong, M.; Solah, V.; Johnson, S.; Meng, X.; Kerr, D.; James, A.; Fenton, H.; Gahler, R.J.; Wood, S. Effects of a viscous-fibre supplemented evening meal and the following un-supplemented breakfast on post-prandial satiety responses in healthy women. *Physiol. Behav.* **2016**, *154*, 34–39. [CrossRef] [PubMed]
45. Kacinik, V.; Lyon, M.R.; Purnama, M.; Reimer, R.A.; Gahler, R.J.; Green, T.J.; Wood, S. Effect of PGX, a novel functional fibre supplement, on subjective ratings of appetite in overweight and obese women consuming a 3-day structured, low-calorie diet. *Nutr. Diab.* **2011**, *1*, e22. [CrossRef] [PubMed]
46. Pal, S.; Ho, S.; Gahler, R.; Wood, S. Effect on body weight and composition in overweight/obese Australian adults over 12 months consumption of two different types of fiber supplementation in a randomized trial. *Nutr. Metab.* **2016**, *13*, 82. [CrossRef] [PubMed]
47. Matulka, R.A.; Lyon, M.R.; Wood, S.; Ann Marone, P.; Merkel, D.J.; Burdock, G.A. The safety of PolyGlycopleX (PGX) as shown in a 90-day rodent feeding study. *Nutr. J.* **2009**, *8*, 1. [CrossRef] [PubMed]

8

Efficacy of Synbiotics in Patients with Slow Transit Constipation

Chao Ding [1,†], Xiaolong Ge [1,†], Xueying Zhang [1], Hongliang Tian [1], Hongkan Wang [2], Lili Gu [1], Jianfeng Gong [1,*], Weiming Zhu [1] and Ning Li [1,*]

[1] Department of General Surgery, Jinling Hospital, Medical School of Nanjing University, Nanjing 210002, China; jinlingh_dc@163.com (C.D.); xiaolongge9118@126.com (X.G.); 15996282291@163.com (X.Z.); kevin_thl@163.com (H.T.); njumedgll@126.com (L.G.); jinlingh_zwm@sina.com (W.Z.)

[2] First Affiliated Hospital, School of Medicine, Zhejiang University, Hangzhou 310003, China; njumedcy@126.com

* Correspondence: jinlingh_gongjf@163.com (J.G.); jinlingh_lining@163.com (N.L.);

† These authors contributed equally to this work.

Abstract: Synbiotic intake may efficiently restore the balance of gut microbiota and improve gastrointestinal functions. The aim of the study was to evaluate the efficacy of a synbiotic in patients with slow transit constipation. A total of 100 patients with slow transit constipation were randomized to receive either a synbiotic or placebo twice daily for 12 weeks. The primary efficacy endpoints were the clinical remission and improvement rates at weeks 4 and 12. Stool frequency and consistency, colonic transit time (CTT), evacuation and abdominal symptoms, patient assessment of constipation symptoms, gastrointestinal quality-of-life index scores, satisfaction scores, and adverse events were also monitored. The clinical remission rates reached 37.5% at week 4 and 45.8% at week 12 in the treatment group, compared to 13.3% at week 4 and 16.7% at week 12 in the placebo group ($p < 0.01$ for both comparisons). Over 12 weeks, 64.6% of the patients who received the synbiotic experienced clinical improvement, compared to 29.2% of the patients in the placebo group ($p < 0.01$). During the intervention period, patients who were treated with the synbiotic exhibited increased stool frequency, improved stool consistency, decreased CTT, and improved constipation-related symptoms. This randomized, placebo-controlled trial suggested that dietary supplementation with a synbiotic improved evacuation-parameters-associated symptoms and colonic motility in patients with slow transit constipation (STC).

Keywords: synbiotic; soluble dietary fiber; slow transit constipation; microbiota

---

1. Introduction

Chronic constipation has become a common, often long-term, functional gastrointestinal disease that influences the quality of life in patients worldwide [1]. According to the Rome III criteria for chronic constipation [2], almost 16% of all adults are affected by chronic constipation worldwide, and it is more prevalent and symptomatic in women and elderly people [3]. Constipation is defined as difficult or infrequent passage of stool, hardness of stool, or a feeling of incomplete evacuation [4]. Clinically, constipation can always be categorized as normal transit constipation (NTC), slow transit constipation (STC), pelvic floor dysfunction, or a defecatory disorder due to assessments of anorectal function and colonic transit time [5]. Among these, STC is the major category and is characterized by a decreased rate of colonic transit [5].

The treatments for chronic constipation are varied, but remain challenging [6]. Most patients with chronic constipation have used laxatives (osmotic or stimulant) or prokinetic agents to alleviate symptoms empirically [7]. Although there is a wide range of medications, many patients are still dissatisfied with their current treatments, according to the results of a long-term survey, due to insufficient efficacy and some adverse effects [8]. Sajid et al. [9] reported that adverse events or side effects such as abdominal cramps, rash, excessive flatulence, and dizziness have occurred in constipated patients who used prucalopride, which is a new pharmacotherapy for chronic constipation. From our clinical experience in constipation, laxatives or other agents could be efficient at the beginning of chronic constipation, but they gradually become largely ineffective. Therefore, novel effective therapies are still needed.

Probiotics are live microorganisms that may benefit human health, and are now used widely to treat some diseases. Cui et al. [10] reported that *Bifidobacteria* intake could play a role in the remission of ulcerative colitis (UC) and that prebiotics, such as dietary fiber, are ingredients in food that may increase the functions of probiotics in the human body. Previous research has suggested that a sufficient intake of dietary fiber with prebiotic effects is necessary for patients with chronic constipation [11–13]. Pectin, one typical kind of dietary fiber, is usually present in the cell walls of fruits, vegetables, and legumes [14]. It is fermented by the intestinal microbiota in the gut and can strongly stimulate the growth and activity of some bacteria, such as *Bifidobacterium* and *Lactobacillus* [14]. Some reports have also shown that therapy with increasing dietary fiber intake, especially soluble fibers, was beneficial for individuals with chronic constipation [15]. Soluble dietary fiber, which includes pectin, is physiologically important [16]. Pectin can be digested into short-chain fatty acids (SCFAs) by intestinal microbiota, which may have effects on motility [17]. Fukumoto et al. [18] reported that SCFAs could stimulate the colon to release serotonin, which is an important factor in colonic motility. In addition, butyrate is used in treating various gastrointestinal motility disorders that are associated with the inhibition of colonic transit [17].

Currently, the combination of prebiotics and probiotics is called synbiotics, and it may have synergistic effects [19]. Morelli et al. [20] suggested that microbiota composition could be modified by synbiotics, which might play a role in gastrointestinal functions. This prospective, randomized study was designed to measure the effects of a symbiotic consisting of *Enterococci*, *Bifidobacteria*, and *Lactobacilli* triple viable bacteria (BIFICO) and pectin on slow transit constipation [10]. This was the first study to assess a specific synbiotic containing triple viable bacteria and pectin in individuals with constipation.

Our objective was to evaluate the clinical efficacy of synbiotic treatment in individuals with slow transit constipation. The primary aim was to assess clinical improvement and remission at weeks 4 and 12. The secondary aim was to assess the frequency of bowel movements, stool consistency, and colonic transit time. Other aims included the assessment of constipation-related symptoms, and the gastrointestinal quality-of-life index.

2. Materials and Methods

2.1. Ethical Issues

This study was registered in the Clinical Trials Database (ID: NCT02844426) and conducted at Jinling Hospital, a teaching hospital of Nanjing University. The current study was approved by the Ethical Committee of Jinling Hospital. All participants provided written informed consent.

2.2. Patients

Patients were eligible if they fulfilled the following criteria:

Inclusion criteria: age $\geq$18 years; body mass index 18.5–25 kg/m^2; chronic constipation was diagnosed according to the Rome III criteria with two or fewer spontaneous, complete bowel movements (SCBMs) per week for a minimum of 6 months [21]; colonic transit time (CTT) >48 h [22]; mild-to-moderate constipation with a Wexner constipation scale score between 16 and 25 [23,24].

Exclusion criteria: Megacolon, intestinal obstruction, inflammatory bowel disease, and cancer; secondary constipation (i.e., due to drugs, endocrine disorders, neurological disorders, metabolic disorders, psychological disorders or abdominal surgery); severe anterior rectocele or full thickness rectorectal intussusception according to defecography; pregnant or lactating women; infection with an enteric pathogen; usage of antibiotics or proton pump inhibitors (PPIs); hepatic, renal, cardiovascular, respiratory or psychiatric disease; and other diseases or factors evaluated by the investigator which could influence intestinal transit or intestinal microbiota [24].

2.3. Study Design

A total of 100 patients were screened for eligibility to participate in our study. The sealed envelope method was used to randomize the participants into either the treatment group or the placebo group. After a week of non-interventional clinical observation, the treatment or placebo group blindly received the synbiotic or placebo twice daily for 12 weeks. The synbiotic (BIFICOPEC) contained 0.63 g of bifid triple viable capsules (BIFICO) [10] and 8 g of soluble dietary fiber (Pectin, provided by Ander Group in Yantai, China) [24]. The placebo group was treated with digestible maltodextrin (CTFH pharmaceutical company, Nanjing, China) by an experienced doctor. These constipated patients were advised to participate in a healthy lifestyle, including proper diet and exercise, and to avoid any other probiotics and dietary fiber during the study period. If patients did not have a bowel movement for 3 or more consecutive days, they were permitted to take up to 20 g of Macrogol 4000 powder (Forlax®, Ipsen, Paris, France). If ineffective, an enema could be used.

During the follow-up, patients were asked to keep daily diaries of their bowel symptoms, including stool consistency, as rated by the Bristol Stool Form Scale (BSFS). The trained physicians, who were blinded to the treatments, assessed the quality of life and constipation-related symptoms of all of the participants at weeks 4 and 12 via phone or e-mail. Adverse events were also monitored during follow-up.

2.4. Outcomes

The primary efficacy endpoints were as follows: (1) Clinical remission rate: the proportion of patients having an average of three or more spontaneous complete bowel movements (SCBMs) per week during the observation period of weeks 4 and 12; and (2) Clinical improvement rate: the proportion of patients with an average increase of one or more SCBMs per week compared with baseline at weeks 4 and 12.

The secondary efficacy endpoints were as follows: (1) Number of bowel movements within one week [24]; (2) Stool consistency according to the BSFS: stool types 1 and 2 indicated constipation, types 3, 4, and 5 indicated a normal consistency, and types 6 and 7 indicated diarrhea [24]; and (3) Colonic transit time (CTT), which was measured at baseline and at weeks 4 and 12 by the Metcalf method [22].

Other endpoints included the following: (1) The Patient Assessment of Constipation Symptoms (PAC-SYM) questionnaire was administered at baseline and at weeks 4 and 12. The questionnaire contained 12 symptoms that were grouped into three subscales for stool, abdominal, and rectal symptoms. For the overall scale and each subscale, the scores ranged from 0 (symptoms absent) to 4 (symptoms very severe) [25]; (2) The Gastrointestinal Quality-of-Life Index (GIQLI) assessment, which was used to evaluate the quality of life in patients with gastrointestinal diseases, comprised 36 questions using a 5-point Likert-type scale ranging from 0 to 4 (0, worst; 4, best) [26]; (3) The satisfaction scoresof constipated patients, which used a 5-point ordinal scale. The score ranged from 1 (extremely unsatisfied) to 5 (extremely satisfied); (4) For evacuation symptoms, patients recorded their perception of straining, lumpy hard stools, the sensation of incomplete evacuation, and the sensation of anorectal blockage according to a 5-point ordinal scale (1, none; 2, mild; 3, moderate; 4, severe; or 5, very severe); (5) Finally, abdominal symptoms were categorized, patients recorded their symptoms of abdominal pain or cramps and bloating or flatulence according to five classifications (1, none; 2, mild; 3, moderate; 4, severe; or 5, very severe).

2.5. Safety Assessments

During treatment and follow-up, patients were advised to record adverse events in daily diaries and to report adverse events immediately. Adverse events could include abdominal pain, flatulence, borborygmus, and other gastrointestinal symptoms.

2.6. Sample Size

The sample size was calculated based on the frequency of evacuation and the standard deviation of the difference as 0.8 between the groups [27]. Therefore, a total sample size of 100 (50 in each group) was sufficient to expect a 95% power with a two-sided significance level of 0.05.

2.7. Statistical Analysis

The results were analyzed with SPSS 19.0 (SPSS, Inc., Chicago, IL, USA). Continuous data were presented as the mean ± standard deviation and categorical data were presented as *n* (%). Paired *t* tests or a repeated measures ANOVA were performed for continuous variables, and for categorical variables; Pearson's chi-square test or the Fisher exact test was performed as appropriate. p values < 0.05 were considered statistically significant for all comparisons.

3. Results

3.1. Baseline Characteristics

In our study, a total of 100 patients were enrolled and randomized into two groups, with 50 participants per group. Seven patients did not complete the study protocol. Therefore, a total of 93 patients, including 48 patients who had received the synbiotic and 45 patients who had received placebo, were included in the final analysis. The patient flow is detailed in Figure 1. The baseline characteristics of patients in the treatment or placebo group are shown in Table 1. Most enrolled patients were females (63.44%) compared to males (36.56%). The disease durations of 7.1 ± 4.2 years and 7.4 ± 3.9 years in the placebo and treatment groups, respectively, were not significantly different. There were also no differences in gender, age, BMI, Wexner score, stool consistency, or colonic transit time.

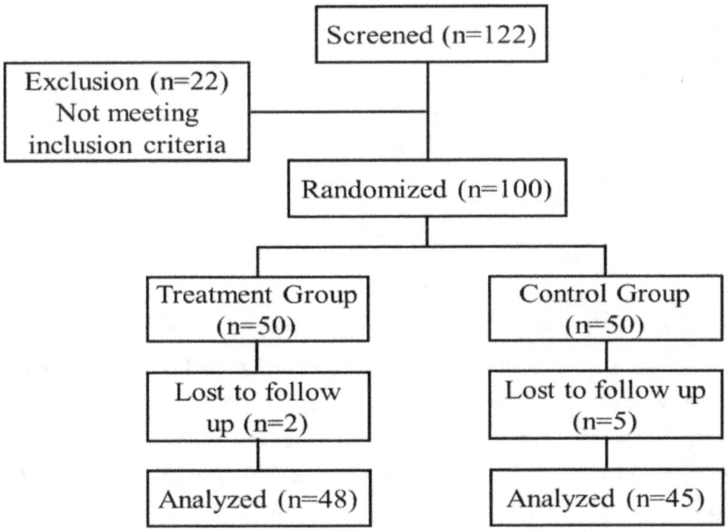

Figure 1. Consolidated standards of reporting trials (CONSORT) flow diagram of patients recruitment and analysis.

Table 1. Baseline demographics in patients received treatment or placebo.

Characteristics	Placebo (n = 45)	Treatment (n = 48)	p Value
Sex (male/female) *	16 (35.6)/29 (64.4)	18 (37.5)/30 (62.5)	0.846
Age (year) †	48.3 ± 11.3	47.2 ± 10.7	0.638
BMI (kg/m^2) †	22.8 ± 1.1	22.6 ± 1.1	0.305
Disease duration (year) †	7.1 ± 4.2	7.4 ± 3.9	0.695
Wexner score †	19.8 ± 2.0	20.0 ± 2.2	0.797
No. of BMs/week †	2.1 ± 0.6	2.2 ± 0.7	0.615
Stool consistency †	2.0 ± 0.6	2.1 ± 0.5	0.366
CTT (h) †	73.0 ± 10.3	71.7 ± 10.8	0.567
Smoker *	3 (6.7)	4 (8.3)	0.761
Alcohol consumer *	6 (13.3)	5 (10.4)	0.663
Regular exercise *	12 (26.7)	14 (29.2)	0.788

BMI, body mass index; BM, bowel movement; CTT, colonic transit time. * Values are expressed as n (%), † values are expressed as the mean ± standard deviation.

3.2. Primary and Secondary Efficacy Endpoints

During the follow-up period, more patients in the synbiotic group achieved a mean of three or more bowel movements per week than in the placebo group at both weeks 4 and 12, and the clinical remission rate in the synbiotic group reached 18% at week 4 and 22% at week 12. There were significant differences in clinical improvement in the synbiotic and the placebo groups at weeks 4 and 12 ($p < 0.01$). After treatment, compared to the placebo group, the number of bowel movements in the synbiotic group improved significantly within one week and reached 4.5 ± 1.6 and 5.1 ± 2.0 at weeks 4 and 12 ($p < 0.001$). In addition, the stool consistency score was statistically significantly increased in the treatment group compared to the placebo group (week 4, 3.2 ± 1.2 vs. 2.5 ± 0.8, $p < 0.001$; week 12, 3.5 ± 1.1 vs. 2.4 ± 0.8, $p < 0.001$). The results of CTT showed that patients who had received the synbiotic treatment had a shorter transit time than did patients in the placebo group at weeks 4 and 12, which could reflect improved intestinal motility. The detailed data are shown in Table 2.

Table 2. Clinical outcomes of treatment vs. placebo groups.

Endpoint	4 Week		12 Week	
	Placebo	Synbiotic	Placebo	Synbiotic
Clinical remission rate (%) †	6 (13.3)	18 (37.5) **	8 (16.7)	22 (45.8) **
Clinical improvement rate (%) †	11 (24.4)	25 (52.1) **	14 (29.2)	31 (64.6) **
No. of BMs/week ‡	2.9 ± 1.1	4.5 ± 1.6 ***	3.1 ± 1.4	5.1 ± 2.0 ***
Stool consistency ‡	2.5 ± 0.8	3.2 ± 1.2 ***	2.4 ± 0.8	3.5 ± 1.1 ***
CTT (h) ‡	68.2 ± 11.3	53.8 ± 10.9 **	70.5 ± 12.1	49.3 ± 11.7 ***

BM, bowel movement; CTT, colonic transit time. † Values are expressed as n (%), ‡ values are expressed as the mean ± SD. ** p value < 0.01; *** p value < 0.001.

3.3. Other Efficacy Results

Treatment with the synbiotic relieved the symptoms of constipated patients. Compared with baseline, the PAC-SYM score significantly decreased in the treatment group at weeks 4 and 12 ($p < 0.001$). However, there was no statistically significant decrease in the PAC-SYM score in the placebo group (Table 3). As shown in Table 3, the GIQLI score in the synbiotic group was 83.5 ± 12.6 before treatment, and it increased to 117.8 ± 15.8 at week 4 ($p < 0.01$) and 126.9 ± 16.5 at week 12 ($p < 0.001$). Although the GIQLI score in the placebo group also improved from 86.3 ± 11.2 to 91.7 ± 12.8 at week 4 and 95.5 ± 15.3 at week 12, no significant difference was found. We also recorded the satisfaction scores of constipated patients during follow-up. Similarly, satisfaction scores in the placebo and treatment groups were analyzed. Our results showed that the score in the treatment group was significantly higher than in the placebo group, not only at week 4, but also at week 12—which indicates that more patients were satisfied with the treatment (Table 3).

In terms of evacuation symptoms, patients in the treatment group reported significantly less straining and fewer lumpy hard stools (Figure 2). No significant improvement was found in the sensation of incomplete evacuation at week 4, but a significantly higher proportion of patients in the treatment group at week 12 reported an improvement in this sensation ($p < 0.05$) (Figure 2). However, there was no significant difference in the sensation of anorectal blockage between groups (Figure 2). For abdominal symptoms, a trend toward improvement was found in the treatment group, but there were no significant differences between the groups (Figure 2). No significant adverse events associated with treatment were reported.

Table 3. Efficacy endpoints.

Week	PAC-SYM †		GIQLI †		Satisfaction Score †	
	Placebo	Synbiotic	Placebo	Synbiotic	Placebo	Synbiotic
Baseline	1.9 ± 0.3	1.9 ± 0.2	86.3 ± 11.2	83.5 ± 12.6	—	—
4 weeks	1.8 ± 0.3	1.4 ± 0.5 **	91.7 ± 12.8	117.8 ± 15.8 **	2.8 ± 1.2	3.5 ± 1.4 *
12 weeks	1.7 ± 0.4	1.2 ± 0.6 ***	95.5 ± 15.3	126.9 ± 16.5 ***	2.9 ± 1.3	3.8 ± 1.4 **

GIQLI, Gastrointestinal Quality-of-Life Index; PAC-SYM, Patient Assessment of Constipation Symptoms. † Values are expressed as the mean ± SD; — indicates not applicable. * p value < 0.05; ** p value < 0.01; *** p value < 0.001.

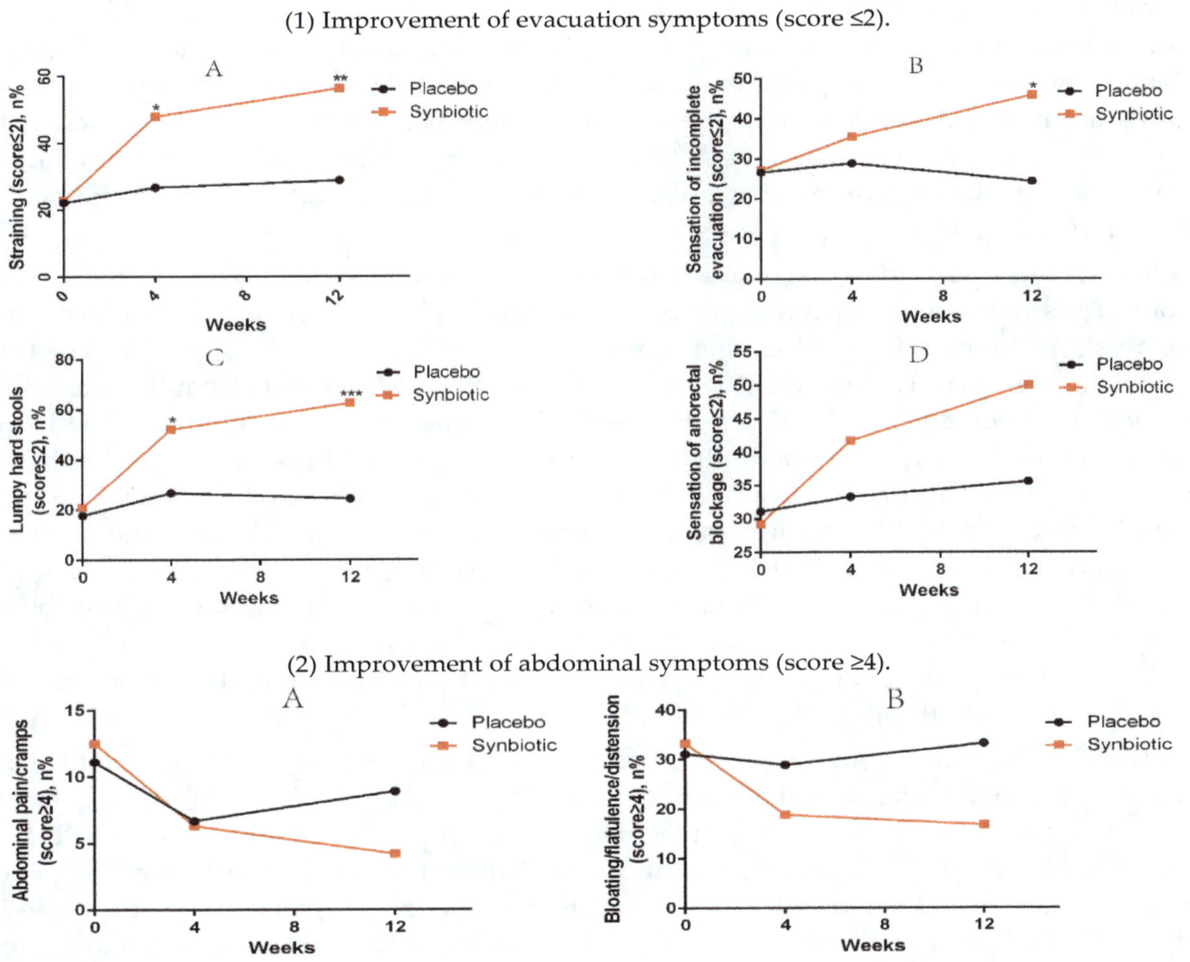

Figure 2. Improvement of constipation-ralated symptoms in the treatment vs. placebo groups. 5-point ordinal scale, 1 indicates none, 2 mild, 3 moderate, 4 severe, and 5 very severe. * p value < 0.05; ** p value < 0.01; *** p value < 0.001. (1) Improvement of evacuation symptoms in treatment vs. placebo groups at baseline, week 4, and week 12; (2) Improvement of abdominal symptoms in treatment vs. placebo groups at baseline, week 4, and week 12.

4. Discussion

This was a prospective randomized trial to evaluate the efficacy of a synbiotic (BIFICOPEC) comprised of probiotics (BIFICO) [10] and soluble dietary fiber (Pectin) in patients with slow transit constipation who met the Rome III criteria. Our study found that 12 weeks of supplementation with probiotics and soluble dietary fiber increased bowel movements, improved the PAC-SYM and GIQLI scores, relieved constipation-related symptoms, and decreased CTT. Finally, the clinical remission and clinical improvement rates reached 45.8% and 64.6%, respectively, at week 12 among patients with mild-to-moderate constipation. No serious treatment-related adverse events were observed during the follow-up period.

Slow transit constipation, which is one type of chronic idiopathic constipation, has an important pathophysiological feature of decreased colonic motility, which could be diagnosed by using radiopaque markers, as occurred in this study [28]. Recently, many researchers have focused on the relationship between intestinal microbiota and constipation and have demonstrated that intestinal microbiota contribute to the pathophysiology of functional gastrointestinal disorders [29]. Parthasarathy et al. [30] suggested that the profile of microbiota in the intestine was associated with colonic transit, and genera from *Firmicutes* was related with faster colonic transit. Zhu et al. [31] reported that, compared with a control group, individuals in a constipation group had a distinct microbiome in the gut. Moreover, the Bristol Stool Scale classification has been widely used to reflect intestinal colon transit time in constipated patients. Vandeputte et al. [32] advised that stool consistency, as evaluated using the Bristol Stool Scale, was strongly correlated with intestinal microbiota. These studies all suggest that gut microbiota contribute to the etiology in constipation. Our previous study [33] reported that the reestablishment of the whole intestinal flora with fecal microbiota transplantation could alleviate the symptoms of slow transit constipation, which might provide a basis for the considerable role of gut microbiota in constipation from the perspective of clinical treatment.

Recently, emerging studies on the individual benefits of probiotics and prebiotics in the treatment of chronic constipation have been reported. Ford et al. [19] reported a systematic review and meta-analysis and showed that probiotics appeared to have beneficial effects in chronic idiopathic constipation (CIC), but only a few RCTs were available for the analysis. Data from RCTs for prebiotics and synbiotics in individuals with CIC are also sparse. Some studies found that prebiotics had a positive effect in constipated patients. Christodoulides et al. [34] suggested that fiber was moderately effective for chronic idiopathic constipation in adults. Suares et al. [35] also reported that soluble fiber might be more beneficial than insoluble fiber in constipated patients in alleviating straining, pain on defecation, improving stool consistency, and other constipation-related symptoms. In addition, research on the changes in intestinal microbiota in individuals with constipation indicated that microbiota other than *Lactobacillus* and *Bifidobacteria* also changed, which might indicate the importance of stability and integration of intestinal microbiota. Therefore, supplementation with both probiotics and prebiotics is better than treatment with probiotics or prebiotics alone.

Pectin is an important soluble dietary fiber that can be fermented by gut microbiota. The most familiar and predominant structural element in pectin is formed by the "smooth" homogalacturonan regions and is composed predominantly of a homopolymer of partially methyl esterified (1–4)-linked α-D-galacturonic acid (GalA) units [12]. The health benefits of pectin might include alterations in the composition of intestinal microbiota and the production of short-chain fatty acids [36,37]. Onumpai et al. [37] reported that pectin could stimulate the activity of *Bifidobacterium* and *Lactobacillus*. Recently, our team also found that fecal microbiota transplantation, in combination with soluble dietary fiber, could improve the symptoms of patients with slow transit constipation, indicating that the regulation of intestinal microecology was associated with constipation [24]. The addition of pectin to the treatment regimen further improved the symptoms in constipated patients. Therefore, pectin may play a beneficial role in constipation.

In contrast, butyrate, which is a byproduct of pectin fermentation by certain microbiota, is necessary for colonic homeostasis and provides energy for intestinal epithelial cells [38]. We chose maltodextrin as a placebo control because maltodextrin is an easily digested carbohydrate, but it is not fermented by intestinal microbiota; thus, it would not affect gut metabolism and microbial ecology [27].

In our study, we provided constipated patients with bifid triple viable capsules and pectin for 12 weeks. Our results revealed an improvement in the number of bowel movements per week, stool consistency, and colonic transit time in constipated patients, which are related to intestinal motility. Intestinal microbiota analysis has already shown that microbiota are associated with colonic transit, stool frequency, and stool consistency in humans [30,32]. During the follow-up, we found that the improvement in stool consistency was the most obvious effect, but a significant improvement in the sensation of incomplete evacuation did not appear until three months after treatment initiation. Harder stools and decreased frequency are associated with a slower colonic transit time, while increased incomplete evacuation is related to outlet obstructive constipation [22]. So the efficacy of synbiotics in constipation might depend on the improvement of intestinal motility through regulating intestinal microecology.

Because pharmacological interventions have limited efficacy and more side effects, traditional treatments have not been able to fully satisfy constipated patients [39]. Prucalopride is a widely used prokinetic agent, but adverse events such as abdominal cramps, headache, skin disorders, and drug dependence have been reported with its use [9]. During our treatment and follow-up, no serious adverse events occurred in the patients. It is found that constipated patients at our hospital prefer to use prebiotics, probiotics, or synbiotics rather than some laxatives.

However, our pilot study does have several limitations. First, this was a single-center study, and the sample size of our trial was relatively small. A multicenter randomized controlled study should be performed to verify these findings. Second, our follow-up period was restricted to 12 weeks. The clinical efficacy of treatment for chronic constipation should be examined in a study with a longer follow-up. Finally, we did not analyze the structural changes in the gut microbiota in constipated patients before and after treatment. Intestinal microbiota analysis might provide us a new perspective to explain the therapeutic mechanism underlying synbiotic treatment.

5. Conclusions

In conclusion, we found that 12 weeks of treatment with a synbiotic that contained pectin as a prebiotic and bifid triple viable capsule (BIFICO) as a probiotic was effective in increasing stool frequency, improving stool consistency, decreasing colonic transit time, and relieving constipation-related symptoms. In addition, synbiotic treatment effectively improved the quality of life in patients with mild-to-moderate constipation. Therefore, additional multicenter randomized clinical trials are needed to confirm these results and assess the role of the regulation of gut microbiota in treatment of constipation.

Acknowledgments: This study was funded by the National Natural Science Foundation of China (81270006) and the National Gastroenterology Research Project (2015BAI13B07). The authors thank Huatong Liu from the Australian National University for checking the entire manuscript for grammar and typographical errors.

Author Contributions: Ning Li, Weiming Zhu and Jianfeng Gong conceived and designed the study; Chao Ding, Xiaolong Ge, Xueying Zhang, and Hongliang Tian performed all required data collection for the study experiment; Hongkan Wang and Lili Gu analyzed the data; Xiaolong Ge and Chao Ding wrote the paper.

References

1. Nelson, A.D.; Camilleri, M.; Chirapongsathorn, S.; Vijayvargiya, P.; Valentin, N.; Shin, A.; Erwin, P.J.; Wang, Z.; Murad, M.H. Comparison of efficacy of pharmacological treatments for chronic idiopathic constipation: A systematic review and network meta-analysis. *Gut* **2016**. [CrossRef] [PubMed]

2. Higgins, P.D.; Johanson, J.F. Epidemiology of constipation in north america: A systematic review. *Am. J. Gastroenterol.* **2004**, *99*, 750–759. [CrossRef] [PubMed]
3. Mugie, S.M.; Benninga, M.A.; Di Lorenzo, C. Epidemiology of constipation in children and adults: A systematic review. *Best Pract. Res. Clin. Gastroenterol.* **2011**, *25*, 3–18. [CrossRef] [PubMed]
4. Rao, S.S.; Rattanakovit, K.; Patcharatrakul, T. Diagnosis and management of chronic constipation in adults. *Nat. Rev. Gastroenterol. Hepatol.* **2016**, *13*, 295–305. [CrossRef] [PubMed]
5. Bharucha, A.E.; Pemberton, J.H.; Locke, G.R., III. American gastroenterological association technical review on constipation. *Gastroenterology* **2013**, *144*, 218–238. [CrossRef] [PubMed]
6. American Gastroenterological Association; Bharucha, A.E.; Dorn, S.D.; Lembo, A.; Pressman, A. American gastroenterological association medical position statement on constipation. *Gastroenterology* **2013**, *144*, 211–217. [CrossRef] [PubMed]
7. Ford, A.C.; Suares, N.C. Effect of laxatives and pharmacological therapies in chronic idiopathic constipation: Systematic review and meta-analysis. *Gut* **2011**, *60*, 209–218. [CrossRef] [PubMed]
8. Camilleri, M.; Kerstens, R.; Rykx, A.; Vandeplassche, L. A placebo-controlled trial of prucalopride for severe chronic constipation. *N. Engl. J. Med.* **2008**, *358*, 2344–2354. [CrossRef] [PubMed]
9. Sajid, M.S.; Hebbar, M.; Baig, M.K.; Li, A.; Philipose, Z. Use of prucalopride for chronic constipation: A systematic review and meta-analysis of published randomized, controlled trials. *J. Neurogastroenterol. Motil.* **2016**, *22*, 412–422. [CrossRef] [PubMed]
10. Cui, H.H.; Chen, C.L.; Wang, J.D.; Yang, Y.J.; Cun, Y.; Wu, J.B.; Liu, Y.H.; Dan, H.L.; Jian, Y.T.; Chen, X.Q. Effects of probiotic on intestinal mucosa of patients with ulcerative colitis. *World J. Gastroenterol.* **2004**, *10*, 1521–1525. [CrossRef] [PubMed]
11. Kaczmarczyk, M.M.; Miller, M.J.; Freund, G.G. The health benefits of dietary fiber: Beyond the usual suspects of type 2 diabetes mellitus, cardiovascular disease and colon cancer. *Metabolism* **2012**, *61*, 1058–1066. [CrossRef] [PubMed]
12. Tian, L.; Bruggeman, G.; van den Berg, M.; Borewicz, K.; Scheurink, A.J.; Bruininx, E.; de Vos, P.; Smidt, H.; Schols, H.A.; Gruppen, H. Effects of pectin on fermentation characteristics, carbohydrate utilization and microbial community composition in the gastrointestinal tract of weaning pigs. *Mol. Nutr. Food Res.* **2016**. [CrossRef] [PubMed]
13. Voderholzer, W.A.; Schatke, W.; Muhldorfer, B.E.; Klauser, A.G.; Birkner, B.; Muller-Lissner, S.A. Clinical response to dietary fiber treatment of chronic constipation. *Am. J. Gastroenterol.* **1997**, *92*, 95–98. [PubMed]
14. Tian, L.; Scholte, J.; Borewicz, K.; Bogert, B.V.; Smidt, H.; Scheurink, A.J.; Gruppen, H.; Schols, H.A. Effects of pectin supplementation on the fermentation patterns of different structural carbohydrates in rats. *Mol. Nutr. Food Res.* **2016**. [CrossRef] [PubMed]
15. Chan, A.O.; Leung, G.; Tong, T.; Wong, N.Y. Increasing dietary fiber intake in terms of kiwifruit improves constipation in chinese patients. *World J. Gastroenterol.* **2007**, *13*, 4771–4775. [CrossRef] [PubMed]
16. Eswaran, S.; Muir, J.; Chey, W.D. Fiber and functional gastrointestinal disorders. *Am. J. Gastroenterol.* **2013**, *108*, 718–727. [CrossRef] [PubMed]
17. Soret, R.; Chevalier, J.; De Coppet, P.; Poupeau, G.; Derkinderen, P.; Segain, J.P.; Neunlist, M. Short-chain fatty acids regulate the enteric neurons and control gastrointestinal motility in rats. *Gastroenterology* **2010**, *138*, 1772–1782. [CrossRef] [PubMed]
18. Fukumoto, S.; Tatewaki, M.; Yamada, T.; Fujimiya, M.; Mantyh, C.; Voss, M.; Eubanks, S.; Harris, M.; Pappas, T.N.; Takahashi, T. Short-chain fatty acids stimulate colonic transit via intraluminal 5-ht release in rats. *Am. J. Physiol. Regul. Integr. Comp. Physiol.* **2003**, *284*, R1269–R1276. [CrossRef] [PubMed]
19. Ford, A.C.; Quigley, E.M.; Lacy, B.E.; Lembo, A.J.; Saito, Y.A.; Schiller, L.R.; Soffer, E.E.; Spiegel, B.M.; Moayyedi, P. Efficacy of prebiotics, probiotics, and synbiotics in irritable bowel syndrome and chronic idiopathic constipation: Systematic review and meta-analysis. *Am. J. Gastroenterol.* **2014**, *109*, 1547–1561. [CrossRef] [PubMed]
20. Morelli, L.; Zonenschain, D.; Callegari, M.L.; Grossi, E.; Maisano, F.; Fusillo, M. Assessment of a new synbiotic preparation in healthy volunteers: Survival, persistence of probiotic strains and its effect on the indigenous flora. *Nutr. J.* **2003**, *2*, 11. [CrossRef] [PubMed]
21. Drossman, D.A. The functional gastrointestinal disorders and the rome iii process. *Gastroenterology* **2006**, *130*, 1377–1390. [CrossRef] [PubMed]

22. Emmanuel, A.; Cools, M.; Vandeplassche, L.; Kerstens, R. Prucalopride improves bowel function and colonic transit time in patients with chronic constipation: An integrated analysis. *Am. J. Gastroenterol.* **2014**, *109*, 887–894. [CrossRef] [PubMed]
23. Agachan, F.; Chen, T.; Pfeifer, J.; Reissman, P.; Wexner, S.D. A constipation scoring system to simplify evaluation and management of constipated patients. *Dis. Colon Rectum* **1996**, *39*, 681–685. [CrossRef] [PubMed]
24. Ge, X.; Tian, H.; Ding, C.; Gu, L.; Wei, Y.; Gong, J.; Zhu, W.; Li, N.; Li, J. Fecal microbiota transplantation in combination with soluble dietary fiber for treatment of slow transit constipation: A pilot study. *Arch. Med. Res.* **2016**, *47*, 236–242. [CrossRef] [PubMed]
25. Frank, L.; Kleinman, L.; Farup, C.; Taylor, L.; Miner, P., Jr. Psychometric validation of a constipation symptom assessment questionnaire. *Scand. J. Gastroenterol.* **1999**, *34*, 870–877. [PubMed]
26. Eypasch, E.; Williams, J.I.; Wood-Dauphinee, S.; Ure, B.M.; Schmulling, C.; Neugebauer, E.; Troidl, H. Gastrointestinal quality of life index: Development, validation and application of a new instrument. *Br. J. Surg.* **1995**, *82*, 216–222. [CrossRef] [PubMed]
27. Waitzberg, D.L.; Logullo, L.C.; Bittencourt, A.F.; Torrinhas, R.S.; Shiroma, G.M.; Paulino, N.P.; Teixeira-da-Silva, M.L. Effect of synbiotic in constipated adult women—A randomized, double-blind, placebo-controlled study of clinical response. *Clin. Nutr.* **2013**, *32*, 27–33. [CrossRef] [PubMed]
28. Li, N.; Jiang, J.; Feng, X.; Ding, W.; Liu, J.; Li, J. Long-term follow-up of the jinling procedure for combined slow-transit constipation and obstructive defecation. *Dis. Colon Rectum* **2013**, *56*, 103–112. [CrossRef] [PubMed]
29. Drossman, D.A. Functional gastrointestinal disorders: History, pathophysiology, clinical features and Rome IV. *Gastroenterology* **2016**, *150*, 1262–1279. [CrossRef] [PubMed]
30. Parthasarathy, G.; Chen, J.; Chen, X.F.; Chia, N.; O'Connor, H.M.; Wolf, P.G.; Gaskins, H.R.; Bharucha, A.E. Relationship between microbiota of the colonic mucosa vs feces and symptoms, colonic transit, and methane production in female patients with chronic constipation. *Gastroenterology* **2016**, *150*, 367–379. [CrossRef] [PubMed]
31. Zhu, L.; Liu, W.; Alkhouri, R.; Baker, R.D.; Bard, J.E.; Quigley, E.M.; Baker, S.S. Structural changes in the gut microbiome of constipated patients. *Physiol. Genom.* **2014**, *46*, 679–686. [CrossRef] [PubMed]
32. Vandeputte, D.; Falony, G.; Vieira-Silva, S.; Tito, R.Y.; Joossens, M.; Raes, J. Stool consistency is strongly associated with gut microbiota richness and composition, enterotypes and bacterial growth rates. *Gut* **2016**, *65*, 57–62. [CrossRef] [PubMed]
33. Tian, H.; Ding, C.; Gong, J.; Ge, X.; McFarland, L.V.; Gu, L.; Wei, Y.; Chen, Q.; Zhu, W.; Li, J.; et al. Treatment of slow transit constipation with fecal microbiota transplantation: A pilot study. *J. Clin. Gastroenterol.* **2016**. [CrossRef] [PubMed]
34. Christodoulides, S.; Dimidi, E.; Fragkos, K.C.; Farmer, A.D.; Whelan, K.; Scott, S.M. Systematic review with meta-analysis: Effect of fibre supplementation on chronic idiopathic constipation in adults. *Aliment. Pharmacol. Ther.* **2016**, *44*, 103–116. [CrossRef] [PubMed]
35. Suares, N.C.; Ford, A.C. Systematic review: The effects of fibre in the management of chronic idiopathic constipation. *Aliment. Pharmacol. Ther.* **2011**, *33*, 895–901. [CrossRef] [PubMed]
36. Dongowski, G.; Lorenz, A.; Proll, J. The degree of methylation influences the degradation of pectin in the intestinal tract of rats and in vitro. *J. Nutr.* **2002**, *132*, 1935–1944. [PubMed]
37. Onumpai, C.; Kolida, S.; Bonnin, E.; Rastall, R.A. Microbial utilization and selectivity of pectin fractions with various structures. *Appl. Environ. Microbiol.* **2011**, *77*, 5747–5754. [CrossRef] [PubMed]
38. Wong, J.M.; de Souza, R.; Kendall, C.W.; Emam, A.; Jenkins, D.J. Colonic health: Fermentation and short chain fatty acids. *J. Clin. Gastroenterol.* **2006**, *40*, 235–243. [CrossRef] [PubMed]
39. Muller-Lissner, S.; Tack, J.; Feng, Y.; Schenck, F.; Specht Gryp, R. Levels of satisfaction with current chronic constipation treatment options in europe - an internet survey. *Aliment. Pharmacol. Ther.* **2013**, *37*, 137–145. [CrossRef] [PubMed]

9

Soluble Fibre Meal Challenge Reduces Airway Inflammation and Expression of GPR43 and GPR41 in Asthma

Isabel Halnes [1], Katherine J. Baines [1], Bronwyn S. Berthon [1], Lesley K. MacDonald-Wicks [2], Peter G. Gibson [1] and Lisa G. Wood [1,*]

1 Centre for Healthy Lungs, Hunter Medical Research Institute, University of Newcastle, Callaghan, NSW 2308, Australia; isabel_h90@hotmail.com (I.H.); Katherine.baines@newcastle.edu.au (K.J.B.); bronwyn.berthon@newcastle.edu.au (B.S.B.); peter.gibson@newcastle.edu.au (P.G.G.)

2 School of Health Sciences, University of Newcastle, Callaghan, NSW 2305, Australia; lesley.wicks@newcastle.edu.au

* Correspondence: lisa.wood@newcastle.edu.au;

Abstract: Short chain fatty acids (SCFAs) are produced following the fermentation of soluble fibre by gut bacteria. In animal models, both dietary fibre and SCFAs have demonstrated anti-inflammatory effects via the activation of free fatty acid receptors, such as G protein-coupled receptor 41 and 43 (GPR41 and GPR43). This pilot study examined the acute effect of a single dose of soluble fibre on airway inflammation—including changes in gene expression of free fatty acid receptors—in asthma. Adults with stable asthma consumed a soluble fibre meal (n = 17) containing 3.5 g inulin and probiotics, or a control meal (n = 12) of simple carbohydrates. Exhaled nitric oxide (eNO) was measured and induced sputum was collected at 0 and 4 h for differential cell counts, measurement of interleukin-8 (IL-8) protein concentration, and GPR41 and GPR43 gene expression. At 4 h after meal consumption, airway inflammation biomarkers, including sputum total cell count, neutrophils, macrophages, lymphocytes, sputum IL-8, and eNO significantly decreased compared to baseline in the soluble fibre group only. This corresponded with upregulated GPR41 and GPR43 sputum gene expression and improved lung function in the soluble fibre group alone. Soluble fibre has acute anti-inflammatory effects in asthmatic airways. Long-term effects of soluble fibre as an anti-inflammatory therapy in asthma warrants further investigation.

Keywords: asthma; prebiotics; G-protein coupled receptor; inflammation; short chain fatty acids

1. Introduction

Asthma is a chronic inflammatory disease of the airways, affecting approximately 300 million people worldwide [1]. In Australia, over two million people are affected [2]. Glucocorticoids are the mainstay of asthma management [3]. However, treatment can predispose individuals to long-term side effects (e.g., osteoporosis, hypertension, insulin resistance, neuropsychiatric effects), and some patients respond poorly [3]. Thus, new ways to treat inflammation in asthma are urgently needed.

While asthma has a significant genetic component, environmental factors also play a role. Epidemiological studies report increased asthma risk with consumption of westernized diets [4–7], which are often high in fat and processed foods, and low in fibre. Dietary fibres are complex carbohydrates found in plant-based foods and are classified based on their solubility in water [8]. Insoluble fibres (e.g., cellulose) are biologically inert substances that assist in the alleviation of constipation by promoting bowel movements [8]. Soluble fibres such as oligosaccharides and fructans (e.g., inulin) act as substrates for fermentation by intestinal microbes [9]. Partial digestion of soluble fibre produces short chain fatty acids (SCFAs), primarily acetate, propionate and butyrate [9]. Butyrate is the preferred fuel source for colonocytes, propionate is mainly metabolized by the liver, while acetate is the main SCFA to enter the circulation where it can act on immune cells and peripheral tissues and potentially elicit anti-inflammatory effects [9,10].

Recently, we reported that fibre intake was inversely associated with lung function and eosinophilic airway inflammation [11,12]. One mechanism potentially linking dietary fibre intake and inflammatory responses, involves the activation of the free fatty acid receptors, G protein-coupled receptor 41 and 43 (GPR41 and GPR43). These are cell surface receptors that are activated by SCFAs on cells of the gastrointestinal tract, as well as immune cells (e.g., eosinophils and neutrophils) and adipocytes [13]. To date, there are no human intervention trials that have assessed how dietary fibre—in particular soluble fibre—can impact airway inflammation. Airway inflammation can be assessed in subjects with asthma by collecting induced sputum (which enables quantification of inflammatory cells) and the use of molecular techniques to measure gene expression to examine mechanistic pathways [14]. Furthermore, sputum can be induced serially, in a safe manner to assess changes in inflammation [15].

We hypothesised that increased intake of soluble fibre would reduce airway inflammation in asthma via activation of free fatty acid receptors. Therefore, in this pilot study, we aimed to investigate the effects of an acute soluble fibre challenge on airway inflammation and free fatty acid receptor activity in asthma.

2. Materials and Methods

2.1. Subjects

Twenty-nine subjects with stable asthma, aged $\geq$18 years and with a body mass index (BMI) between 18 and 30 kg/m^2 were recruited from the John Hunter Hospital Asthma Clinic, NSW, Australia, from existing study volunteer databases and by advertisement. A subset of data from these participants has previously been reported [16]. Asthma stability was confirmed, defined as no exacerbation, respiratory tract infection, or oral corticosteroids in the past four weeks. Asthma control was assessed using the seven-item Asthma Control Questionnaire (ACQ-7) [17]. Clinical asthma pattern (intermittent, mild, moderate, or severe persistent) was determined according to the Global Initiative for Asthma (GINA) guidelines [18]. Subjects were excluded from the study if they were current smokers or had any respiratory-related illness other than asthma on presentation. This trial was conducted at the Hunter Medical Research Institute, Newcastle, Australia according to the guidelines laid down in the Declaration of Helsinki, and all procedures involving human subjects were approved by the Hunter New England Human Research Ethics Committee (HREC) (06/10/25/5.03, 11/06/15/4.02) and registered with the University of Newcastle HREC. Written informed consent was obtained from all subjects. The trial was registered with the Australian and New Zealand Clinical Trials Registry (number ACTRN12607000236493) prior to the study commencing.

2.2. Study Design

All subjects fasted for 12 h, withheld short acting β_2-agonist medications (for 12 h) and long acting β_2-agonist medications (for 24 h), and underwent exhaled nitric oxide (eNO, Ecomedics CLD 88sp, Ecomedics, Duernten, Switzerland), spirometry, and hypertonic saline challenge with combined sputum induction, and then consumed the study meal (soluble fibre n = 17, control n = 12) within 15 min. Four hours after meal consumption, eNO, spirometry, and sputum induction were repeated. The soluble fibre meal consisted of commercial probiotic yoghurt (Vaalia, low fat, 175 g), containing 806 kJ, the soluble fibre inulin (3.5 g), and the probiotics *Lactobacillus acidophilus* strain LA5, *Bifidobacterium lactis* strain Bb12, and *Lactobacillus rhamnosus* strain GG, each at a concentration of $\geq 10^8$ colony forming units. The control meal consisted of an isocaloric meal of 200 g plain mashed potato.

2.3. Hypertonic Saline Challenge

Baseline spirometry (Minato Autospiro AS-600; Minato Medical Science, Osaka, Japan) was performed to measure lung function, and predicted values for forced expiratory volume in one second (FEV_1) and forced vital capacity (FVC) were calculated using NHANES (National Health and Nutrition Examination Survey) III data, which accounts for gender, age, and height [19]. Using predicted values for FEV_1 and FVC allows for interpretation of actual lung function values (L) as a percent of expected values developed from reference data in healthy populations [20]. Combined bronchial provocation and sputum induction with nebulized (ULTRA-NEBTM ultrasonic nebulizer, Model 2000; DeVilbiss, Tipton, West Midlands, United Kingdom) hypertonic saline (4.5%) were performed as previously described [21]. If FEV_1 dropped below 15% of baseline, subjects were considered to have airway hyperresponsiveness (AHR). The response of all subjects to hypertonic saline was also described by the dose response slope (DRS, the percent decline in FEV_1 per mL hypertonic saline).

2.4. Sputum Processing

Sputum was selected from saliva [21,22], dispersed with dithiothreitol, and a total cell count of leukocytes and viability were performed. Cytospins were prepared, stained (May-Grunwald Geimsa), and a differential cell count obtained from 400 non-squamous cells. The remaining solution was centrifuged ($400\times g$, 10 min, 4 °C) and the cell-free supernatant was aspirated and stored at −80 °C. For GPR41 and GPR43 gene expression analysis, 100 μL of selected sputum was added to Buffer RLT (Qiagen, Hilden, Germany) and stored at −80 °C until RNA extraction.

2.5. Sputum Supernatant Measurements

The concentration of interleukin 8 (IL-8) was determined by Enzyme-linked Immunosorbent Assay (ELISA) using R&D Systems Human CXCL8/IL-8 DuoSet Ancillary Reagent ELISA kit (R&D Systems, Minneapolis, MN, USA). IL-8 has been previously validated for assessment in induced sputum [23,24].

2.6. RNA Extraction and cDNA Synthesis

Total RNA was extracted from sputum samples stored in Buffer RLT using the RNeasy Mini Kit (Qiagen) as per kit instructions. Sputum RNA was quantitated using the Quant-iT RiboGreen RNA Assay Kit (Invitrogen, Eugene, OR, USA), whereby fluorescence was measured by FLUOstar OPTIMA spectrometer (BMG LabTech, Ortenberg, Germany). Genomic DNA was removed via treatment with DNase I (Life Technologies, Scoresby, Australia) and cDNA was generated via reverse transcription from 200ng of RNA using the High Capacity cDNA Reverse Transcription Kit, as per kit instructions (Applied Biosystems, Forster City, CA, USA).

2.7. mRNA Quantification by Real-Time qRT-PCR

Taqman gene expression assays for GPR41 and GPR43 were purchased as proprietary pre-optimised reagents (Applied Biosystems) and combined with cDNA and Taqman master mix in duplicate singleplex quantitative real-time polymerase chain reactions (qRT-PCR) (ABI 7500 Real time PCR system). 18S ribosomal RNA was utilised as the housekeeping reference gene. Relative fold change in gene expression after the soluble fibre and control meal challenge was calculated using $2^{-\Delta\Delta Ct}$ relative to the housekeeping gene 18S rRNA (ΔCt) and the baseline ($\Delta\Delta$Ct).

2.8. Statistical Analysis

Data were analysed with STATA 11 (StataCorp, College Station, TX, USA) and reported as mean $\pm$ standard error of mean (SEM) for parametric and median (interquartile range, IQR) for nonparametric data. Data was tested for normality using the D'Agostino–Pearson omnibus normality test. To compare baseline characteristics between groups, normally distributed variables were analysed using Students t-tests, and non-parametric variables were analysed using the Wilcoxon rank sum test. Categorical variables were analysed by Fisher's exact test. Within-group changes were compared using Wilcoxon matched-pairs signed rank test, and between group changes were analysed using the Wilcoxon rank sum test. Significance was accepted if $p < 0.05$.

3. Results

3.1. Baseline Characteristics

Twenty-nine subjects with stable asthma were included in the study, allocated to the soluble fibre (n = 17) or control group (n = 12). The clinical characteristics at baseline were similar between the two groups (Table 1).

Table 1. Baseline clinical characteristics.

Clinical Characteristic	Soluble Fibre Group (n = 17)	Control Group (n = 12)	p *
Gender Male n (%)	7 (41)	6 (50)	0.716
Female n (%)	10 (59)	6 (50)	
Age (years)	42.1 ± 3.4	40.4 ±4.6	0.770
BMI (kg/m^2)	24.9 ± 0.7	26.6 ± 0.7	0.099
Ex-smokers n (%)	6 (35)	3 (25)	0.694
ACQ-7 (units)	0.7 ± 0.1	0.7 ± 0.2	0.941
Atopy n (%)	14 (82)	8 (67)	0.403
AHR n (%)	10 (59]	5 (41.7)	0.462
DRS (%ΔFEV$_1$/mL), med [IQR]	2.2 [0.4, 6.4]	0.6 [0.2, 2.4]	0.109
ICS dose † (μg/day), med [IQR]	1000 [400, 1000]	1000 [563, 1000]	0.679

Data are means ± SEM unless otherwise stated. BMI: body mass index; ACQ: 7-item asthma control questionnaire; AHR: airway hyperresponsiveness; DRS: dose–response slope (% fall in forced expiratory volume in one second (FEV$_1$)/mL saline); ICS: inhaled corticosteroids. * Difference between soluble fibre and control groups. † Beclomethasone equivalents.

3.2. Airway Inflammatory Markers

There was no difference in airway inflammation at baseline between groups; however, the response to the soluble fibre and control meals was different (Table 2, Figure 1). Following the control meal, there were no changes in airway inflammation. Within the soluble fibre group, there was a significant decrease in sputum total cell count which was significantly different to the control group (Figure 1a). Sputum neutrophils (Figure 1b), macrophages (Figure 1d), lymphocytes, sputum IL-8 (Figure 1c), and eNO (Figure 1f) also decreased significantly in the soluble fibre group at 4 h compared to baseline, though these changes were not significantly different between the control and intervention groups.

Table 2. Airway inflammation at baseline and change at 4 h following soluble fibre or control meal challenge ^.

Airway Inflammation	Soluble Fibre Group		$p^{\dagger}$	Control Group		$p^{\dagger}$	p^*
	0 h	Δ4 h		0 h	Δ4 h		
Sputum (n)	16	14		10	9		
TCC ($\times10^6$/mL)	3.7 [2.2, 6.3]	−2.0 [−2.8, −1.1]	0.013	3.0 [1.4, 6.0]	0.2 [−0.8, 1.4]	0.833	0.037
Neutrophils ($\times10^4$/mL)	76.2 [54.6, 249.4]	−67.5 [−158.0, −6.4]	0.033	92.4 [7.2, 342.7]	−1.1 [−94.9, 105.1]	1.000	0.148
Eosinophils ($\times10^4$/mL)	3.3 [1.3, 16.0]	−1.2 [−5.8, 1.8]	0.490	2.4 [0.0, 4.5]	2.6 [−1.7, 6.7]	0.440	0.393
Macrophages ($\times10^4$/mL)	144.0 [93.0, 386.3]	−99.1 [−244.6, −12.2]	0.030	124.5 [104.5, 211.5]	3.4 [−47.6, 85.1]	0.779	0.117
Lymphocytes ($\times10^4$/mL)	1.6 [0.2, 7.1]	−1.4 [−3.9, −0.3]	0.002	4.1 [0.4, 6.7]	2.1 [−1.5, 3.9]	0.401	0.034
Sputum IL-8 (ng/mL)	5.7 [3.9, 9.7]	−1.9 [−7.6, −1.1]	0.005	3.7 [3.0, 22.6]	−1.3 [−10.1, 1.2]	0.208	0.539
Exhaled NO (ppb)	17.5 [14.5, 70.5]	−3.4 [−7.9, −0.6]	0.028	14.9 [11.0, 51.0]	−1.9 [−4.6, 1.0]	0.170	0.301

TCC: total cell count; NO: nitric oxide; ppb: parts per billion. ^ Data are nonparametric, presented as median [quartile 1, quartile 3], within-group changes analyzed by Wilcoxon matched pairs signed-rank test, and group comparison performed using Wilcoxon rank-sum test. † Difference in change from 0 to 4 h within group. * Difference in change from 0 to 4hrs between the soluble fibre and control group.

Table 3. Sputum mRNA gene expression at baseline, 4 h, and fold change at 4 h following soluble fibre or control meal challenge ^.

Gene	Soluble Fibre Group (n = 8)			$p^{\dagger}$	Control Group (n = 4)			$p^{\dagger}$	p^*
	0 h	4 h	FC		0 h	4 h	FC		
GPR43	0.07 [0.05, 0.29]	0.79 [0.26, 2.01]	6.26 [1.66, 13.5]	0.124	1.53 [0.29, 3.64]	0.24 [0.17, 0.27]	0.31 [0.07, 0.67]	0.068	0.007
GPR41	0.07 [0.04, 0.35]	1.70 [0.14, 5.18]	5.15 [3.96, 22.9]	0.161	1.27 [0.80, 1.42]	0.58 [0.41, 1.22]	0.41 [0.31, 2.37]	0.715	0.027

GPR: G protein-coupled receptor; FC: fold change. ^ Data are nonparametric, presented as median [quartile 1, quartile 3], within-group changes analyzed by Wilcoxon matched pairs signed-rank test and group comparison performed using Wilcoxon rank-sum test. † Difference in change from 0 to 4 h within group. * Difference in fold change between the soluble fibre and control group.

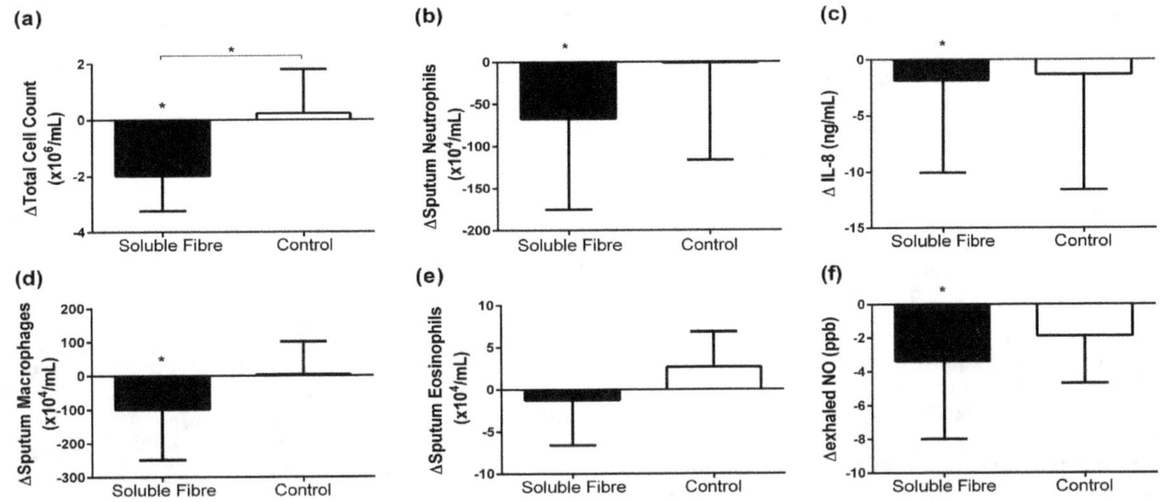

Figure 1. Change in airway inflammatory markers: (**a**) sputum total cell count; (**b**) sputum neutrophils; (**c**) sputum interleukin 8 (IL-8); (**d**) sputum macrophages; (**e**) sputum eosinophils; (**f**) exhaled nitric oxide 4 h following soluble fibre challenge (soluble fibre group) or control meal challenge (control group). Data expressed as median (IQR) and analyzed by Wilcoxon matched pairs signed-rank for within group and Wilcoxon rank-sum for between group comparisons. * $p < 0.05$.

3.3. *GPR41 and GPR43 Sputum Gene Expression*

GPR41 and GPR43 gene expression fold change in sputum was compared between the two groups after the soluble fibre and the control meals. Both GPR43 and GPR41 expression were significantly upregulated following the soluble fibre meal compared to the control meal (Table 3, Figure 2).

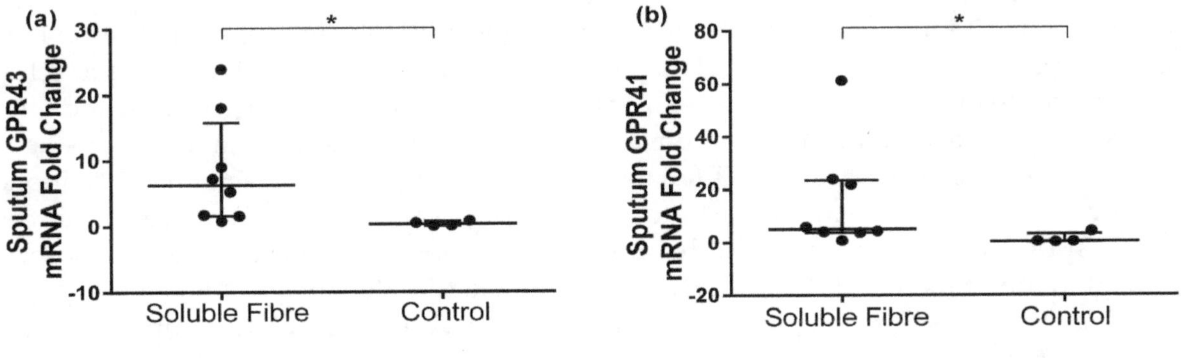

Figure 2. Change in sputum (**a**) GPR43 and (**b**) GPR41 gene expression 4 h following soluble fibre challenge (soluble fibre group $n = 8$) or control meal challenge (control group $n = 4$). Data expressed as median (IQR) and analyzed by Wilcoxon rank-sum test.* $p < 0.05$.

3.4. *Lung Function*

At baseline, forced vital capacity (FVC % predicted) was lower in the control group, but both groups were within normal range (80–120) of percentage predicted FVC [25]. FEV_1 and FEV_1/FVC improved 4 h following the soluble fibre meal, while no changes in lung function were seen following the control meal (Table 4, Figure 3). There were no significant differences in lung function changes between groups.

Table 4. Lung function at baseline and change at 4 h following soluble fibre or control meal challenge.

Lung Function	Soluble Fibre Group		p †	Control Group		p †	p *
	0 h	Δ4 h		0 h	Δ4 h		
(n)	17	17		12	12		
FEV_1 (L) ^	2.7 [2.2, 3.6]	0.1 [0.0, 0.2]	0.022	2.9 [2.0, 3.5]	0.1 [−0.1, 0.2]	0.347	0.341
FEV_1 (% predicted) #	82.4 ± 4.4	4.0 ± 1.6	0.024	77.7 ± 6.8	1.0 ± 1.4	0.506	0.190
FVC (L) ^	4.1 [3.4, 4.7]	0.0 [−0.1, 0.1]	0.331	4.0 [3.5, 4.9]	0.01 [−0.04, 0.1]	0.503	0.595
FVC (% predicted) #	98.9 ± 3.4 §	1.6 ± 1.2	0.193	86.9 ± 4.5	−0.2 ± 1.0	0.859	0.285
FEV_1/FVC (%) #	69.2 ± 2.5	3.8 ± 1.1	0.002	71.9 ± 4.6	1.2 ± 0.7	0.101	0.070

FEV_1: forced expiratory volume in 1 s; FVC: forced vital capacity. ^ Data are nonparametric, presented as median [quartile 1, quartile 3], within-group changes analyzed by Wilcoxon matched pairs signed-rank test and group comparison performed using Wilcoxon rank-sum test. # Data are normally distributed and presented as means ± SEMs, within group changes analyzed by paired t-test and group comparison performed using two-sample t-test. § $p < 0.05$ versus control group at baseline. † Difference in change from 0 to 4 h within group. * Difference in change from 0 to 4 h between the soluble fibre and control group.

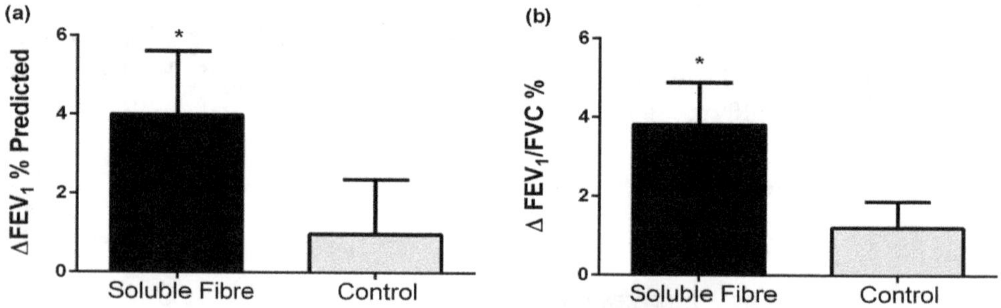

Figure 3. Change in lung function (**a**) FEV_1% predicted and (**b**) FEV_1/FVC % 4 h following soluble fibre challenge (soluble fibre group) or control meal challenge (control group). Data expressed as mean ± SEMs and analyzed by two-sample t-test. * $p < 0.05$.

4. Discussion

To gain a better understanding of the effects of soluble fibre on airway inflammation in people with asthma, this pilot study examined changes in airway inflammatory biomarkers at 4 h versus baseline (0 h), following a soluble fibre or control meal. We observed significant reductions in airway inflammation four hours after the consumption of a single dose of soluble fibre (3.5 g inulin). This was characterised by decreases in sputum total cell count, neutrophils, macrophages, lymphocytes, sputum IL-8 and eNO. When compared to the control subjects, we also found significantly upregulated GPR41 and GPR43 sputum cell gene expression in the soluble fibre group. We also observed an improvement in lung function (FEV_1 and FEV_1/FVC) in the soluble fibre group.

Several studies in the general population have reported an inverse relationship between dietary fibre intake and systemic inflammation [26,27]. We have previously extended these observations by demonstrating that dietary fibre is also inversely associated with eosinophilic airway inflammation in asthma [12]. The current study suggests that a key mechanism driving the anti-inflammatory actions of soluble fibre is the activation of free fatty acid receptors. The soluble fibre inulin is partially fermented by commensal bacteria in the colon, providing the substrate for production of physiologically active by-products, including the SCFAs: acetate, propionate, and butyrate. Our observations suggest that fermentation of inulin leads to activation of GPR41 and GPR43 in immune cells in the airways, which results in a reduction in airway inflammation. While we did not observe a reduction in airway eosinophils in the current study, we did observe a decrease in eNO, which is a marker of eosinophilic inflammation [28].

Our observations support findings from animal models, which have shown that GPR43/41 stimulation by SCFAs is necessary for the resolution of airway inflammation. In an allergic airways model, GPR43-deficient mice showed more severe inflammation, with increased inflammatory cell numbers in the lung lining fluid and higher levels of eosinophil peroxidase activity and inflammatory cells in lung tissue [29]. In another study in mice with allergic airways disease [30], a fibre-rich diet changed the composition of the gut microbiota by increasing proportions of the Bacteroidaceae and Bifidobacteriaceae families, which are potent fermenters of soluble fibre into SCFA. Increased circulating SCFA levels were observed and airway inflammation was attenuated, with dendritic cells having an impaired ability to activate Th2 effector cells in the lung [30]. Consequently, in mice fed either a high fibre diet or directly administered with acetate or propionate in their drinking water, airway inflammation could not be sustained; after an allergen challenge, cellular infiltration (eosinophils), IL-4, IL-5, IL-13, and IL-17A levels were reduced in the lungs and AHR improved. The effects were dependent on GPR41, but not GPR43. This highlights the importance of measuring both free fatty acid receptors in order to understand their anti-inflammatory actions.

This is the first study to examine the effects of SCFAs on inflammation in human airways. The majority of previous studies in humans that have looked at the role of SCFAs have examined gut inflammation, predominantly ulcerative colitis where sodium butyrate is administered either orally (using capsules with slow release coating to release butyrate into the colon), or through enemas [10]. We are interested in the effects of SCFAs on inflammation in peripheral tissues, in particular the lungs [31]. Certainly, it has previously been shown that soluble fibre can affect inflammation in the circulation. In a randomized, double-blind, placebo-controlled crossover study on inflammation and gut microbiota following soluble fibre supplementation, improvements in the composition and metabolic activity of gut microbiota—such as increased production of butyrate—was seen after two and four weeks [32]. In addition, significant reductions in circulating pro-inflammatory mediators such as tumour necrosis factor-alpha (TNF-α), IL-6, and IL-8 were observed [32]. We sought to extend our investigations to the airways, and have shown that a single dose of soluble fibre can modulate airway inflammation. This was associated with an improvement in lung function, and hence appears to be clinically important.

The single meal challenge design that we employed mimics many previous studies that have shown that a single meal high in carbohydrates and/or fat causes postprandial systemic inflammation [33]. We have also previously shown that a single high fat mixed meal increases airway inflammation within 4 h [16]. This is biologically plausible, as it is known that at 4 h after the consumption of inulin, the SCFAs acetate, propionate, and butyrate are all elevated compared to baseline in plasma [34]. Nonetheless, a clinical trial of longer duration is warranted to determine what clinical effects would occur with chronic supplementation.

As the importance of SCFAs in human health is being increasingly recognized, further research is required to assess changes that occur in circulating SCFA levels and inflammation following the intake of various types of soluble fibres. In addition, research is also needed to determine the optimal delivery form for increasing circulating SCFAs. In animal studies, SCFAs are often administered directly through the drinking water of animals, however oral delivery of SCFA is not optimal for humans, as the majority of acetate delivered orally is oxidized, with plasma levels only remaining elevated for 60 min [35]. Hence, supplementation with soluble fibre (as we have done in this study) is a useful strategy to increase circulating SCFA levels [34].

From our study, we are unable to determine whether SCFA reach the lungs, and this is an important area for future research. Previous animal studies have shown that SCFA are not detectable in lung tissue following soluble fibre supplementation [30]. Hence, it appears likely that effects of SCFA on immune function initially occur systemically. Supporting this hypothesis, it has been reported that mice treated with propionate have altered haematopoiesis in bone marrow, characterised by changes in the types of dendritic cell (DC) precursors generated, which have greater phagocytic ability but reduced ability to promote Th2 responses once in the lungs [30].

A limitation of this study is the small sample size; however, this was adequate for us to demonstrate, for the first time, that soluble fibre can reduce airway inflammation in people with asthma. Another potential limitation is the short duration of the study, as the soluble fibre was delivered as a single meal. Nonetheless, the chronic effects of soluble fibre on airway inflammation in asthma are likely to be even greater, as in addition to activation of free fatty acid receptors, gut microbial changes will also be induced, which further enhance SCFA production [36]. Hence, long-term studies of soluble fibre supplementation are warranted.

5. Conclusions

In summary, we have shown that a single dose of soluble fibre was able to significantly reduce airway inflammation in stable asthma. The long-term benefits of increasing soluble fibre intake are likely to have a greater impact on inflammation, as soluble fibre also enhances the growth of SCFA-producing gut bacteria, which will further enhance the production of beneficial SCFAs. Supplementing with a prebiotic such as inulin has the potential to be widely accepted and adopted, and could potentially reduce the amount of inhaled glucocorticoids required for treatment. As such, this approach provides a less costly strategy for managing asthma, as well as lowering the risk of asthma patients experiencing adverse side effects due to pharmacological treatment.

Acknowledgments: The authors would like to acknowledge the research participants and the HMRI Respiratory Research clinical team including Amber Smith, Joanne Smart, Hayley Scott and the laboratory team including Bridgette Donati, Michelle Gleeson, Kellie Fakes and Naomi Fibbens for assistance with collection, processing and analysis of samples. This trial was supported by a National Health and Medical Research Council of Australia Project Grant and a Hunter Medical Research Institute project grant sponsored by the Piggott family.

Author Contributions: I.H. conducted the laboratory work and statistical analysis and contributed to drafting the manuscript, K.J.B. contributed to the conception and design of the study, analysis, interpretation of data and revising the manuscript, B.S.B. contributed to the data acquisition, interpretation of data and revising the manuscript, P.G.G. contributed to the conception and design of the study, analysis, interpretation of data and revising the manuscript, L.K.M.-W. contributed to the study design, interpretation of data and revising the manuscript, L.G.W. had overall responsibility for the conception and design of the study, analysis, interpretation of data, revising the manuscript and obtaining funding for the work.

References

1. Masoli, M.; Fabian, D.; Holt, S.; Beasley, R. Global initiative for asthma (GINA) program. The global burden of asthma: Executive summary of the GINA dissemination committee report. *Allergy* **2004**, *59*, 469–478. [CrossRef] [PubMed]
2. Australian Centre for Asthma Monitoring. Asthma in Australia 2011. In *AIHW Asthma Series No. 4. Cat. No. ACM 22*; Australian Institute of Health and Welfare (AIHW): Canberra, Australia, 2011.
3. Barnes, P.J.; Adcock, I.M. Glucocorticoid resistance in inflammatory diseases. *Lancet* **2009**, *373*, 1905–1917. [CrossRef]
4. Wickens, K.; Barry, D.; Friezema, A.; Rhodius, R.; Bone, N.; Purdie, G.; Crane, J. Fast foods—Are they a risk factor for asthma? *Allergy* **2005**, *60*, 1537–1541. [CrossRef] [PubMed]
5. Hijazi, N.; Abalkhail, B.; Seaton, A. Diet and childhood asthma in a society in transition: A study in urban and rural Saudi Arabia. *Thorax* **2000**, *55*, 775–779. [CrossRef] [PubMed]
6. Carey, O.J.; Cookson, J.B.; Britton, J.; Tattersfield, A.E. The effect of lifestyle on wheeze, atopy, and bronchial hyperreactivity in Asian and white children. *Am. J. Respir. Crit. Care Med.* **1996**, *154*, 537–540. [CrossRef] [PubMed]
7. Huang, S.-L.; Pan, W.-H. Dietary fats and asthma in teenagers: Analyses of the first Nutrition and Health Survey in Taiwan (NAHSIT). *Clin. Exp. Allergy* **2001**, *31*, 1875–1880. [CrossRef] [PubMed]
8. Rolfes, S.R.; Pinna, K.; Whitney, E. *Understanding Normal and Clinical Nutrition*, 8th ed.; Wadsworth: Belmont, CA, USA, 2009.
9. Ganapathy, V.; Thangaraju, M.; Prasad, P.D.; Martin, P.M.; Singh, N. Transporters and receptors for short-chain fatty acids as the molecular link between colonic bacteria and the host. *Curr. Opin. Pharmacol.* **2013**, *13*, 869–874. [CrossRef] [PubMed]
10. Vinolo, M.A.R.; Rodrigues, H.G.; Nachbar, R.T.; Curi, R. Regulation of Inflammation by Short Chain Fatty Acids. *Nutrients* **2011**, *3*, 858–876. [CrossRef] [PubMed]

11. Root, M.M.; Houser, S.M.; Anderson, J.J.; Dawson, H.R. Healthy Eating Index 2005 and selected macronutrients are correlated with improved lung function in humans. *Nutr. Res.* **2014**, *34*, 277–284. [CrossRef] [PubMed]
12. Berthon, B.S.; Macdonald-Wicks, L.K.; Gibson, P.G.; Wood, L.G. Investigation of the association between dietary intake, disease severity and airway inflammation in asthma. *Respirology* **2013**, *18*, 447–454. [CrossRef] [PubMed]
13. Brown, A.J.; Goldsworthy, S.M.; Barnes, A.A.; Eilert, M.M.; Tcheang, L.; Daniels, D.; Muir, A.I.; Wigglesworth, M.J.; Kinghorn, I.; Fraser, N.J.; et al. The Orphan G protein-coupled receptors GPR41 and GPR43 are activated by propionate and other short chain carboxylic acids. *J. Biol. Chem.* **2003**, *278*, 11312–11319. [CrossRef] [PubMed]
14. Baines, K.J.; Simpson, J.L.; Wood, L.G.; Scott, R.J.; Gibson, P.G. Transcriptional phenotypes of asthma defined by gene expression profiling of induced sputum samples. *J. Allergy Clin. Immunol.* **2011**, *127*, 153–160. [CrossRef] [PubMed]
15. Fahy, J.V.; Liu, J.; Wong, H.; Boushey, H.A. Analysis of cellular and biochemical constituents of induced sputum after allergen challenge: A method for studying allergic airway inflammation. *J. Allergy Clin. Immunol.* **1994**, *93*, 1031–1039. [CrossRef]
16. Wood, L.G.; Garg, M.L.; Gibson, P.G. A high fat challenge increases airway inflammation and impairs bronchodilator recovery in asthma. *J. Allergy Clin. Immunol.* **2011**, *127*, 1133–1140. [CrossRef] [PubMed]
17. Juniper, E.F.; Bousquet, J.; Abetz, L.; Bateman, E.D. Identifying 'well-controlled' and 'not well-controlled' asthma using the Asthma Control Questionnaire. *Respir. Med.* **2006**, *100*, 616–621. [CrossRef] [PubMed]
18. Global Initiative for Asthma (GINA). Global Strategy for Asthma Management and Prevention 2012 (Update). Available online: http://wwwginasthmaorg (accessed on 30 July 2012).
19. Hankinson, J.; Odencrantz, J.; Fedan, K. Spirometric reference values from a sample of the general U.S. population. *Am. J. Respir. Crit. Care Med.* **1999**, *159*, 179–187. [CrossRef] [PubMed]
20. Stanojevic, S.; Wade, A.; Stocks, J. Reference values for lung function: Past, present and future. *Eur. Respir. J.* **2010**, *36*, 12–19. [CrossRef] [PubMed]
21. Gibson, P.G.; Wlodarczyk, J.W.; Hensley, M.J.; Gleeson, M.; Henry, R.L.; Cripps, A.W.; Clancy, R.L. Epidemiological Association of Airway Inflammation with Asthma Symptoms and Airway Hyperresponsiveness in Childhood. *Am. J. Respir. Crit. Care Med.* **1998**, *158*, 36–41. [CrossRef] [PubMed]
22. Gibson, P.G.; Henry, R.L.; Thomas, P. Noninvasive assessment of airway inflammation in children: Induced sputum, exhaled nitric oxide, and breath condensate. *Eur. Respir. J.* **2000**, *16*, 1008–1015. [PubMed]
23. Simpson, J.L.; Scott, R.J.; Boyle, M.J.; Gibson, P.G. Differential proteolytic enzyme activity in eosinophilic and neutrophilic asthma. *Am. J. Respir. Crit. Care Med.* **2005**, *172*, 559–565. [CrossRef] [PubMed]
24. Wood, L.G.; Garg, M.L.; Simpson, J.L.; Mori, T.A.; Croft, K.D.; Wark, P.A.B.; Gibson, P.G. Induced Sputum 8-Isoprostane Concentrations in Inflammatory Airway Diseases. *Am. J. Respir. Crit. Care Med.* **2005**, *171*, 426–430. [CrossRef] [PubMed]
25. Altalag, A.; Road, J.; Wilcox, P. *Pulmonary Function Tests in Clinical Practice*; Springer: London, UK, 2009.
26. Ma, Y.; Griffith, J.A.; Chasan-Taber, L.; Olendzki, B.C.; Jackson, E.; Stanek, E.J.; Li, W.; Pagoto, S.L.; Hafner, A.R.; Ockene, I.S. Association between dietary fiber and serum C-reactive protein. *Am. J. Clin. Nutr.* **2006**, *83*, 760–766. [PubMed]
27. Ajani, U.A.; Ford, E.S.; Mokdad, A.H. Dietary fiber and C-reactive protein: Findings from national health and nutrition examination survey data. *J. Nutr.* **2004**, *134*, 1181–1185. [PubMed]
28. Taylor, D.R.; Pijnenburg, M.W.; Smith, A.D.; Jongste, J.C.D. Exhaled nitric oxide measurements: Clinical application and interpretation. *Thorax* **2006**, *61*, 817–827. [CrossRef] [PubMed]
29. Maslowski, K.M.; Vieira, A.T.; Ng, A.; Kranich, J.; Sierro, F.; Yu, D.; Schilter, H.C.; Rolph, M.S.; Mackay, F.; Artis, D.; et al. Regulation of inflammatory responses by gut microbiota and chemoattractant receptor GPR43. *Nature* **2009**, *461*, 1282–1286. [CrossRef] [PubMed]
30. Trompette, A.; Gollwitzer, E.S.; Yadava, K.; Sichelstiel, A.K.; Sprenger, N.; Ngom-Bru, C.; Blanchard, C.; Junt, T.; Nicod, L.P.; Harris, N.L.; et al. Gut microbiota metabolism of dietary fiber influences allergic airway disease and hematopoiesis. *Nat. Med.* **2014**, *20*, 159–166. [CrossRef] [PubMed]
31. De Filippo, C.; Cavalieri, D.; Di Paola, M.; Ramazzotti, M.; Poullet, J.B.; Massart, S.; Collini, S.; Pieraccini, G.; Lionetti, P. Impact of diet in shaping gut microbiota revealed by a comparative study in children from Europe and rural Africa. *Proc. Natl. Acad. Sci. USA* **2010**, *107*, 14691–14696. [CrossRef] [PubMed]

32. Macfarlane, S.; Cleary, S.; Bahrami, B.; Reynolds, N.; Macfarlane, G.T. Synbiotic consumption changes the metabolism and composition of the gut microbiota in older people and modifies inflammatory processes: A randomised, double-blind, placebo-controlled crossover study. *Aliment. Pharmacol. Ther.* **2013**, *38*, 804–816. [CrossRef] [PubMed]
33. Nappo, F.; Esposito, K.; Cioffi, M.; Giugliano, G.; Molinari, A.M.; Paolisso, G.; Marfella, R.; Giugliano, D. Postprandial endothelial activation in healthy subjects and in Type 2 diabetic patients: Role of fat and carbohydrate meals. *J. Am. Coll. Cardiol.* **2002**, *39*, 1145–1150. [CrossRef]
34. Tarini, J.; Wolever, T.M. The fermentable fibre inulin increases postprandial serum short-chain fatty acids and reduces free-fatty acids and ghrelin in healthy subjects. *Appl. Physiol. Nutr. Metab.* **2010**, *35*, 9–16. [CrossRef] [PubMed]
35. Smith, G.I.; Jeukendrup, A.E.; Ball, D. Sodium acetate induces a metabolic alkalosis but not the increase in fatty acid oxidation observed following bicarbonate ingestion in humans. *J. Nutr.* **2007**, *137*, 1750–1756. [PubMed]
36. Roberfroid, M.B. Introducing inulin-type fructans. *Br. J. Nutr.* **2005**, *93*, S13–S25. [CrossRef] [PubMed]

10

Intra Amniotic Administration of Raffinose and Stachyose Affects the Intestinal Brush Border Functionality and Alters Gut Microflora Populations

Sarina Pacifici [1], Jaehong Song [2], Cathy Zhang [3], Qiaoye Wang [4], Raymond P. Glahn [5], Nikolai Kolba [5] and Elad Tako [5,*]

[1] Department of Animal Sciences, Cornell University, Ithaca, NY 14853, USA; sjp233@cornell.edu
[2] Department of Biological Sciences, Cornell University, Ithaca, NY 14853, USA; js2833@cornell.edu
[3] Division of Nutritional Sciences, Cornell University, Ithaca, NY 14853, USA; cz223@cornell.edu
[4] Department of Food Science and Technology, Cornell University, Ithaca, NY 14853, USA; yw696@cornell.edu
[5] USDA-ARS, Robert W. Holley Center for Agriculture and Health, Cornell University, Ithaca, NY 14853, USA; rpg3@cornell.edu (R.P.G.); nk598@cornell.edu (N.K.)
* Correspondence: et79@cornell.edu;

Abstract: This study investigates the effectiveness of two types of prebiotics—stachyose and raffinose—which are present in staple food crops that are widely consumed in regions where dietary Fe deficiency is a health concern. The hypothesis is that these prebiotics will improve Fe status, intestinal functionality, and increase health-promoting bacterial populations in vivo (*Gallus gallus*). By using the intra-amniotic administration procedure, prebiotic treatment solutions were injected in ovo (day 17 of embryonic incubation) with varying concentrations of a 1.0 mL pure raffinose or stachyose in 18 MΩ H_2O. Four treatment groups (50, 100 mg·mL^{-1} raffinose or stachyose) and two controls (18 MΩ H_2O and non-injected) were utilized. At hatch the cecum, small intestine, liver, and blood were collected for assessment of the relative abundance of the gut microflora, relative expression of Fe-related genes and brush border membrane functional genes, hepatic ferritin levels, and hemoglobin levels, respectively. The prebiotic treatments increased the relative expression of brush border membrane functionality proteins ($p < 0.05$), decreased the relative expression of Fe-related proteins ($p < 0.05$), and increased villus surface area. Raffinose and stachyose increased the relative abundance of probiotics ($p < 0.05$), and decreased that of pathogenic bacteria. Raffinose and stachyose beneficially affected the gut microflora, Fe bioavailability, and brush border membrane functionality. Our investigations have led to a greater understanding of these prebiotics' effects on intestinal health and mineral metabolism.

Keywords: raffinose; stachyose; brush border membrane; iron; prebiotics

---

1. Introduction

Iron (Fe) deficiency is the most common nutrient deficiency worldwide, affecting between 30% and 40% of the world's population [1,2]. Those who suffer from this condition can experience fatigue, cognitive impairment, and death [3]. The prevalence of Fe deficiency in these geographical regions can be attributed to the populations' consumption of low-diversity plant-based diets including cereals and legumes, which contain low amounts of bioavailable Fe as well as compounds such as polyphenols that further inhibit Fe absorption [4,5]. Dietary Fe deficiency and other dietary mineral deficiencies stem from a lack of essential nutrients in staple food crops, and thus health sectors have turned to various agricultural interventions as potential solutions. A form of intervention that shows great promise is biofortification. Biofortification refers to the use of traditional breeding practices to bring about significant increases in bioavailable micronutrients in the edible portions of food crops [6,7]. Once biofortified, the seedlings of staple foods crops can be distributed to farmers who are already experienced in growing these particular crops. In fact, biofortified crops are found to have a multitude of agronomic benefits for farmers due to their high micronutrient stores, including disease resistance, improved seed viability, greater seedling vigor, lower seeding rate requirements, and faster root establishment—all of which lead to increased productivity relative to the original seedlings [7]. Another sustainable aspect of this solution is that once biofortified varieties are grown, they will not continue to require government attention or funding [7].

However, a major challenge associated with biofortification of staple food crops—namely cereal grains and legume seeds—in developing regions is that they contain factors such as polyphenols and phytic acid that inhibit the absorption of Fe [8]. When these crops are biofortified via conventional breeding, there is the potential for these inhibitory factors to increase along with Fe [9–11]. Despite containing inhibitory factors, cereal grains and legumes also carry other substances, referred to as promoters, which have the potential to counteract the effects of these inhibitory factors. Thus, one prospective solution to the aforementioned dilemma is to increase the content of these promoter substances to counteract the negative effects of the inhibitory factors such as polyphenols [9]. One of the most notable of these promoter substances is the prebiotic [9,12].

Prebiotics are polysaccharides that have been shown to enhance the growth and activities of probiotics, or beneficial gut microflora. These compounds are capable of surviving acidic and enzymatic digestion in the small intestine, and thus can be fermented by probiotics that reside in the colon/cecum [6]. The fermentation of prebiotics by probiotics leads to the production of short-chain fatty acids, which lower intestinal pH, inhibiting the growth of potentially pathogenic bacterial populations and improving the absorption of minerals such as Fe [7]. Raffinose and stachyose were chosen as the prebiotics for investigation in this study, since they are found in high concentrations in lentils and chickpeas [8], which are staple crops consumed by populations in which Fe deficiency is a health concern [5]. Previously, we demonstrated the effects of the wheat prebiotics arabinoxylans and fructans on intestinal probiotics [12] as a potential approach to improving Fe bioavailability in staple food crops and gut health.

In the current study, raffinose and stachyose effects were studied in vivo by utilizing the poultry model (*Gallus gallus*). The broiler chicken is a fast-growing animal with sensitivities to dietary deficiencies of trace minerals such as Fe [13], and is very receptive to dietary manipulations [9,12–14]. Additionally, there is >85% homology between gene sequences of human and chicken intestinal genes such as DMT1, DcytB, ZnT1, and Ferroportin [15]. Thus, one objective of this study is to assess the effects of intra-amniotic raffinose and stachyose administration on Fe status in vivo (*Gallus gallus*), an animal model that has been used to investigate the physiological effects of various nutritional solutions [16,17]. Specifically, the expression of Fe metabolism-related genes (DMT1, the major Fe intestinal transporter; DcytB, Fe reductase; and Ferroportin, the major intestinal enterocyte Fe exporter), in the duodenum (the major Fe absorption site). The second objective in using this model is to assess the effects of raffinose and stachyose on brush border membrane (BBM) development and functionality using biomarkers for BBM absorptive ability such as the relative expressions of aminopeptidase (AP), sucrase isomaltase (SI), and sodium glucose cotransporter-1 (SGLT1), as well as the surface areas of the intestinal villi. The third objective is to evaluate the effects of the intra-amniotic administration of these prebiotics on intestinal bacterial populations by measuring the relative abundances of probiotic health-promoting populations bacteria such as *Bifidobacterium* and *Lactobacillus* versus those of potentially pathogenic bacteria such as *E. coli* and *Clostridium*.

The goal in investigating these effects is to determine whether raffinose and stachyose may be candidates for biofortification in staple food crops. If they demonstrate the ability to improve Fe status, BBM functionality, and intestinal bacterial populations, breeding lentils and chickpeas for increased stachyose and raffinose content may potentially eliminate the need for exogenous Fe supplementation by increasing the bioavailability of Fe in these crops. The distribution of biofortified crop seedlings would serve as a sustainable means of combating malnutrition in developing regions where dietary Fe deficiency is common.

2. Materials and Methods

2.1. Animals and Design

Cornish cross-fertile broiler chicken eggs (n = 120) were obtained from a commercial hatchery (Moyer's chicks, Quakertown, PA, USA). The eggs were incubated under optimal conditions at the Cornell University Animal Science poultry farm incubator.

2.2. Intra-Amniotic Administration

All animal protocols were approved by Cornell University Institutional Animal Care and Use committee (ethic approval code: 2007-0129). Pure stachyose and raffinose in powder form were separately diluted in 18 MΩ H_2O to determine the concentrations necessary to maintain an osmolarity value of less than 320 Osm to ensure that the chicken embryos would not be dehydrated upon injection of the solution. This intra-amniotic administration procedure followed that of Tako et al. [12]. On day 17 of embryonic incubation, eggs containing viable embryos were weighed and divided into 6 groups (n = 12) with an approximately equal weight distribution. The intra-amniotic treatment solution (1 mL per egg) was injected with a 21-gauge needle into the amniotic fluid, which was identified by candling. After injection, the injection sites were sealed with cellophane tape. The six groups were assigned as follows: 1. 5% stachyose (in 18 MΩ H_2O); 2. 10% stachyose (in 18 MΩ H_2O); 3. 5% raffinose (in 18 MΩ H_2O); 4. 10% raffinose (in 18 MΩ H_2O); 5. 18 MΩ H_2O; 6. non-injected. Eggs were placed in hatching baskets such that each treatment was equally represented at each incubator location.

2.3. Tissue Collection

On the day of hatch (day 21), birds were euthanized by CO_2 exposure. The small intestines, ceca, blood, and livers were quickly removed from the carcasses and placed in separate tubes for storage. The samples were immediately frozen in liquid nitrogen and then stored in a −80 °C freezer until analysis.

2.4. Isolation of Total RNA

Total RNA was extracted from 30 mg of small intestine (duodenal) tissue using Qiagen RNeasy Mini Kit. RNA was quantified by absorbance at 260–280 nm. Integrity of the 28S and 18S rRNA was verified by 1.5% agarose gel electrophoresis followed by ethidium bromide staining.

2.5. Gene Expression Analysis

As was previously described [9,12,13], RT-PCR was carried out with primers chosen from the fragments of chicken duodenal tissues. After the completion of PCR, the results were run under gel electrophoresis on 2% agarose gel stained with ethidium bromide for separation of the target genes (DMT1, Ferroportin, DcytB, AP, SI, SGLT1). Quantity One 1D analysis software (Bio-Rad, Hercules, CA, USA) was utilized to quantify the resulting bands. Highly conserved tissue-specific 18S rRNA was used as internal standard to normalize the results.

2.6. Bacterial Analysis

As was previously described [18–20], the contents of the ceca were placed into a sterile 50 mL tube containing 9 mL of sterile phosphate-buffered saline (PBS) and homogenized by vortexing with glass beads. Debris was removed by centrifugation. For DNA purification, the pellet was treated with lysozyme. The bacterial genomic DNA was isolated using a Wizard Genomic DNA purification kit. Primers for *Lactobacillus*, *Bifidobacterium*, *Clostridium*, and *E. coli* were designed according to previously published data by Zhu et al. in 2002 [19]. The universal primers—which identify all known strains of bacteria in the intestine—were prepared with the invariant region in the 16S rRNA of bacteria, and were used as internal standard to normalize the results. The DNA samples underwent PCR, and the amplified results were loaded on 2% agarose gel stained with ethidium bromide and underwent electrophoresis for separation. Then, the bands were quantified using Quantity One 1-D analysis software (Bio-Rad, Hercules, CA, USA). Abundance of individual bacterial gene expression was measured relative to the universal primer product, where the total bacteria equaled 100%.

2.7. Assessment of Liver Ferritin

As was previously described [9,14], the collected liver samples were treated similarly to the procedures described in a previous study by Passaniti et al. in 1989 [21]. Approximately 0.25 g of liver sample was diluted into 0.5 mL of 50 mM Hepes buffer (pH 7.4) and homogenized on ice using an UltraTurrax homogenizer at maximum speed (5000× *g*) for 2 min. Each homogenate was subjected to heat treatment for 10 min at 75 °C to aid isolation of ferritin. The samples were immediately cooled on ice for 30 min after heat treatment, centrifuged at 13,000× *g* for 30 min until a clear supernatant was obtained, and the pellet containing insoluble denatured proteins was discarded. Native polyacrylamide gel electrophoresis was utilized for separation technique. Six percent separating gel and 5% stacking gel were prepared for the procedure. A constant 100 V voltage was administered throughout the process. The resulting gels were then treated with two specific stains: potassium ferricyanide ($K_3Fe(CN)_6$)—a stain specific for Fe—and Coomassie blue G-250 stain, specific for protein in general. The Fe-stained bands represented ferritin levels, and were compared to the corresponding bands in the Coomasie-stained gel to calculate relative abundance of ferritin (ferritin-to-total-protein ratio). Gels were scanned by using the Bio-Rad densitometer and measured using the Quantity-One 1-D analysis program (Bio-Rad, Hercules, CA, USA). Horse spleen ferritin was used as a standard to calibrate ferritin/Fe concentrations. Ferritin saturation levels were measured by calculating relative percentage of Fe present in the protein to the maximum number of Fe atoms that can be present per molecule of ferritin (approximately 4500 Fe atoms) [22].

2.8. Blood Analysis and Hb Measurements

Blood was collected using micro-hematocrit heparinized capillary tubes (Fisher Scientific, Waltham, MA, USA). Blood Hb concentrations were determined spectrophotometrically using the cyanmethemoglobin method (H7506-STD, Pointe Scientific Inc., Canton, MI, USA) following the kit manufacturer's instructions.

2.9. Morphological Examination of the Intestinal Villi

As was previously described [17], intestinal samples (duodenal region as the main intestinal Fe absorption site) at day of hatch from each treatment were fixed in fresh 4% (*vol*/*vol*) buffered formaldehyde, dehydrated, cleared, and embedded in paraffin. Serial sections were cut at 5 μm and placed on glass slides. Sections were deparaffinized in xylene, rehydrated in a graded alcohol series, stained with hematoxylin and eosin, and examined by light microscopy. Morphometric measurements of villus height and width were performed with an Olympus light microscope using EPIX XCAP software. Villus surface area was calculated from villus height and width at half height.

2.10. Goblet Cell Diameter

Morphometric measurements of goblet cell diameter were performed with an Olympus light microscope using EPIX XCAP software.

2.11. Statistical Analysis

Results were analyzed by one-way multiple analysis of variance (MANOVA) using the JMP software (SAS Institute Inc., Cary, NC, USA). Differences between treatments were compared by Tukey's test, and values were statistically different at $p < 0.05$ (values in the text are means $\pm$ SEM).

3. Results

3.1. Intestinal Content Bacterial Genera- and Species-Level Analysis

The relative abundance of both *Bifidobacterium* and *Lactobacillus*—which are known to be probiotics—significantly ($p < 0.05$) increased in the presence of both concentrations of stachyose and raffinose. The relative abundance of *E. coli* did not significantly ($p > 0.05$) increase or decrease in the presence of the prebiotic treatment solutions compared to the controls. *Clostridium*'s relative abundance significantly ($p < 0.05$) decreased in the presence of both concentrations of stachyose and raffinose compared to the controls (Figure 1). These results indicate that stachyose and raffinose improved gut health by promoting the survival of probiotics and limiting the existence of potentially pathogenic bacterial populations. The presence of these probiotics was expected to give rise to an increase in short-chain fatty acid production and an increase in Fe solubility, and in turn, Fe bioavailability.

3.2. BBM Functional Genes

The relative expressions of AP, SI, and SGLT1 were all significantly ($p < 0.05$) up-regulated in the presence of both concentrations of stachyose and raffinose (Figure 2). The up-regulation of the expression of BBM functional genes signifies increased absorptive ability of the BBM, which indicates improved functionality and gut health [23].

3.3. Fe Metabolism Genes

The relative expressions of DcytB, DMT1, and ferroportin were all significantly ($p < 0.05$) down-regulated in the presence of both concentrations of stachyose and raffinose (Figure 2). The down-regulation of these genes is in turn suggested to be an indicator of Fe-replete conditions. This is a potential biomarker for improved Fe status.

3.4. Cecum-to-Body-Weight Ratio

The cecum-to-bodyweight ratios were significantly ($p < 0.05$) higher in the prebiotic treatment groups compared to the controls. The ceca of subjects that received stachyose and raffinose increased, indicating an increase in their content of bacterial populations (Table 1).

3.5. Morphometric Data for Villi

The villus surface areas significantly ($p < 0.05$) increased in the presence of both concentrations of stachyose and raffinose (Table 2). This serves as a mechanical measurement of BBM absorptive ability and improvement in BBM functionality and gut health by indicating that the introduction of stachyose and raffinose enhanced proliferation of enterocytes.

3.6. Goblet Cell Diameters

The goblet cell diameters significantly ($p < 0.05$) increased in the presence of both concentrations of stachyose and raffinose (Table 2).

3.7. Liver Ferritin and Hb

There were no significant ($p > 0.05$) differences in ferritin or Hb values between treatment groups. The lack of a significant difference in these physiological measurements of Fe status between groups is posited to be because there was not enough Fe in the environment to create a significant change (Table 3).

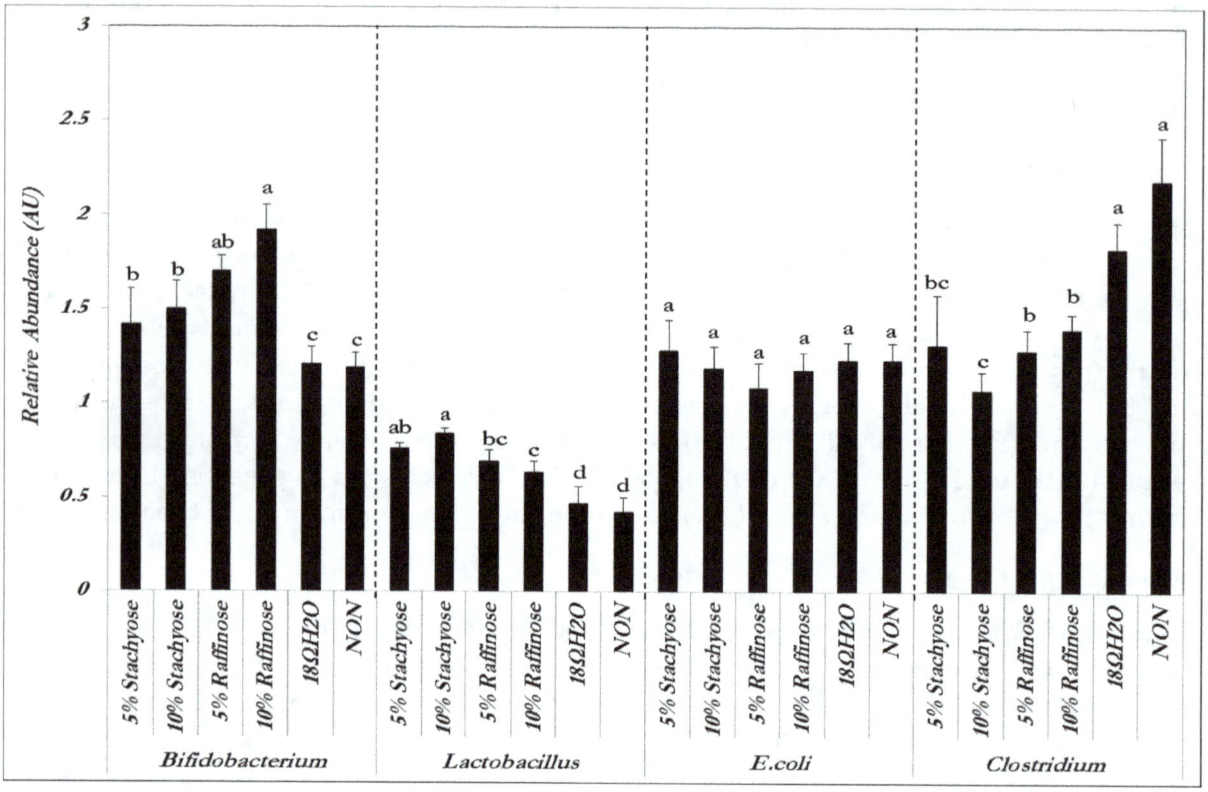

Figure 1. Genera and species-level bacterial populations (AU) from cecal contents measured on the day of hatch. Values are means ± SEM, $n = 8$. Per bacterial category, treatment groups not indicated by the same letter are significantly different ($p < 0.05$).

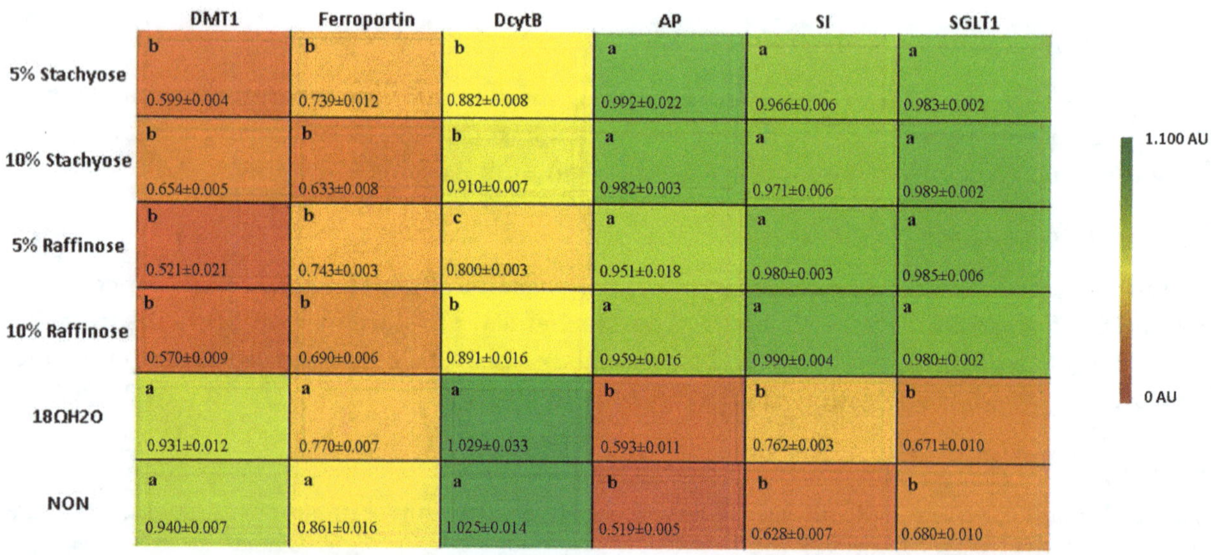

Figure 2. Duodenal mRNA expression (in AU) of measured brush border membrane (BBM) functional and Fe metabolism genes on the day of hatch. Values are means ± SEM, $n = 8$. Standard errors are represented by vertical bars. Per gene, treatments groups not indicated by the same letter are significantly different ($p < 0.05$). AP: aminopeptidase; SI: sucrase isomaltase; SGLT1: sodium glucose cotransporter-1.

Table 1. Cecum-to-body weight ratio (%). Values are means ± SEM, $n = 12$. [a,b] Treatment groups not indicated by the same letter are significantly different ($p < 0.05$).

Treatment Group	Cecum/Body Weight Ratio (%)
5% Stachyose	1.67 ± 0.21 [a]
10% Stachyose	1.63 ± 0.18 [a]
5% Raffinose	1.83 ± 0.20 [a]
10% Raffinose	1.55 ± 0.13 [a]
18ΩH_2O	1.35 ± 0.08 [b]
Non-injected	1.22 ± 0.07 [b]

Table 2. Effect of intra-amniotic administration of experimental solutions on the duodenal small intestinal villus surface area (mm^2) and goblet cells diameter (μm). Values are means ± SEM, $n = 6$. [a–e] Treatment groups not indicated by the same letter are significantly different ($p < 0.05$).

Treatment Group	Villus Surface Area (mm^2)	Goblet Cell Diameter (μm)
5% Stachyose	459.2 ± 32.09 [a,b]	18.2 ± 0.143 [c]
10% Stachyose	493.8 ± 10.31 [a]	19.1 ± 0.152 [b]
5% Raffinose	467.5 ± 35.55 [a,b]	22.5 ± 0.180 [a]
10% Raffinose	425.2 ± 24.04 [b,c]	19.5 ± 0.156 [b]
18ΩH_2O	384.4 ± 14.16 [c]	15.4 ± 0.123 [d]
Non-injected	353.1 ± 13.24 [c]	13.2 ± 0.105 [e]

Table 3. Liver Ferritin protein amounts (AU) and blood hemoglobin (Hb) concentrations (g/dL). Values are means ± SEM, $n = 10$. [a] Treatment groups not indicated by the same letter are significantly different ($p < 0.05$).

Treatment Group	Ferritin (AU)	Hb (g/dL)
5% Stachyose	0.48 ± 0.09 [a]	10.7 ± 0.54 [a]
10% Stachyose	0.48 ± 0.08 [a]	11.1 ± 0.55 [a]
5% Raffinose	0.47 ± 0.10 [a]	10.5 ± 0.68 [a]
10% Raffinose	0.48 ± 0.09 [a]	11.0 ± 0.56 [a]
18ΩH_2O	0.47 ± 0.09 [a]	10.4 ± 0.42 [a]
Non-injected	0.47 ± 0.07 [a]	10.3 ± 0.65 [a]

4. Discussion

This study utilized the *Gallus gallus* model, as it is a fast growing animal with relatively high mineral requirements, and hence can develop deficiency considerably quickly [13]. Previous studies have shown that intra-amniotic administration is useful for investigating the effects of specific nutrients at particular stages of intestinal development [16,17,24]. According to Ludwiczek et al., intracellular Fe concentrations play a role in regulating Fe absorption into the enterocytes and are beneficial to bacteria within the cecum [25].

There was an increased abundance of both *Lactobacillus* ($p < 0.05$) and *Bifidobacterium* ($p < 0.05$), and a decrease in *Clostridium* in the cecal contents of the birds that received the prebiotic treatments. However, there were no significant differences for *E. coli* between the groups ($p > 0.05$), and likewise a lack of significant differences within and between the raffinose and stachyose groups ($p > 0.05$) of same bacterial species (Figure 1). As previously mentioned, *Lactobacillus* and *Bifidobacterium* are known probiotics, whereas *Clostridium* is a potentially pathogenic genus and *E. coli* can be either pathogenic or beneficial, depending on the strain [20,26,27]. *Lactobacillus* and *Bifidobacterium* both produce short chain fatty acids (SCFA), potentially increasing Fe bioavailability and reducing the abundance of pathogenic bacteria that utilize dietary Fe in the colon [28,29]. Other prebiotic compounds such as inulin have been shown to enhance the proliferation of selected beneficial colonic microflora [26,30]. *Bifidobacterium* and *Lactobacillus* have an advantage over other intestinal microorganisms due to their β-1,2-glycosidase activity that allows them to break down prebiotics, resulting in their proliferation and possibly leading to greater SCFA production [18–20]. Therefore, it is reasonable to suspect that the intra-amniotic administration of stachyose and raffinose may improve Fe status by inducing a more efficient Fe uptake and intestinal transferring. In addition to the more efficient Fe uptake, the cecum-to-bodyweight ratios were higher in the prebiotic treatment groups versus the control groups ($p < 0.05$), indicating that the cecal content of chickens that received intra-amniotic prebiotic solutions was greater than those that did not. This observation is used as an indicator for a potential increase in cecal bacterial populations (Table 1) [12].

In addition, the expressions of duodenal (the major Fe absorption site) Fe metabolism-related proteins (DMT1, the major Fe intestinal transporter; DcytB, Fe reductase; and Ferroportin, the major intestinal enterocyte Fe exporter), was decreased in treatment groups receiving the raffinose and stachyose solutions versus controls ($p < 0.05$) (Figure 2). These results are comparable to those of a previous study conducted on late-term broiler embryos and hatchlings, in which treatment groups with improved Fe status expressed significantly less Fe-related proteins [31]. The results suggest that the increased Fe bioavailability led to Fe-sufficient conditions, meaning an increase in Fe metabolism-related transporters and enzymes were not required (as a compensatory mechanism). Furthermore, there was no significant differences ($p > 0.05$) between the two raffinose administered groups in DMT1 and ferroportin; whereas DcytB actually showed a significant decrease ($p < 0.05$) in the 10% versus 5% raffinose (Figure 2). One reasonable explanation is that SCFA produced from bacteria increases Fe^{3+} solubility, resulting in more bioavailable Fe that led to the decreased DcytB expression [16].

The significant increase in the expression of the BBM functionality genes (AP, SI, SGLT1, $p < 0.05$) is in agreement with the morphometric measurements, indicating that intra-amniotic administration of raffinose and stachyose improved BBM functionality and potentially enhanced the absorptive and digestive capacity of the villi (Table 2). As is evident in the current study, it was previously suggested that dietary prebiotics increase probiotics' butyrate production, which may lead to cellular (enterocyte) proliferation. It was also demonstrated that birds that received intra-amniotic administration of carbohydrates developed villi with greater surface areas compared to the untreated birds [32]. Scholz-Ahrens et al. (2007) and Preidis et al. (2012) support these results by concluding that some of their respective prebiotics increase cellular proliferation, which causes the increase in villi surface area [33,34]. Additionally, we also measured an increase in goblet cell diameter, which suggests an increased production of mucus that coats the intestinal lumen and effects bacterial composition and function [35,36].

Overall, the up-regulation of BBM functional proteins, down-regulation of Fe metabolism proteins, in addition to the increase in the relative abundance of beneficial probiotics, intestinal villi surface area, and goblet cell diameters, suggest that stachyose and raffinose are promising in their potential for improving Fe status and BBM functionality.

5. Conclusions

The current research validates the need for future studies that could incorporate these plant origin prebiotics in long-term feeding trials. The potential breeding of staple food crops such as lentils and chickpeas for increased stachyose and raffinose contents may serve as a sustainable means of combating malnutrition in developing regions, which is a strategy that has been proven effective in wheat [12]. This study served as a preliminary step to provide a greater understanding of the way that various prebiotics can alleviate dietary deficiencies.

Author Contributions: E.T. led the research conceived and designed the experiment, wrote and edited the manuscript, N.K., S.P. and Q.W. collected and analyzed the data and wrote the initial draft of the paper. J.S., C.Z. and R.G. analyzed the data. All authors critically reviewed the final draft.

Abbreviations

Fe	iron
Hb	hemoglobin
DMT1	divalent metal transporter 1
DcytB	duodenal cytochrome B
AP	amino peptidase
SI	sucrose isomaltase
SGLT-1	sodium glucose transporter 1
BBM	brush border membrane

References

1. World Health Organization. *Iron Deficiency Anemia: Assessment, Prevention and Control: A Guide for Programme Managers*; World Health Organization: Geneva, Switzerland, 2001; pp. 15–21.
2. World Health Organization. *The Global Prevalence of Anaemia in 2011*; World Health Organization: Geneva, Switzerland, 2015; pp. 3–6.
3. Pollitt, E.; Soemantri, A.G.; Yunis, F.; Scrimshaw, N.S. Cognitive effects of iron-deficiency Anaemia. *Lancet* **1985**, *325*, 158. [CrossRef]
4. Johnson, C.R.; Thavarajah, D.; Combs, G.F.; Thavarajah, P. Lentil (*Lens culinaris* L.): A prebiotic-rich whole food legume. *Food Res. Int.* **2013**, *51*, 107–113. [CrossRef]
5. Dwivedi, S.; Sahrawat, K.; Puppala, N.; Ortiz, R. Plant prebiotics and human health: Biotechnology to breed prebiotic-rich nutritious food crops. *Electron. J. Biotechnol.* **2014**, *17*, 238–245. [CrossRef]
6. Nestel, P.; Bouis, H.E.; Meenakshi, J.V.; Pfeiffer, W. Biofortification of staple food crops. *J. Nutr.* **2006**, *136*, 1064–1067. [PubMed]
7. Welch, R.M.; Graham, R.D. Breeding for micronutrients in staple food crops from a human nutrition perspective. *J. Exp. Bot.* **2004**, *55*, 353–364. [CrossRef] [PubMed]
8. Wiesinger, J.A.; Cichy, K.A.; Glahn, R.P.; Grusak, M.A.; Brick, M.A.; Thompson, H.J.; Tako, E. Demonstrating a Nutritional Advantage to the Fast-Cooking Dry Bean (*Phaseolus vulgaris* L.). *J. Agric. Food Chem.* **2016**, *64*, 8592–8603. [CrossRef] [PubMed]
9. Tako, E.; Beebe, S.E.; Reed, S.; Hart, J.J.; Glahn, R.P. Polyphenolic compounds appear to limit the nutritional benefit of biofortified higher iron black bean (*Phaseolus vulgaris* L.). *Nutr. J.* **2014**, *13*, 1. [CrossRef] [PubMed]
10. Petry, N.; Egli, I.; Zeder, C.; Walczyk, T.; Hurrell, R. Polyphenols and phytic acid contribute to the low iron bioavailability from common beans in young women. *J. Nutr.* **2010**, *140*, 1977–1982. [CrossRef] [PubMed]
11. Petry, N.; Egli, I.; Gahutu, J.B.; Tugirimana, P.L.; Boy, E.; Hurrell, R. Phytic acid concentration influences iron bioavailability from biofortified beans in Rwandese women with low iron status. *J. Nutr.* **2014**, *144*, 1681–1687. [CrossRef] [PubMed]
12. Tako, E.; Glahn, R.P.; Knez, M.; Stangoulis, J.C. The effect of wheat prebiotics on the gut bacterial population and iron status of iron deficient broiler chickens. *Nutr. J.* **2014**, *13*, 1. [CrossRef] [PubMed]
13. Tako, E.; Rutzke, M.A.; Glahn, R.P. Using the domestic chicken (*Gallus gallus*) as an in vivo model for iron bioavailability1. *Poult. Sci.* **2010**, *89*, 514–521. [CrossRef] [PubMed]
14. Tako, E.; Reed, S.M.; Budiman, J.; Hart, J.J.; Glahn, R.P. Higher iron pearl millet (*Pennisetum glaucum* L.) provides more absorbable iron that is limited by increased polyphenolic content. *Nutr. J.* **2015**, *14*, 1. [CrossRef] [PubMed]
15. Hillier, L.W.; Miller, W.; Birney, E.; Warren, W.; Hardison, R.C.; Ponting, C.P.; Bork, P.; Burt, D.W.; Groenen, M.A.M.; Delany, M.E.; et al. Sequence and comparative analysis of the chicken genome provide unique perspectives on vertebrate evolution. *Nature* **2004**, *432*, 695–716. [CrossRef] [PubMed]
16. Tako, E.; Glahn, R.P. Intra-amniotic administration and dietary inulin affect the iron status and intestinal functionality of iron-deficient broiler chickens. *Poult. Sci.* **2012**, *91*, 1361–1370. [CrossRef] [PubMed]
17. Tako, E.; Ferket, P.; Uni, Z. Changes in chicken intestinal zinc exporter mRNA expression and small intestinal functionality following intra-amniotic zinc-methionine administration. *J. Nutr. Biochem.* **2005**, *16*, 339–346. [CrossRef] [PubMed]

18. Hartono, K.; Reed, S.; Ankrah, N.A.; Glahn, R.P.; Tako, E. Alterations in gut microflora populations and brush border functionality following intra-amniotic daidzein administration. *RSC Adv.* **2015**, *5*, 6407–6412. [CrossRef]
19. Zhu, X.Y.; Zhong, T.; Pandya, Y.; Joerger, R.D. 16S rRNA-Based Analysis of Microbiota from the Cecum of Broiler Chickens. *Appl. Environ. Microbiol.* **2002**, *68*, 124–137. [CrossRef] [PubMed]
20. Tako, E.; Glahn, R.P.; Welch, R.M.; Lei, X.; Yasuda, K.; Miller, D.D. Dietary inulin affects the expression of intestinal enterocyte iron transporters, receptors and storage protein and alters the microbiota in the pig intestine. *Br. J. Nutr.* **2008**, *99*, 472–480. [CrossRef] [PubMed]
21. Passaniti, A.; Roth, T.F. Purification of chicken liver ferritin by two novel methods and structural comparison with horse spleen ferritin. *Biochem. J.* **1989**, *258*, 413–419. [CrossRef] [PubMed]
22. Mete, A.; van Zeeland, Y.R.A.; Vaandrager, A.B.; van Dijk, J.E.; Marx, J.J.M.; Dorrestein, G.M. Partial purification and characterization of ferritin from the liver and intestinal mucosa of chickens, turtledoves and mynahs. *Avian Pathol.* **2005**, *34*, 430–434. [CrossRef] [PubMed]
23. Reed, S.; Qin, X.; Ran-Ressler, R.; Brenna, J.; Glahn, R.; Tako, E. Dietary zinc deficiency affects blood linoleic acid: Dihomo-γ-linolenic acid (LA:DGLA) ratio; a sensitive physiological marker of zinc status in vivo (*Gallus gallus*). *Nutrients* **2014**, *6*, 1164–1180. [CrossRef] [PubMed]
24. Smirnov, A.; Tako, E.; Ferket, P.R.; Uni, Z. Mucin gene expression and mucin content in the chicken intestinal goblet cells are affected by in ovo feeding of carbohydrates. *Poult. Sci.* **2006**, *85*, 669–673. [CrossRef] [PubMed]
25. Ludwiczek, S.; Theurl, I.; Artner-Dworzak, E.; Chorney, M.; Weiss, G. Duodenal HFE expression and hepcidin levels determine body iron homeostasis: Modulation by genetic diversity and dietary iron availability. *J. Mol. Med.* **2004**, *82*, 373–382. [CrossRef] [PubMed]
26. Gibson, G.; Beatty, E.; Wang, X.; Cummings, J.H. Selective stimulation of Bifidobacteria in the Human Colon by Oligofructose and Inulin. *Gastroenterology* **1995**, *108*, 975–982. [CrossRef]
27. Roberfroid, M.; Van Loot, J.; Gibson, G. The bifidogenic nature of chicory inulin and its hydrolysis products. *J. Nutr.* **1998**, *128*, 11–19. [PubMed]
28. Patterson, J.K.; Lei, X.G.; Miller, D.D. The pig as an experimental model for elucidating the mechanisms governing dietary influence on mineral absorption. *Exp. Biol. Med.* **2008**, *233*, 651–664. [CrossRef] [PubMed]
29. Gibson, G.R.; Rastall, R.A. *Prebiotics: Development & Application*; John Wiley & Sons: Chichester, UK; Hoboken, NJ, USA, 2006.
30. Tzortzis, G.; Goulas, A.K.; Gibson, G.R. Synthesis of prebiotic galactooligosaccharides using whole cells of a novel strain, Bifidobacterium bifidum NCIMB 41171. *Appl. Microbiol. Biotechnol.* **2005**, *68*, 412–416. [CrossRef] [PubMed]
31. Tako, E.; Glahn, R.P. Iron status of the late term broiler (*Gallus gallus*) embryo and hatchling. *Int. J. Poul. Sci.* **2011**, *10*, 42–48. [CrossRef]
32. Tako, E.; Ferket, P.R.; Uni, Z. Effects of in ovo feeding of carbohydrates and beta-hydroxy-beta-methylbutyrate on the development of chicken intestine. *Poult. Sci.* **2004**, *83*, 2023–2028. [CrossRef] [PubMed]
33. Scholz-Ahrens, K.; Ade, P.; Marten, B.; Weber, P.; Timm, W.; Acil, Y.; Gluer, C.; Schrezenmeir, J. Prebiotics, probiotics, and synbiotics affect mineral absorption, bone mineral content, and bone structure. *J. Nutr.* **2007**, *137*, 838S–846S. [PubMed]
34. Preidis, G.A.; Saulnier, D.M.; Blutt, S.E.; Mistretta, T.-A.; Riehle, K.P.; Major, A.M.; Venable, S.F.; Finegold, M.J.; Petrosino, J.F.; Conner, M.E.; et al. Probiotics stimulate enterocyte migration and microbial diversity in the neonatal mouse intestine. *FASEB J.* **2012**, *26*, 1960–1969. [CrossRef] [PubMed]
35. Ouwehand, A.C.; Derrien, M.; de Vos, W.; Tiihonen, K.; Rautonen, N. Prebiotics and other microbial substrates for gut functionality. *Curr. Opin. Biotechnol.* **2005**, *16*, 212–217. [CrossRef] [PubMed]
36. Deplancke, B.; Gaskins, H.R. Microbial modulation of innate defense: Goblet cells and the intestinal mucus layer. *Am. J. Clin. Nutr.* **2001**, *73*, 1131S–1141S. [PubMed]

11

Butyrate Inhibits Cancerous HCT116 Colon Cell Proliferation but to a Lesser Extent in Noncancerous NCM460 Colon Cells

Huawei Zeng [1,*], David P. Taussig [1], Wen-Hsing Cheng [2], LuAnn K. Johnson [1] and Reza Hakkak [3,4]

1 United States Department of Agriculture, Agricultural Research Service, Grand Forks Human Nutrition Research Center, Grand Forks, ND 58203, USA; dtaussig@gmail.com (D.P.T.); luann.johnson@ars.usda.gov (L.K.J.)
2 Department of Food Science, Nutrition and Health Promotion, Mississippi State University, Starkville, MS 39762, USA; wcheng@fsnhp.msstate.edu
3 Departments of Dietetics and Nutrition, University of Arkansas for Medical Sciences, Little Rock, AR 72205, USA; RHakkak@uams.edu
4 Arkansas Children Research Institute, Little Rock, AR 72202, USA
* Correspondence: huawei.zeng@ars.usda.gov;

Abstract: Butyrate, an intestinal microbiota metabolite of dietary fiber, exhibits chemoprevention effects on colon cancer development. However, the mechanistic action of butyrate remains to be determined. We hypothesize that butyrate inhibits cancerous cell proliferation but to a lesser extent in noncancerous cells through regulating apoptosis and cellular-signaling pathways. We tested this hypothesis by exposing cancerous HCT116 or non-cancerous NCM460 colon cells to physiologically relevant doses of butyrate. Cellular responses to butyrate were characterized by Western analysis, fluorescent microscopy, acetylation, and DNA fragmentation analyses. Butyrate inhibited cell proliferation, and led to an induction of apoptosis, genomic DNA fragmentation in HCT116 cells, but to a lesser extent in NCM460 cells. Although butyrate increased H3 histone deacetylation and p21 tumor suppressor expression in both cell types, p21 protein level was greater with intense expression around the nuclei in HCT116 cells when compared with that in NCM460 cells. Furthermore, butyrate treatment increased the phosphorylation of extracellular-regulated kinase 1/2 (p-ERK1/2), a survival signal, in NCM460 cells while it decreased p-ERK1/2 in HCT116 cells. Taken together, the activation of survival signaling in NCM460 cells and apoptotic potential in HCT116 cells may confer the increased sensitivity of cancerous colon cells to butyrate in comparison with noncancerous colon cells.

Keywords: apoptosis; butyrate; colon cancer; cell proliferation; microbiota

---

1. Introduction

Colon cancer is the third most frequently occurring cancer in men and women in the United States. In 2016 about 134,490 people are predicted to be diagnosed with colorectal cancer in the US, and it is likely that half the Western population will develop at least one colorectal tumor by the age of 70 years [1,2]. It has been reported that high intake of dietary fiber and resistant starches reduces the risk of colon cancer in human populations and animal models [3,4]. This effect may be related to butyrate, a short chain fatty acid (SCFA), which is produced in the colonic lumen by the bacterial fermentation of dietary fiber [3–6]. Colonic luminal SCFA concentration can reach 10 mmol/L when humans consume diets containing moderate levels of fiber [7,8]. Conceivably, there is continuous butyrate exposure in the colonic epithelium, and butyrate may exert several anticarcinogenic effects through the modulation of colon cell proliferation and apoptosis [9–12].

A successful chemoprevention agent should have a minimal effect on normal cells but a strong inhibitory effect on cell proliferation and carcinogenic pathways in cancer cells. While much has been studied on the effect of butyrate on colon cancer cells, little is known about its effect on noncancerous cells, which is essential for understanding butyrate's anticancer properties. Several studies have shown that histone deacetylase (HDAC) activity represses transcriptional activity by condensing the chromatin package leading to an epigenetically mediated silencing of tumor suppressor genes like p21 [13,14]. Butyrate is an HDAC inhibitor (HDACi) and a potential anti-tumor agent. HDACi strongly activates the expression of the cyclin-dependent kinase inhibitor p21, a tumor suppressor [13,15]. In addition, previous data have shown that the extracellular-regulated kinase 1/2 (ERK1/2) and myelocytomatosis (c-Myc) signaling pathways are both required to drive cell cycle progression during cell proliferation [16–18]; c-Myc may also modulate p21 expression [19,20]. To study the effects of butyrate on these signaling pathways related to colon cancer proliferation, two human colon cell lines were employed in this study. The NCM460 colon cell line is an epithelial cell line which is noncancerous and derived from normal colon mucosa [21]. This cell line has not been infected or transfected with any genetic information, and is widely used because there are few other noncancerous colon cell lines [21]. Although there are several cancerous colon cell lines (e.g., HCT116, HT29, and Caco-2) available, most of these cell lines are derived from adenocarcinoma, and only the HCT116 cell line is derived from carcinoma [22,23]. It is known that adenocarcinoma develops in glands whereas carcinoma originates in the epithelial tissue, and there are differences between colorectal carcinoma and advanced adenomas [24]. Given the fact that NCM460 and HCT116 cells were both originally derived from (male adult) colon epithelial tissues and are the same cell subtypes, we believe that NCM460 and HCT116 cells are the best cell-line pair to use in our present study.

In view of the critical role of butyrate in colon cancer prevention [3–6], we hypothesize that butyrate inhibits cancerous cell proliferation but to a lesser extent in noncancerous colon cells through signaling pathways regulating apoptosis and cellular survival [21,22]. Colon crypt cells divide rapidly and travel to the top of the epithelium where they differentiate, proliferate, and undergo cell cycle progression and apoptosis within 48 h. Thus, we focused on the effects of butyrate on colon cell growth and apoptosis for up to 48 h in the present study whereas signaling molecules were examined at early time points (e.g., 1.5 h) to limit the bystander effect.

2. Materials and Methods

2.1. Cell Cultures

HCT116 colorectal carcinoma cells were obtained from American Type Culture Collection and maintained in Dulbecco's Modified Eagle Medium (DMEM) (Invitrogen, Carlsbad, CA, USA) with 10% fetal bovine serum (FBS; Sigma Chemical Co., St. Louis, MO, USA). The nontransformed, noncancerous colon NCM460 cells derived from human normal colon mucosa [21,25] were maintained in M3 Base medium (INCELL Corp., San Antonio, TX, USA) with 10% FBS. Sodium butyrate (purity > 98.5%) was purchased from Sigma Chemical Corporation (St. Louis, MO, USA). Stock cells were passaged twice weekly at ~<80% confluency in Ca-Mg-free Hanks' balanced salt solution (Sigma Chemical Co., St. Louis, MO, USA) containing 0.25% trypsin (Invitrogen) and 1 mmol/L ethylenediamine tetra-acetic acid (EDTA). Cell viability was determined by trypan blue exclusion based on hemocytometer counts and cells were incubated in a humidified chamber at 36.5 °C with 5% CO_2. Cultures were tested and found to be mycoplasma free [26]. HCT116 cells at passages 22–40 and NCM460 cells at passages 34–50 were used. Importantly, both HCT116 and NCM460 cell lines were grown in DMEM medium with 10% FBS in all subsequent assays.

2.2. Cell Count/Growth Assay

HCT116 and NCM460 cell lines were both cultured in DMEM medium with 10% FBS, harvested with 0.25% trypsin (Invitrogen) and 1 mmol/L EDTA, and resuspended in 1 mL medium. Cells were then diluted 1:2 (or 1:4) in 0.2% trypan blue and counted in duplicate using a hemocytometer. At least 200 cells per sample were counted.

2.3. Apoptosis Analysis

Apoptosis was analyzed using a Guava Nexin™ Kit (Guava Technologies, Inc. Hayward, CA, USA). HCT116 and NCM460 cell lines were tryspinized, and then suspended in growth media (DMEM with 10% FBS). Annexin V is a calcium-dependent phospholipid binding protein with high affinity to phosphatidylserine (PS), which has translocated from the internal to external side of the cell membrane upon induction of apoptosis. The cell impermeant dye 7-amino-actinomycin D (7-AAD) is included in the assay kit as an indicator of membrane structural integrity [27]. Therefore, [Annexin V (+), 7-AAD (−)] cells are in the early stages of apoptosis, and [Annexin V (+) and 7-AAD (+)] cells are in the late stages of apoptosis. At least 2000 single cell events per sample were analyzed by the Guava PCA System (Hayward, CA, USA).

2.4. DNA Fragmentation Assay

Each DNA sample was extracted from about 1,000,000 cells by overnight incubation at 50–55 °C in a lysis buffer (50 mmol/L Tris-HCl, pH 8.0, 10 mmol/L EDTA, 150 mmol/L NaCl, 100 μg/mL proteinase K). These DNA samples were recovered by isopropanol precipitation, resuspended in Tris-EDTA-RNase (6 units/mL), analyzed using 1.9% agarose gels, and visualized by ethidium bromide staining. The intensity signals of genomic DNA fragmentation were analyzed by the UVP Bioimaging Systems (Upland, CA, USA).

2.5. Western Blotting Analysis

After butyrate treatment for 1.5 or 15 h, adherent cells were scraped, pooled with the detached cells in 5 mL media, and then these cells were collected by centrifugation at 350× g for 10 min at 4 °C. At least four independent experimental cell sample sets were collected. The cell pellet (about 1,000,000 cells) was washed once in ice-cold PBS and lysed in a cell lysis buffer (20 mmol/L Tris-HCT, pH 7.5, 150 mmol/L NaCl, 1 mmol/L Na2EDTA, 1 mmol/L EGTA, 1% Triton, 2.5 mmol/L sodium pyrophosphate, 1 mmol/L Na_3VO_4, 1 μg/mL leupeptin, 1 mmol/L phenylmethylsulfonyl fluoride) (Cell Signaling Technology, Inc., Danvers, MA, USA). After 15 s sonication, the cell lysate was centrifuged at 14,000× g for 30 min at 4 °C. The supernatant was designated as whole cell protein extract and kept at −80 °C. The protein concentration was quantified by the Bradford dye-binding assay (Bio-Rad laboratories, Richmond, CA, USA). Protein extracts with equal amount (~40 μg) were resolved over 4%–20% Tris-glycine gradient gels under denaturing and reducing conditions and electroblotted onto polyvinylidene difluoride (PVDF) membranes (Invitrogen, Carlsbad, CA, USA). Membrane blots were blocked in phosphate-buffered saline (PBS)—0.05% Tween (v/v) supplemented with 1% (wt/v) nonfat dry milk (BioRad, Hercules, CA, USA) overnight at 4 °C. Membranes were probed with antibodies against c-Myc (Epitomics, Inc., Burlingame, CA, USA), phosphorylated ERK1/2 (p-ERK1/2), ERK1/2, acetyl-Histone H3 (Lys9), and p21 antibodies (Cell Signaling Technology, Inc., Danvers, MA, USA), and then incubated with an anti-mouse/rabbit (1:3000 dilution) horseradish peroxidase (HRP)-conjugated secondary antibody (Cell Signaling Technology, Inc., Danvers, MA, USA) in blocking solution for 1 h at room temperature. Blots were washed as above and proteins were incubated with an ECL plus kit (Amersham Pharmacia Biotech, Piscataway, NJ, USA) and imaged by the Molecular Dynamics Image-Quant system (Sunnyvale, CA, USA).

2.6. Immunfluorescent Staining

HCT116 and NCM460 colon cells were seeded on microscope slides (about 200,000 cells per cell culture chamber slide) in DMEM media supplemented with 10% FBS under an atmosphere of 5% CO_2 at 37 °C overnight. For the observation of p21 and its nuclear localization, the cells were pretreated with butyrate for 15 h. After the treatment, cells were fixed using 4% paraformaldehyde for 15 min, they were permeabilized with ice-cold 100% methanol for 10 min at −20 °C with PBS rinse for 5 min. Cells were then blocked with 10% goat serum (Sigma Chemical Corporation, St. Louis, MO, USA) for 1 h, and then incubated with an anti-p21 antibody (Cell Signaling Technology, Inc., Danvers, MA, USA) overnight at 4 °C. Cells, after washing with PBS, were incubated with anti-rabbit Immunoglobulin G (IgG, H and L), F(ab′)$_2$ Fragment (Alexa Fluor® 488 Conjugate) (green fluorescence) (Cell Signaling Technology, Inc., Danvers, MA, USA) for 1 h at room temperature with propidium iodide (PI) (25 μg/mL). Finally, fluoroshield with PI (Sigma Chemical Corporation, St. Louis, MO, USA), an aqueous mounting medium, was used for preserving fluorescence and producing a red fluorescence as counter stain for overall cell morphology. The fluorescence images and intensity quantification of at least more 2000 cells (per sample) were analyzed by Nikon E400 microscope and Image Pro Plus version 9.1 (North Central Instruments, Plymouth, MN, USA).

2.7. Statistical Analysis

Results are given as means ± SDs. The concentration of butyrate needed to inhibit cell growth by 50% (IC_{50}) was estimated by fitting a three-parameter logistic model to percent inhibition using concentration as the independent variable. The resulting model was used to predict the concentration at which 50% inhibition was expected to occur. Proc NLIN in SAS was used to fit the model. The HCT116 and NCM460 data for 24 h and 48 h were analyzed by two-way analysis of variance with cell type (HCT116 or NCM460), treatment concentration, and their interaction as fixed effects and experiment as a blocking factor. Data were log-transformed prior to analysis in order to test whether changes were proportional across treatment concentrations. Dunnett's multiple comparison procedure was used to compare individual HCT116 or NCM460 group means with their respective control group (untreated cells). The Proc Mixed procedure in SAS v. 9.4 (SAS Institute, Inc., Cary, NC, USA) was used for all analyses. Differences with a p value < 0.05 were considered statistically significant.

3. Results

3.1. Differential Effects of Butyrate (NaB) on Cell Growth

The cell growth rate was inhibited in a dose-dependent manner with a maximum of 58% at 24 h, and 84% at 48 h, respectively, in HCT116 cells treated with 0.5, 1, 1.5, or 2 mmol/L NaB when compared with that of untreated cells (Figure 1). In contrast, the cell growth rate was inhibited to a lesser extent in a dose-dependent manner with a maximum of 38% at 24 h, and 47% at 48 h, respectively, in NCM460 cells treated with 0.5, 1, 1.5, or 2 mmol/L NaB when compared with that of untreated cells (Figure 1). At 48 h, the IC50 of butyrate to inhibit HCT116 cell growth was 0.91 mmol/L, and the 95% confidence interval around this estimate was (0.81, 1.02). In contrast, the IC50 of butyrate to inhibit NCM460 cell growth was greater than 2 mmol/L; we could not precisely determine the value because 2 mmol/L was the highest concentration of NaB used in this study (Figure 1B).

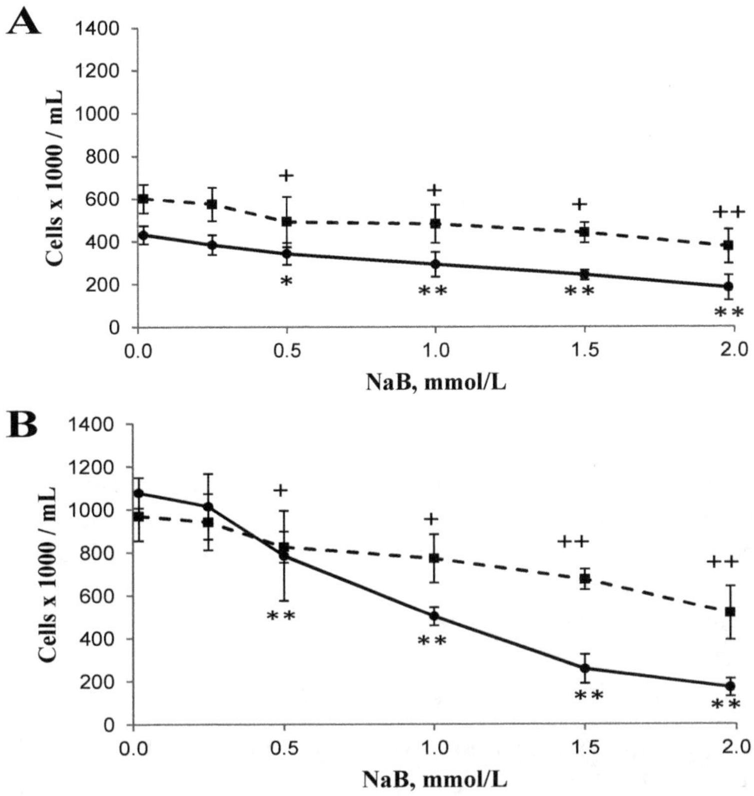

Figure 1. Effect of sodium butyrate (NaB) treatment for (**A**) 24 h and (**B**) 48 h on the growth of cancerous HCT116 (solid lines) and non-cancerous NCM460 (dashed lines) colon cells. Values are means ± SD, $n = 5$ to 6. There was a significant interaction between cell type and concentration at 24 h ($p = 0.01$) and at 48 h ($p < 0.0001$) by two-way ANOVA. * Different from HCT116 control (0 mmol/L NaB); * $p < 0.05$, ** $p < 0.0001$. + Different from NCM460 control (0 mmol/L NaB); $^{+}$ $p < 0.05$, $^{++}$ $p < 0.0001$.

3.2. Differential Effects of Butyrate (NaB) on Apoptosis

Apoptotic cells (including both early and late apoptosis) were increased in a dose-dependent manner with a maximum 1.7 fold increase at 24 h, and 5.4 fold increase at 48 h, respectively, in HCT116 cells treated with 1, 1.5, or 2 mmol/L NaB when compared with that of untreated cells (Figure 2). In contrast, apoptotic cells were increased in a dose-dependent manner with a maximum 0.2 fold increase at 24 h, and 0.4 fold increase at 48 h, respectively, in NCM460 cells treated with 1, 1.5, or 2 mmol/L NaB when compared with that of untreated cells (Figure 2). Furthermore, the early and late apoptotic cells were also increased in a dose-dependent manner, respectively. The percentage of early apoptotic cells was greater ($p < 0.05$) in HCT116 cells treated with 1, 1.5, or 2 mmol/L NaB when compared with that of untreated cells (9.05 ± 5.07, 16.05 ± 5.76, 21.63 ± 6.84 vs. 2.36 ± 0.75, respectively) at 48 h. The percentage of early apoptotic cells was greater ($p < 0.05$) in NCM460 cells treated with 0.5, 1, 1.5, or 2 mmol/L NaB when compared to untreated cells (5.23 ± 1.45, 6.21 ± 1.86, 6.37 ± 2.04, 6.59 ± 1.83 vs. 3.91 ± 1.27) at 48 h. Similarly, the percentage of late apoptotic cells was greater ($p < 0.05$) in HCT116 cells treated with 1, 1.5, or 2 mmol/L NaB when compared with that of untreated cells (8.89 ± 2.76, 13.48 ± 2.78, 17.09 ± 3.09 vs. 3.70 ± 1.36, respectively) at 48 h. In contrast, in NCM460 cells, the percentage of late apoptotic cells was greater ($p < 0.05$) only in cells treated with the highest concentration of NaB (2 mmol/L) when compared to untreated cells (7.93 ± 1.02 vs. 6.49 ± 1.20) at 48 h.

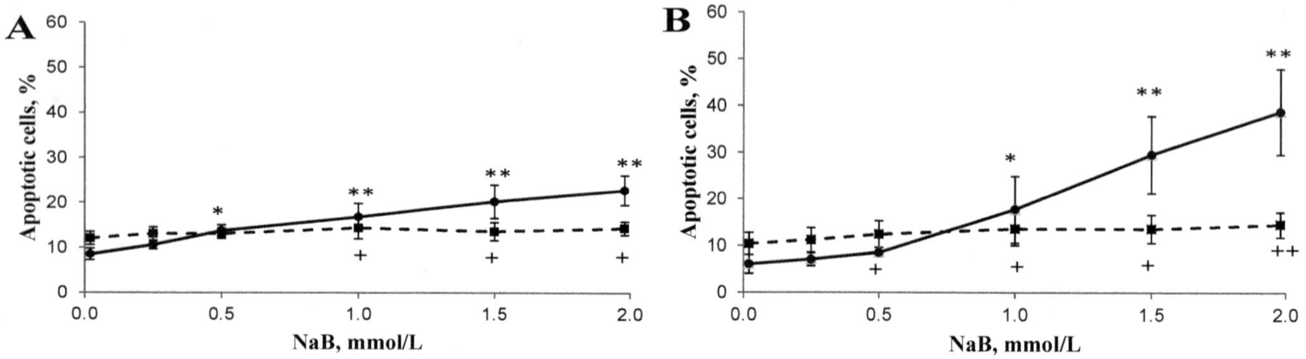

Figure 2. Effect of sodium butyrate (NaB) treatment for (**A**) 24 h and (**B**) 48 h on the apoptosis (including both early and late apoptosis) of cancerous HCT116 (solid lines) and non-cancerous NCM460 (dashed lines) colon cells. Values are means $\pm$ SD, $n = 5$ to 6. There was a significant interaction between cell type and concentration at 24 h ($p < 0.0001$) and at 48 h ($p < 0.0001$) by two-way ANOVA. * Different from HCT116 control (0 mmol/L NaB); * $p < 0.05$, ** $p < 0.0001$. + Different from NCM460 control (0 mmol/L NaB); $^{+}$ $p < 0.05$, $^{++}$ $p < 0.0001$.

3.3. *Differential Effects of Butyrate (NaB) on DNA Fragmentation*

The intensity of genomic DNA fragmentation was increased by 1.3 and 2.1 fold in HCT116 cells treated with 1.5 or 2 mmol/L NaB, respectively, for 15 h (Figure 3B) but not 1.5 h (Figure 3A) when compared with that of untreated cells (Figure 3). There was no NaB-induced genomic DNA fragmentation at 1.5 or 15 h in NCM460 cells.

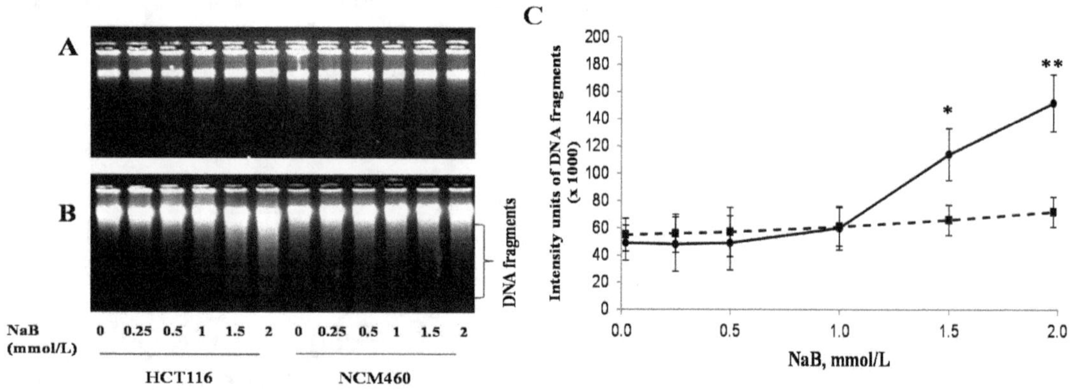

Figure 3. Effect of sodium butyrate (NaB) on the genomic DNA fragmentation of cancerous HCT116 and non-cancerous NCM460 colon cells. A representative DNA image showing DNA fragmentation at (**A**) 1.5 h; (**B**) 15 h; (**C**) the intensity signals of genomic DNA fragmentation (at 15 h) of cancerous HCT116 (solid lines) and non-cancerous NCM460 (dashed lines) colon cells were analyzed by the UVP Bioimaging Systems (there was no DNA fragmentation at 1.5 h). Values are means $\pm$ SD, $n = 4$. There was a significant interaction between cell type and concentration ($p < 0.0001$) by two-way ANOVA. * Different from HCT116 control (0 mmol/L NaB); * $p < 0.05$, ** $p < 0.0001$.

3.4. *Differential Effects of Butyrate (NaB) on Signaling Molecules*

While the p-ERK1/2 level was decreased dose-dependently at 15 h after treatment with NaB in HCT116 cells, the opposite trend was observed in NCM460 cells (Figure 4). Except for the p21 level at 1.5 h in HCT116 cells, there were NaB dose-dependent increases in levels of p21 and acetyl-H3 at

Lys 9 at 1.5 and 15 h in both HCT116 and NCM460 cells (Figure 4). Except for the level of acetyl-H3 at Lys 9 in HCT116 cells, the extent of p21 and acetyl-H3 at Lys 9 induction was greater at 15 h than 1.5 h in both types of cells. In contrast, there were NaB dose-dependent decreases in c-Myc protein level at 1.5 and 15 h in HCT116 cells and 15 h in NCM460 cells (Figure 4). The β-actin and total ERK1/2 protein levels did not differ at 1.5 and 15 h in HCT116 and NCM460 cells because of NaB treatment (Figure 4).

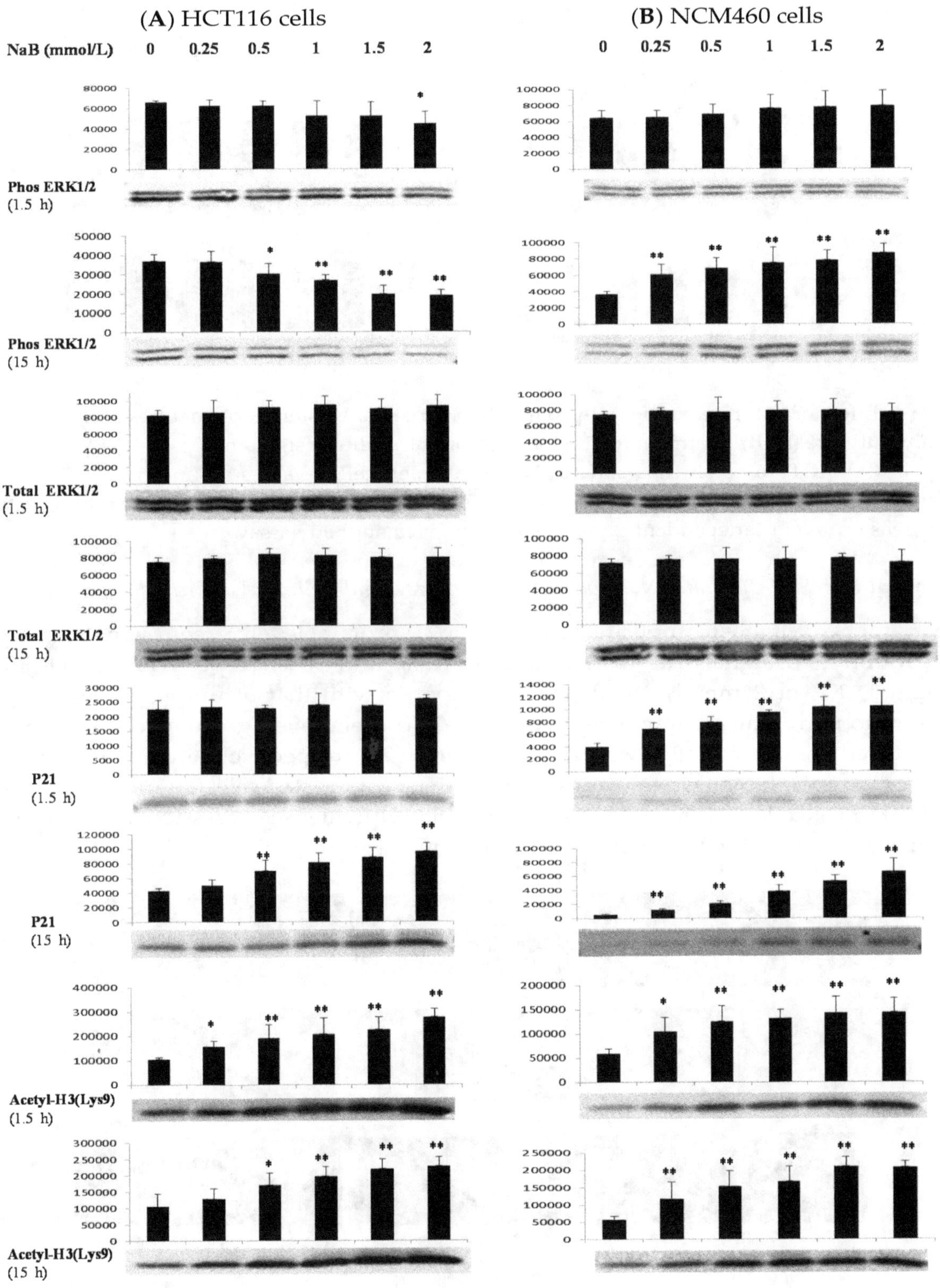

Figure 4. *Cont.*

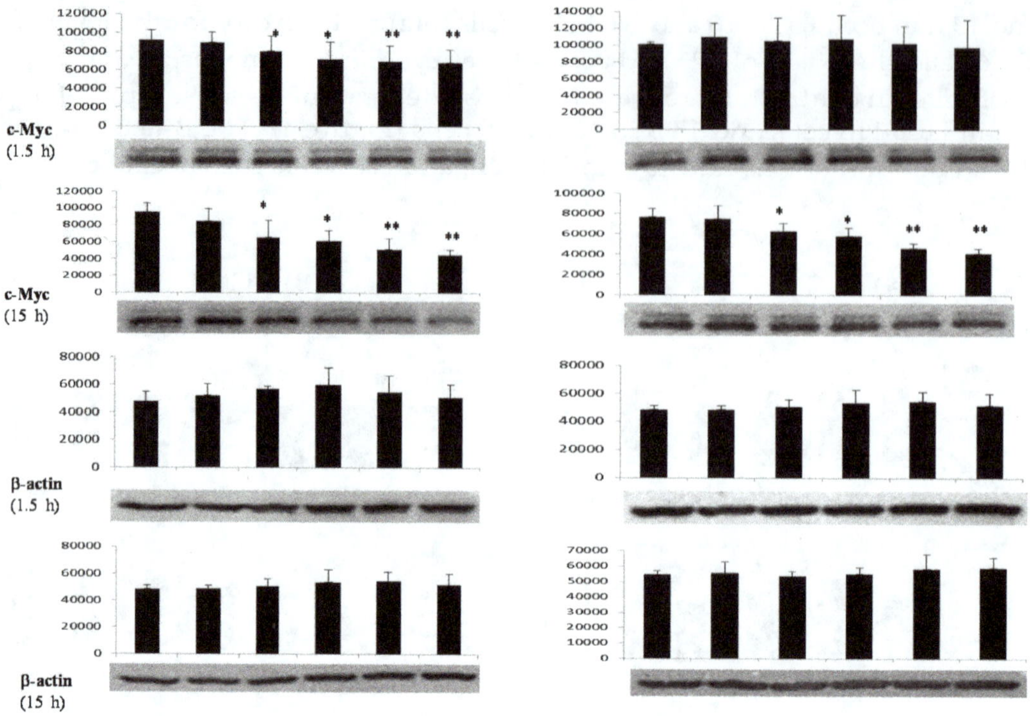

Figure 4. Effect of butyrate on the cell-proliferation proteins. Western blot analyses of the effects of sodium butyrate (NaB) treatment for 1.5 h or 15h on intracellular signaling proteins (densitometric units) in (**A**) HCT116 colon cells and (**B**) NCM460 colon cells. Values are means ± SD, $n = 4$, * Different from control (0 mmol/L NaB); * $p < 0.05$, ** $p < 0.0001$. A representative Western blotting image was from four independent experiments for a given antibody assay.

3.5. Differential Effects of Butyrate (NaB) on p21 Protein Level and Cellular Localization

The ratio percentage (composite image) of p21 protein level (green signals) vs. overall cell background (red signals) at 15 h was 69%, 81%, and 93%, respectively, in HCT116 cells treated with 1, 1.5, or 2 mmol/L NaB when compared with that of untreated cells. To a lesser extent, the ratio percentage (composite image) of p21 protein level (green signals) vs. overall cell background (red signals) at 15 h was 42%, 56%, and 62%, respectively, in NCM460 cells treated with 1, 1.5, or 2 mmol/L NaB when compared with that of untreated cells (Figure 5A,B). In addition, the overall p21 protein level (green signals) was greater with intense expression around the nuclei in HCT116 cells when compared with that in NCM460 cells (Figure 5C,D).

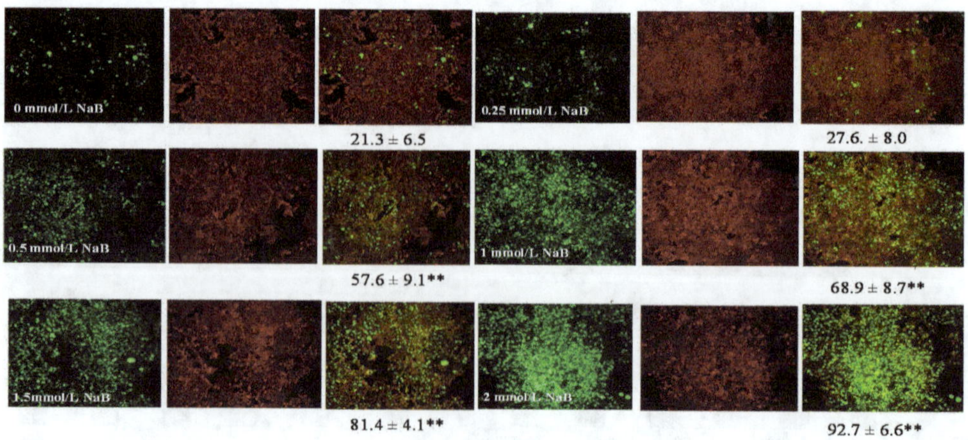

(**A**)

Figure 5. *Cont.*

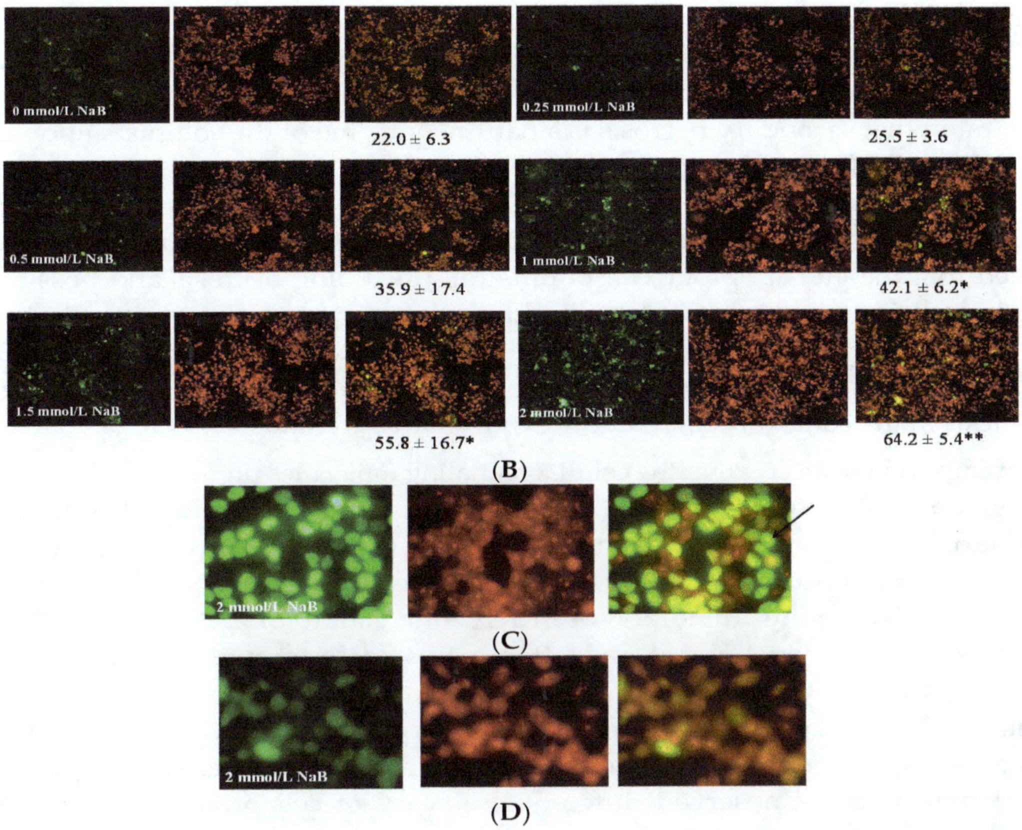

Figure 5. Effect of sodium butyrate (NaB) treatment for 15 h on p21 protein level and distribution at cellular level in HCT116 and NCM460 colon cells. Each sample consists three images: image 1, cells were labeled with anti-p21 antibody, and followed by anti-Rabbit IgG (H and L), $F(ab')_2$ Fragment (Alexa Fluor® 488 Conjugate) (green signals); image 2, cells were mounted by fluoroshield with PI as counter staining for overall cell morphology-background (red signals); image 3, the p21 protein image was superimposed on the respective overall cell morphology-background image to generate the composite image (orange signals). (**A**) HCT cells at 200× magnification; (**B**) NCM460 cells at 200× magnification; (**C**) HCT116 cells with intense p21 expression around the nucleus (arrow) at 1000× magnification; (**D**) NCM460 cells at 1000× magnification. For panel (**A**,**B**) composite images, the area of p21 protein level (green signals) in percentage when compared with that of overall cell morphology-background (red signals). Values are means ± SD, $n = 4$. There was a significant interaction between cell type and concentration ($p < 0.001$) by two-way ANOVA. * Different from control (0 mmol/L NaB); * $p < 0.05$, ** $p < 0.0001$.

4. Discussion

Butyrate has been shown to abrogate the S-phase cell cycle checkpoint, and exhibits colon cancer preventive effects through cell proliferation regulation [5,6,28–30]. As there are few reports concerning the apoptotic potential, we propose that butyrate plays differential roles in the cell proliferation of noncancerous NCM460 cell and cancerous HCT116 colon cells through cellular signaling modulation. Thus, examining molecular effects of butyrate on cell proliferation/apoptosis in cancerous and noncancerous colon cells is expected to shed light on butyrate's anticancer mechanism.

It has been reported that butyrate at mmol/L levels in the colon is well within physiological concentrations [7,8]. Our data showed that butyrate (0.25 to 2 mmol/L) was much more effective on inhibiting cell proliferation in cancerous (HCT116) colon cells than in noncancerous (NCM460) colon cells (Figure 1). Similarly, we found, for the first time, that butyrate was effective in inducing apoptosis/DNA fragmentation in HCT116 cells but not NCM460 cells (Figures 2 and 3). This observation suggests that the stronger DNA fragmentation and apoptotic potential may confer the increased sensitivity of cancerous colon cells to butyrate in terms of cell proliferation when compared with that of noncancerous colon cells. In our present apoptosis assay, 7-AAD was excluded from live, healthy cells and early apoptotic cells, but permeated late apoptotic or necrotic cells [27]. It has been demonstrated that secondary necrosis is a natural outcome of the complete apoptotic program (e.g., late apoptotic cells) [31]. Although lactate dehydrogenase (LDH), a cytoplasmic enzyme, is widely used to detect necrosis and secondary necrosis based on plasma membrane leakage, the measurement of 7-AAD positive cells is a powerful approach to directly detect leaky membrane cells [31,32]. As our results showed that the late apoptotic cell population (including necrosis and possible secondary necrosis) was greatly increased in HCT116 cells but to a lesser extent in NCM460 cells due to butyrate treatment, it is conceivable that necrotic cell death may evoke inflammatory responses [32,33]. In the future, clinical samples from patients are needed to examine the impact of inflammatory responses on host pathogenesis in the context of high or low exposure to butyrate.

The other important aspect is that the cellular signaling molecules underlying the differential effect of butyrate remain to be determined. The ERK1/2 pathway plays a pivotal role in cell proliferation as it is an important cellular signaling component that translates various extracellular signals into intracellular responses through phosphorylation cascades [18,34–36]. Moreover, cell-cycle arrest by PD184352 or U0126 requires inhibition of ERK1/2 activation [37]. Thus, the ERK1/2 pathway is recognized as a pro-survival signal and often activated by growth factors [18,34,35]. In this study, butyrate up-regulated ERK1/2 phosphorylation in NCM460 cells (Figure 4). In contrast, butyrate inhibited ERK1/2 phosphorylation in HCT116 cells, which is consistent with the previous report [38] (Figure 4). The opposing effect of butyrate on cell survival signals provides an important mechanistic insight into the observed differential efficacy of cell proliferation and apoptosis in cancerous and noncancerous colon cells.

Appropriate control over cell cycle and proliferation depends on many factors. Cyclin-dependent kinase (CDK) inhibitor p21 (also known as p21 (WAF1/Cip1)) is one of these factors that promotes both cell cycle arrest and proliferation in response to a variety of stimuli [39–41]. To provide further mechanistic insights, we examined p21 protein expression, which is known to be the most critical effector of butyrate-induced growth arrest in colon cancer cells [39,42] (Figure 4). Butyrate is known to induce general histone acetylation, specifically, hyperacetylation of the H3 and other species through inhibition of the histone deacetylase enzyme [42,43]. Previous studies have shown that histone hyperacetylation is at least partly responsible for the induction of p21 [42,44]. In addition, the nuclear protein c-Myc, a central regulator of cellular proliferation, activates a multitude of pathways to repress p21 at the transcriptional and post-transcriptional levels [19,20]. We found that butyrate increased histone H3 acetylation at 1.5 and 15 h while it decreased c-Myc expression only at 15 h in NCM460 cells (Figure 4). However, p21 expression was increased at 1.5 and 15 h in NCM460 cells. Therefore, our results suggest that butyrate-related histone acetylation (compared with c-Myc) plays a major role in p21 expression because we could only detect the increase of histone H3 acetylation and p21 but not c-Myc expression in NCM460 cells in early molecular events at 1.5 h.

The other important aspect of p21 function is that, depending on intracellular localization, p21 is involved in different signaling cascades [39–41]. It is generally believed that nuclear p21 is a negative regulator of cell proliferation and a tumor suppressor while cytoplasmic p21 facilitates cell proliferation and inhibits apoptosis [39–41]. In addition to high p21 levels in HCT116 cells (Figure 5A,B), our cellular immunofluorescent staining data demonstrated that butyrate-induced p21 protein was located in or surrounding the nuclei of HCT116 cells to a greater extent when compared with that of NCM460 cells (Figure 5C,D). This observation indicates that butyrate induces p21 expression, and may exacerbate the negative role of p21 in HCT116 cell proliferation when compared with that of NCM460 cells. Therefore, butyrate treatment leads to the significant induction of apoptosis and inhibition of cell proliferation in cancerous HCT116 colon cells, but to a lesser extent in the noncancerous NCM460 colon cells. To extrapolate these mechanistic data to all colon cancer cell types and disease stages, we are planning to test other pairs of noncancerous and cancerous colon cell lines. However, there are very limited noncancerous colon cell lines available, which is a challenge. The other approach would be to evaluate clinical samples from patients with possible high or low exposure to butyrate.

Colon carcinogenesis consists of initiation, promotion, and progression phases [45,46]. Suppression of apoptosis and promotion of colonocyte proliferation are key cellular carcinogenic events as a consequence of dysregulation of molecular signal cascades [46]. Taken together, our findings on the differential roles of butyrate in cell proliferation and the activation of ERK1/2, histone hyperacetylation, and c-Myc, p21 protein abundance and intracellular location in cancerous HCT116 and noncancerous NCM460 colon cells may, at least in part, account for the selective potential of butyrate's anticancer colon cancer action.

Acknowledgments: We greatly appreciate Emily Fair, Mary Briske-Anderson, Brenda Skinner, Kay Keehr, Bryan Safratowich, and Laura Idso for the technical support. This work was funded by the US Department of Agriculture, Agricultural Research Service, Research Project 3062-51000-050-00D.

Author Contributions: H.Z., W.-H.C. and R.H. conceived and designed the experiments; H.Z. and D.P.T. performed the experiments; H.Z. and L.K.J. analyzed the data; H.Z., W.-H.C. and R.H. wrote the paper.

References

1. American Cancer Society. *Cancer Facts & Figures*; American Cancer Society: Atlanta, GA, USA, 2016.
2. Simon, K. Colorectal cancer development and advances in screening. *J. Clin. Interv. Aging* **2016**, *11*, 967–976.
3. Perrin, P.; Pierre, F.; Patry, Y.; Champ, M.; Berreur, M.; Pradal, G.; Bornet, F.; Meflah, K.; Menanteau, J. Only fibres promoting a stable butyrate producing colonic ecosystem decrease the rate of aberrant crypt foci in rats. *Gut* **2001**, *48*, 53–61. [CrossRef] [PubMed]
4. Zeng, H.; Lazarova, D.L.; Bordonaro, M. Mechanisms linking dietary fiber, gut microbiota and colon cancer prevention. *World J. Gastrointest. Oncol.* **2014**, *6*, 41–51. [CrossRef] [PubMed]
5. Lazarova, D.L.; Bordonaro, M. Vimentin, colon cancer progression and resistance to butyrate and other HDACis. *J. Cell. Mol. Med.* **2016**, *20*, 989–993. [CrossRef] [PubMed]
6. Bultman, S.J. The microbiome and its potential as a cancer preventive intervention. *Semin. Oncol.* **2016**, *43*, 97–106. [CrossRef] [PubMed]
7. Fleming, S.E.; O'Donnell, A.U.; Perman, J.A. Influence of frequent and long-term bean consumption on colonic function and fermentation. *Am. J. Clin. Nutr.* **1985**, *41*, 909–918. [PubMed]
8. Fleming, S.E.; Marthinsen, D.; Kuhnlein, H. Colonic function and fermentation in men consuming high fiber diets. *J. Nutr.* **1983**, *113*, 2535–2544. [PubMed]
9. Leonel, A.J.; Alvarez-Leite, J.I. Butyrate: Implications for intestinal function. *Curr. Opin. Clin. Nutr. Metab. Care* **2012**, *15*, 474–479. [CrossRef] [PubMed]
10. Brown, D.G.; Rao, S.; Weir, T.L.; O'Malia, J.; Bazan, M.; Brown, R.J.; Ryan, E.P. Metabolomics and metabolic pathway networks from human colorectal cancers, adjacent mucosa, and stool. *Cancer Metab.* **2016**, *4*, 11. [CrossRef] [PubMed]
11. Zeng, H.; Davis, C.D. Down-regulation of proliferating cell nuclear antigen gene expression occurs during cell cycle arrest induced by human fecal water in colonic HT-29 cells. *J. Nutr.* **2003**, *133*, 2682–2687. [PubMed]
12. Hu, G.X.; Chen, G.R.; Xu, H.; Ge, R.S.; Lin, J. Activation of the AMP activated protein kinase by short-chain fatty acids is the main mechanism underlying the beneficial effect of a high fiber diet on the metabolic syndrome. *Med. Hypotheses* **2010**, *74*, 123–126. [CrossRef] [PubMed]
13. Ocker, M.; Schneider-Stock, R. Histone deacetylase inhibitors: Signalling towards $p21^{cip1/waf1}$. *Int. J. Biochem. Cell Biol.* **2007**, *39*, 1367–1374. [CrossRef] [PubMed]
14. Bi, G.; Jiang, G. The molecular mechanism of HDAC inhibitors in anticancer effects. *Cell. Mol. Immunol.* **2006**, *3*, 285–290. [PubMed]
15. Chen, H.P.; Zhao, Y.T.; Zhao, T.C. Histone deacetylases and mechanisms of regulation of gene expression. *Crit. Rev. Oncog.* **2015**, *20*, 35–47. [CrossRef] [PubMed]
16. Jones, S.M.; Kazlauskas, A. Growth-factor-dependent mitogenesis requires two distinct phases of signalling. *Nat. Cell Biol.* **2001**, *3*, 165–172. [CrossRef] [PubMed]

17. Karslioglu, E.; Kleinberger, J.W.; Salim, F.G.; Cox, A.E.; Takane, K.K.; Scott, D.K.; Stewart, A.F. cMyc is a principal upstream driver of beta-cell proliferation in rat insulinoma cell lines and is an effective mediator of human beta-cell replication. *Mol. Endocrinol.* **2011**, *25*, 1760–1772. [CrossRef] [PubMed]
18. Sun, Y.; Liu, W.Z.; Liu, T.; Feng, X.; Yang, N.; Zhou, H.F. Signaling pathway of MAPK/ERK in cell proliferation, differentiation, migration, senescence and apoptosis. *J. Recept. Signal Transduct. Res.* **2015**, *35*, 600–604. [CrossRef] [PubMed]
19. Gartel, A.L.; Ye, X.; Goufman, E.; Shianov, P.; Hay, N.; Najmabadi, F.; Tyner, A.L. Myc represses the p21(WAF1/CIP1) promoter and interacts with Sp1/Sp3. *Proc. Natl. Acad. Sci. USA* **2001**, *98*, 4510–4515. [CrossRef] [PubMed]
20. Wang, Z.; Liu, M.; Zhu, H.; Zhang, W.; He, S.; Hu, C.; Quan, L.; Bai, J.; Xu, N. Suppression of p21 by c-Myc through members of miR-17 family at the post-transcriptional level. *Int. J. Oncol.* **2010**, *37*, 1315–1321. [PubMed]
21. Moyer, M.P.; Manzano, L.A.; Merriman, R.L.; Stauffer, J.S.; Tanzer, L.R. NCM460, a normal human colon mucosal epithelial cell line. *In Vitro Cell. Dev. Biol. Anim.* **1996**, *32*, 315–317. [CrossRef] [PubMed]
22. Brattain, M.G.; Fine, W.D.; Khaled, F.M.; Thompson, J.; Brattain, D.E. Heterogeneity of malignant cells from a human colonic carcinoma. *Cancer Res.* **1981**, *41*, 1751–1756. [PubMed]
23. Megna, B.W.; Carney, P.R.; Nukaya, M.; Geiger, P.; Kennedy, G.D. Indole-3-carbinol induces tumor cell death: Function follows form. *J. Surg. Res.* **2016**, *204*, 47–54. [CrossRef] [PubMed]
24. De Meij, T.G.; Larbi, I.B.; van der Schee, M.P.; Lentferink, Y.E.; Paff, T.; Terhaar Sive Droste, J.S.; Mulder, C.J.; van Bodegraven, A.A.; de Boer, N.K. Electronic nose can discriminate colorectal carcinoma and advanced adenomas by fecal volatile biomarker analysis: Proof of principle study. *Int. J. Cancer* **2014**, *134*, 1132–1138. [CrossRef] [PubMed]
25. Zhao, D.; Keates, A.C.; Kuhnt-Moore, S.; Moyer, M.P.; Kelly, C.P.; Pothoulakis, C. Signal transduction pathways mediating neurotensin-stimulated interleukin-8 expression in human colonocytes. *J. Biol. Chem.* **2001**, *276*, 44464–44471. [CrossRef] [PubMed]
26. Chen, T.R. In situ detection of mycoplasma contamination in cell cultures by fluorescent Hoechst 33258 stain. *Exp. Cell Res.* **1977**, *104*, 255–262. [CrossRef]
27. Schmid, I.; Krall, W.J.; Uittenbogaart, C.H.; Braun, J.; Giorgi, J.V. Dead cell discrimination with 7-amino-actinomycin D in combination with dual color immunofluorescence in single laser flow cytometry. *Cytometry* **1992**, *13*, 204–208. [CrossRef] [PubMed]
28. Zeng, H.; Briske-Anderson, M. Prolonged butyrate treatment inhibits the migration and invasion potential of HT1080 tumor cells. *J. Nutr.* **2005**, *135*, 291–295. [PubMed]
29. Saldanha, S.N.; Kala, R.; Tollefsbol, T.O. Molecular mechanisms for inhibition of colon cancer cells by combined epigenetic-modulating epigallocatechin gallate and sodium butyrate. *Exp. Cell Res.* **2014**, *324*, 40–53. [CrossRef] [PubMed]
30. Gospodinov, A.; Popova, S.; Vassileva, I.; Anachkova, B. The inhibitor of histone deacetylases sodium butyrate enhances the cytotoxicity of mitomycin C. *Mol. Cancer Ther.* **2012**, *11*, 2116–2126. [CrossRef] [PubMed]
31. Silva, M.T. Secondary necrosis: The natural outcome of the complete apoptotic program. *FEBS Lett.* **2010**, *584*, 4491–4499. [CrossRef] [PubMed]
32. Chan, F.K.; Moriwaki, K.; De Rosa, M.J. Detection of necrosis by release of lactate dehydrogenase activity. *Methods Mol. Biol.* **2013**, *979*, 65–70. [PubMed]
33. Kono, H.; Rock, K.L. How dying cells alert the immune system to danger. *Nat. Rev. Immunol.* **2008**, *8*, 279–289. [CrossRef] [PubMed]
34. Meloche, S.; Pouysségur, J. The ERK1/2 mitogen-activated protein kinase pathway as a master regulator of the G1- to S-phase transition. *Oncogene* **2007**, *26*, 3227–3239. [CrossRef] [PubMed]
35. Xia, Z.; Dickens, M.; Raingeaud, J.; Davis, R.J.; Greenberg, M.E. Opposing effects of ERK and JNK-p38 MAP kinases on apoptosis. *Science* **1995**, *270*, 1326–1331. [CrossRef] [PubMed]
36. Park, J.I. Growth arrest signaling of the Raf/MEK/ERK pathway in cancer. *Front. Biol. (Beijing)* **2014**, *9*, 95–103. [CrossRef] [PubMed]
37. Squires, M.S.; Nixon, P.M.; Cook, S.J. Cell-cycle arrest by PD184352 requires inhibition of extracellular signal-regulated kinases (ERK) 1/2 but not ERK5/BMK1. *Biochem. J.* **2002**, *366*, 673–680. [CrossRef] [PubMed]

38. Davido, D.J.; Richter, F.; Boxberger, F.; Stahl, A.; Menzel, T.; Lührs, H.; Löffler, S.; Dusel, G.; Rapp, U.R.; Scheppach, W. Butyrate and propionate downregulate ERK phosphorylation in HT-29 colon carcinoma cells prior to differentiation. *Eur. J. Cancer Prev.* **2001**, *10*, 313–321. [CrossRef] [PubMed]
39. Karimian, A.; Ahmadi, Y.; Yousefi, B. Multiple functions of p21 in cell cycle, apoptosis and transcriptional regulation after DNA damage. *DNA Repair* **2016**, *42*, 63–71. [CrossRef] [PubMed]
40. Romanov, V.S.; Pospelov, V.A.; Pospelova, T.V. Cyclin-dependent kinase inhibitor p21(Waf1): Contemporary view on its role in senescence and oncogenesis. *Biochemistry (Mosc.)* **2012**, *77*, 575–584. [CrossRef] [PubMed]
41. Parveen, A.; Akash, M.S.; Rehman, K.; Kyunn, W.W. Dual Role of p21 in the Progression of Cancer and Its Treatment. *Crit. Rev. Eukaryot. Gene Expr.* **2016**, *26*, 49–62. [CrossRef] [PubMed]
42. Archer, S.Y.; Meng, S.; Shei, A.; Hodin, R.A. p21(WAF1) is required for butyrate-mediated growth inhibition of human colon cancer cells. *Proc. Natl. Acad. Sci. USA* **1998**, *95*, 6791–6796. [CrossRef] [PubMed]
43. Pham, T.X.; Lee, J. Dietary regulation of histone acetylases and deacetylases for the prevention of metabolic diseases. *Nutrients* **2012**, *4*, 1868–1886. [CrossRef] [PubMed]
44. Nian, H.; Delage, B.; Pinto, J.T.; Dashwood, R.H. Allyl mercaptan, a garlic-derived organosulfur compound, inhibits histone deacetylase and enhances Sp3 binding on the P21WAF1 promoter. *Carcinogenesis* **2008**, *29*, 1816–1824. [CrossRef] [PubMed]
45. Gatenby, R.A.; Vincent, T.L. An evolutionary model of carcinogenesis. *Cancer Res.* **2003**, *63*, 6212–6220. [PubMed]
46. Rajamanickam, S.; Agarwal, R. Natural products and colon cancer: Current status and future prospects. *Drug Dev. Res.* **2008**, *69*, 460–471. [CrossRef] [PubMed]

12

Exercise and Beta-Glucan Consumption (*Saccharomyces cerevisiae*) Improve the Metabolic Profile and Reduce the Atherogenic Index in Type 2 Diabetic Rats (HFD/STZ)

Eric Francelino Andrade [1,*], Andressa Ribeiro Veiga Lima [2], Ingrid Edwiges Nunes [3], Débora Ribeiro Orlando [4], Paula Novato Gondim [1], Márcio Gilberto Zangeronimo [1], Fernando Henrique Ferrari Alves [2] and Luciano José Pereira [2]

1 Department of Veterinary Medicine, Federal University of Lavras, Mail Box 3037, Lavras 37200-000, Brazil; pngondim@hotmail.com (P.N.G.); zangeronimo@prpg.ufla.br (M.G.Z.)
2 Department of Health Sciences, Federal University of Lavras, Mail Box 3037, Lavras 37200-000, Brazil; andressaveigalima@outlook.com (A.R.V.L.); fernando.ferrari@dsa.ufla.br (F.H.F.A.); lucianojosepereira@dsa.ufla.br (L.J.P.)
3 Department of Animal Sciences, Federal University of Lavras, Mail Box 3037, Lavras 37200-000, Brazil; inunes2611@gmail.com
4 Department of Agricultural Sciences, Federal University of Jequitinhonha and Mucuri Valleys, Rua Vereador João Narciso, 1380—Bairro Cachoeira, Unaí 3861-000, Brazil; debora.ribeiro@ufvjm.edu.br
* Correspondence: ericfrancelinoandrade@gmail.com;

Abstract: Physical activity and the ingestion of dietary fiber are non-drug alternatives commonly used as adjuvants to glycemic control in diabetic individuals. Among these fibers, we can highlight beta-glucans. However, few studies have compared isolated and synergic effects of physical exercise and beta-glucan ingestion, especially in type 2 diabetic rats. Therefore, we evaluated the effects beta-glucan (*Saccharomyces cerevisiae*) consumption, associated or not to exercise, on metabolic parameters of diabetic Wistar rats. The diabetes *mellitus* (DM) was induced by high-fat diet (HFD) associated with a low dose of streptozotocin (STZ—35 mg/kg). Trained groups were submitted to eight weeks of exercise in aquatic environment. In the last 28 days of experiment, animals received 30 mg/kg/day of beta-glucan by gavage. Isolated use of beta-glucan decreased glucose levels in fasting, Glycated hemoglobin (HbA1c), triglycerides (TAG), total cholesterol (TC), low-density lipoprotein (LDL-C), the atherogenic index of plasma. Exercise alone also decreased blood glucose levels, HbA1c, and renal lesions. An additive effect for reducing the atherogenic index of plasma and renal lesions was observed when both treatments were combined. It was concluded that both beta-glucan and exercise improved metabolic parameters in type 2 (HFD/STZ) diabetic rats.

Keywords: dietary fibers; glycemic control; metabolic profile

---

1. Introduction

Diabetes *mellitus* (DM) is a metabolic disorder characterized by chronic hyperglycemia, caused by the absence or reduction in insulin production (type 1 DM) as well as the resistance to the action of this hormone, featuring type 2 DM [1]. About 90% of DM cases are of type 2, and this fact is associated with increased incidence of obesity and obesity in the general population, especially in developing nations [2,3]. In addition, DM may predispose to diseases, such as retinopathy, nephropathy, neuropathy and heart disease, further aggravating the health condition of patients [2,4].

Glycemic control in diabetic patients can be achieved through the use of exogenous insulin and/oral hypoglycemic drugs [5]. However, the interaction between medications could cause side effects, and does not prevent the diseases associated with DM, making necessary the search for non-pharmacological alternatives to assist in the maintenance of blood sugar levels [4,6]. In this sense, the practice of physical exercise and diet therapy has been recommended as a treatment or therapeutic adjuvant [7]. Physical exercise increases the uptake and utilization of circulating glucose and improves insulin sensitivity [8]. The ingestion of some dietary fibers has also been reported to show antihyperglycemic action—mainly by reducing the absorption of carbohydrates and lipids in the intestine. Among these fibers, we can highlight beta-glucans that are polysaccharides found in the composition of cereal, fungi, bacteria and some grass cell walls [9].

The chemical structure of beta-glucan varies according to its origin [10]. Beta-glucans found in plants and cereals are linear and have branchings with β-1,3/1,4-type glycosidic linkages (soluble with low molecular weight), while those found in yeasts and fungi have β-1,3/1,6-type glycosidic linkages (insoluble with high molecular weight) [11]. These conformations make beta-glucans exhibit distinct physicochemical characteristics, such as molecular mass and solubility [12,13]. Cereal beta-glucans are reported to show metabolic potential, while those from fungi and yeast increase immune response [10,14,15]. Although fungi beta-glucans are recognized to modulate the immune response [16], recent studies from our group have also demonstrated interesting metabolic effects of yeast beta-glucans (*Saccharomyces cereviseae*) [10,17,18].

Considering the previously known effects of both exercise and the beta-glucan on glycemic control and metabolism, it is necessary to investigate the concomitant action of these agents in the treatment of type DM. In addition, there is a shortage of studies evaluating such effects in type 2 diabetes model. Thus, the present study aimed to evaluate the effects of beta-glucan (*Saccharomyces cerevisiae*), associated or not to physical exercise, on the metabolic parameters of type 2 diabetic rats (HFD/STZ).

2. Materials and Methods

2.1. Animals

This study was approved by the Ethics Committee on Animal Use of Federal University of Lavras (CEUA protocol 002/2015). The animals were kept in accordance with the Guide to the Care and Use of Experimental Animals (1993). The number of animals per group was kept at a minimum for ethical reasons but still enough to reach statistical significance. Thus, a power calculation test was performed to determine the sample size. The sample size was determined to provide 80% power to recognize a significant difference of 20% among groups and a standard deviation of 15% with a 95% confidence interval ($\alpha = 0.05$).

We used adult male Wistar rats (*Rattus norvegicus albinos*)—from the Animal Laboratory of the Federal University of Lavras (UFLA). Animals weighed 195.0 ± 15.7 g at the beginning of the study. Initially, rats were submitted to seven days of acclimatization in polypropylene boxes (dimensions 41 cm × 34 cm × 17.5 cm), containing wood shavings (for absorbing urine and water). Six animals were placed in each box. Throughout the experimental period, the rodents remained under controlled temperature (22 ± 2 °C), humidity (45% ± 15%) and luminosity (12–12 h light-dark cycle) conditions. High-fat diet and water were provided ad libitum throughout the experiment.

2.2. Induction of Diabetes Mellitus

At the end of the acclimatization period, all animals were submitted to type 2 diabetes induction protocol as described by Wang et al. [19]. The animals received high-fat diet (HFD—25% fat, 48% carbohydrates and 20% protein) for 28 days. Then, a low dose of streptozotocin (dissolved in citrate buffer—pH = 4.5) was injected intraperitoneally (STZ—35 mg/kg). Blood glucose levels were measured 48 h after STZ injection. Rats with blood glucose levels above 200 mg/dL [19] were considered diabetic. This model mimic advanced stages of type 2 diabetes in humans [19,20]. Rats that did not reach these glucose values were excluded from the experiment. Glycemia was checked weekly to ensure that diabetes was not reversed.

After diabetes induction, animals were randomly divided into four groups containing six animals each. A completely randomized experimental design in a 2 × 2 factorial scheme was used: with or without exercise and with or without beta-glucan.

2.3. Physical Training

After an acclimatization period, an adaptation to the aquatic environment was performed. Animals undergoing physical training remained for two hours daily, during seven days, in a polyethylene tank with a total capacity of 300 L, containing five centimeters of water at a temperature of approximately 32 ± 2 °C. The purpose of this acclimatization was to reduce stress against the aquatic environment, without causing, however, changes arising from the physical training [21].

In the following week, animals were submitted to progressive swimming sessions with time increments. This phase consisted of swimming without load, in 50 cm of water (in order to avoid animal tail contact with the bottom of the tank), where the animals swam 10 min in the first day, increasing 10 min daily until the end of six days, when each animal was swimming for 60 uninterrupted minutes without load [22].

In the subsequent eight weeks, the animals swam for 60 min daily, five times a week with a load of 5% of their body weight. This load causes improvement in the animals' endurance capacity, characterizing moderate intensity aerobic exercise [22]. After training sessions, we dried the animals with absorbent towels, before returning them to their cages [21].

2.4. Administration of Beta-Glucans

Simultaneously with training, in the last 28 days of the experiment, the animals in beta-glucan groups received a experimental solution and controls received saline—both by gavage. Beta-glucan solutions that contained 30 mg/kg of powder diluted in 0.3 mL saline solution prepared daily.

Beta-glucan used in the present study were derived from yeast *Saccharomyces cerevisiae*, with structural β-1,3/1,6 conformation. The beta-glucan powder presented the following composition: β-glucans—Min. 60.0%; Crude Protein—Max. 8.0%; pH (solution 2%) 4.0–7.0; Ash—Max. 10.0 g/100 g. Distribution of particle size: mean—41 μm; <20 μm 19%; 20–50 μm 43%; 50–100 μm 28%; 100–200 μm 10%; >200 μm 0%; Fluidity (seconds)—70.2; Angle of repose (degrees) 31.2; Compressibility 37%; Water retention capacity (mean) 7.4; and Solubility rate in water 7.9. The solutions were always administered daily in the morning. In animals under physical training, gavage was always performed with a minimum of 45 min before exercise, as described in previous studies [21,23].

2.5. Collection of Biological Material and Assessment of the Atherogenic Index of Plasma

At the end of the experimental period (eight weeks), the animals fasted for eight hours. Euthanasia was conducted by cardiac puncture under anesthesia (sodium thiopental 50 mg/kg ip). Glycated hemoglobin (HbA1c) and other blood biochemical parameters such as glucose, triacylglycerols (TAG), high density lipoprotein (HDL-C) and total cholesterol (TC) were determined using commercial kits (Labtest Diagnostica®, Belo Horizonte, Brazil and Gold analyzes diagnoses®, Belo Horizonte, Brazil) as described by Amr and Abeer [24]. The low-density lipoprotein (LDL) + very-low-density lipoprotein cholesterol (VLDL-C) levels of each animal were obtained by using the following equation: total cholesterol − HDL-C = LDL + VLDL-C [25]. Additionally, the animals' atherogenic index of plasma was calculated using the equation: log (TG)/(HDL-C), which is used as a significant predictor of atherosclerosis [26]. This index was used because type 2 diabetes increases one's chances of developing atherosclerosis [27].

2.6. Lee Index Assessment and Chemical Composition of the Body

The Lee index was calculated dividing the cubic root of body weight (grams) by the naso-anal length (cm) [18,28]. Internal organs, skin, head, feet and tail were removed from the animals and the clean carcasses were weighed and processed. Percentages of water, protein, fat and mineral matter present in the carcasses were evaluated by the meat FoodScan™ NIR analyzer (near-infra-red) (Foss, Warrington, UK) as performed by Vickers et al. [29]. This evaluation method of carcass composition has been considered as the gold standard [29].

2.7. Histological Analysis

Fragments of the right kidney and liver were fixed in 10% buffered formalin for 48 h, and then processed routinely for preparation of histological slices, which were then colored with hematoxylin-eosin [30]. An experienced veterinary pathologist conducted all histopathologic analysis (blind about experimental treatments). Tissue integrity, as well as the presence of alterations, were considered in the evaluations. Liver tissue ratings were assigned according to the presence and/or degree of steatosis as follows: no change—1; discreet—2; light—3; moderate—4; and severe—5. Steatosis was classified according to the presence of vacuoles in hepatocytes. Staining was performed with Periodic acid-Schiff (PAS) indicating accumulation of lipids or glycogen.

Similarly, the presence of renal lesions was scored as: no change—1; mild degeneration—2; low degeneration—3; moderate degeneration—4; marked degeneration 5. We observed the presence of alterations in the proximal and distal convoluted tubules, and the presence of calcifications in the glomerulus.

2.8. Statistical Analysis

Data were subjected to analysis of variance (two-way ANOVA) and means were compared by Tukey test ($p < 0.05$). Nonparametric data of liver and kidney damage scores were analyzed by the Kruskal–Wallis test ($p < 0.05$). We performed all analyses using statistical program Sisvar (version 5.3, Universidade Federal de Lavras, Lavras, Minas Gerais, Brazil) [31].

3. Results

Animals submitted to physical training, or consuming beta-glucan isolated and in association, presented lower fast blood glucose and HbA1c levels than diabetic animals (Table 1). Serum levels of TAG, TC and LDL-C were significantly reduced in animals consuming beta-glucan, independently of physical training. In addition, HDL-C levels were higher in animals treated with beta-glucan. Exercise did not significantly alter this parameter (Table 1). The atherogenic index of plasma in animals treated with beta-glucan was lower in comparison to without treatment. An additive effect of beta-glucan and physical exercise was observed for the atherogenic index of plasma. Blood parameters and atherogenic index of plasma means and standard deviations are presented in Table 1.

All treatments promoted similar results in the percentage of protein, fat and water in animals' carcasses. An increase in the percentage of mineral matter was observed in groups under physical training and beta-glucan consumption, with an extra increase when both treatments were associated. Exercise promoted a decrease in the Lee index compared to controls, with similar results among the other groups (Figure 1).

Liver histopathology slices revealed similar signs of steatosis in all groups (Table 2). Likewise, hydropic degeneration was found in the renal tissue from all groups. The degree of these lesions was attenuated by both physical exercise and beta-glucan ingestion (Table 3). Figures 2 and 3 represent, respectively, hepatic steatosis and renal degeneration in the different experimental groups.

Table 1. Biochemical parameters and atherogenic index of plasma in type 2 diabetic rats (high-fat diet/streptozotocin) submitted to physical training and treated beta-glucan (30 mg/kg/day).

	Beta-Glucan	Physical Training	
		Without	With
Glucose (mg/dL)	Without	371.0 (±21.4) [A,a]	335.0 (±10.4) [b]
	With	311.0 (±25.0) [b]	327.5 (±42.6)
HbA1c (mg/dL)	Without	9.4 (±0.4) [A,a]	8.8 (±0.3) [B]
	With	8.33 (±0.1) [b]	8.8 (±0.4)
Triacylglycerols (mg/dL)	Without	105.8 (±11.1) [a]	99.7 (±2.2) [a]
	With	71.5 (±7.2) [b]	57.5 (±12.8) [b]
Total cholesterol (mg/dL)	Without	88.8 (±22.9) [a]	85.4 (±9.4) [a]
	With	65.1 (±3.3) [b]	63.8 (±7.2) [b]
HDL-C (mg/dL)	Without	34.33 (±3.8) [a]	37.7 (±6.9)
	With	42.66 (±5.2) [b]	44.26 (±4.0)
LDL-C (mg/dL)	Without	34.6 (±20.1) [a]	33.4 (±5.8) [a]
	With	10.95 (±3.4) [b]	19.6 (±4.9) [b]
Atherogenic index of plasma	Without	1.6 (±0.6) [a]	1.3 (±0.2) [a]
	With	0.6 (±0.1) [A,b]	0.4 (±0.1) [B,b]

[a,b] Means followed by different letters in columns indicate significant differences between groups with and without beta-glucan treatment ($p < 0.05$); [A,B] Means followed by different letters in lines indicate significant difference between groups with and without physical training ($p < 0.05$).

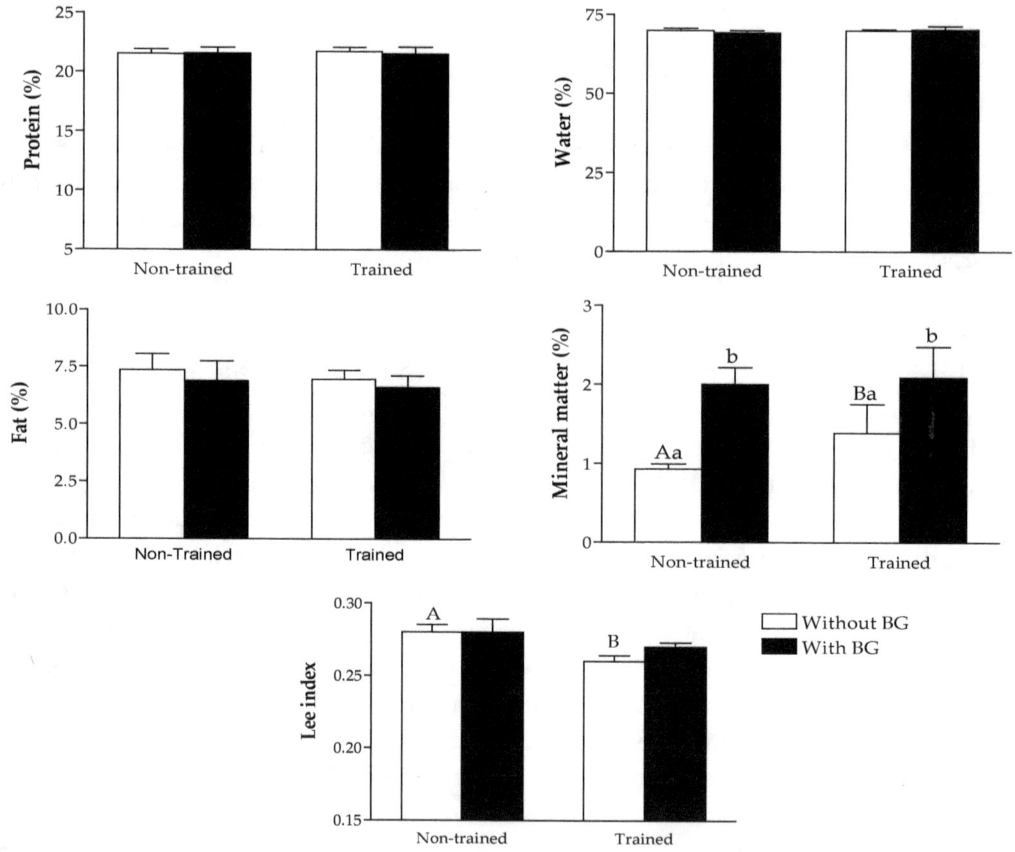

Figure 1. Chemical body composition (water, protein, fat and mineral matter) and Lee index of type 2 diabetic rats (high-fat diet/streptozotocin) submitted to physical training and treated with beta-glucan (30 mg/kg/day). [A,B] Significant difference between trained and non-trained groups; [a,b] Significant difference between groups with and without beta-glucans.

Table 2. Degree of hepatic steatosis in type 2 diabetic rats (HFD/STZ) submitted to physical training and/or treated with beta-glucans (30 mg/kg/day).

Group	Score of Steatosis				
	*	**	***	****	*****
A	0	3	0	3	0
B	1	3	2	0	0
C	2	3	0	1	0
D	1	5	0	0	0

* No change. ** Discreet Degeneration; *** Mild degeneration; **** Moderate degeneration; ***** Marked degeneration; A: diabetes *mellitus*; B: diabetes *mellitus* + beta-glucan; C: diabetes *mellitus* + exercise; D: diabetes *mellitus* + beta-glucan + exercise.

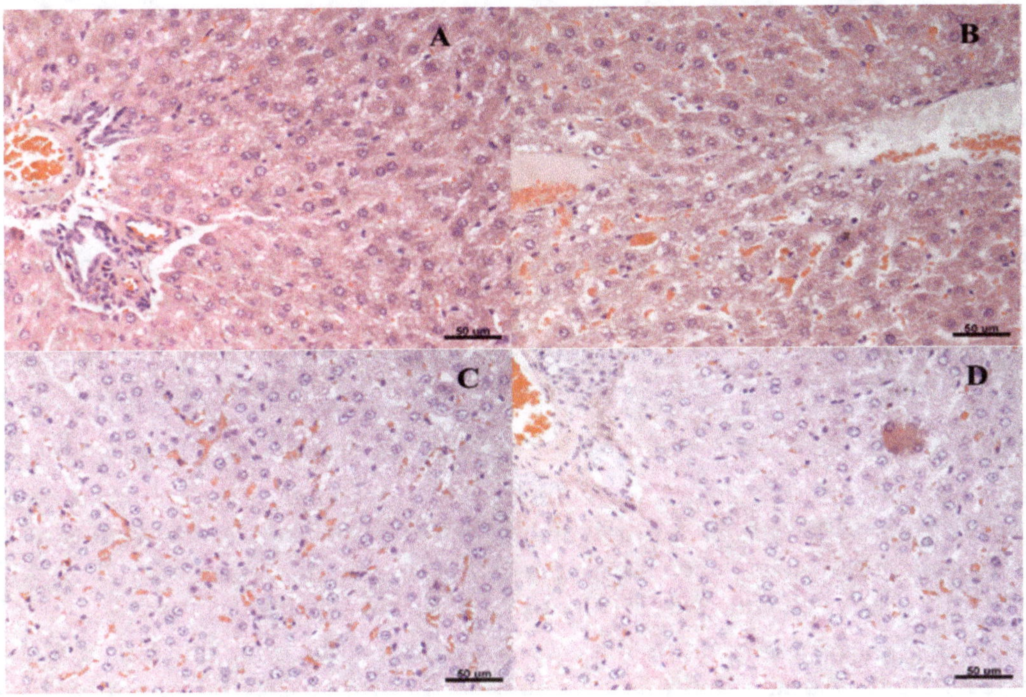

Figure 2. Histological representation (hematoxylin and eosin—20×) of degrees of hepatic steatosis in type 2 diabetic rats (HFD/STZ) submitted to physical training and/or treated with beta-glucans (30 mg/kg/day). (**A**) diabetes *mellitus*; (**B**) diabetes *mellitus* + beta-glucan; (**C**) diabetes *mellitus* + exercise; (**D**) diabetes *mellitus* + beta-glucan + exercise.

Table 3. Degree of renal degeneration in type 2 diabetic rats (HFD/STZ) submitted to physical training and/or treated with beta-glucans (30 mg/kg/day).

	Score of Renal Degeneration				
Group	*	**	***	****	*****
A	0	0	0	2	4
B	0	0	0	6	0
C	0	0	1	5	0
D #	0	0	1	5	0

* No change; ** Discreet Degeneration; *** Mild degeneration; **** Moderate degeneration; ***** Marked degeneration; # Difference compared to the DM group; A: diabetes *mellitus*; B: diabetes *mellitus* + beta-glucan; C: diabetes *mellitus* + exercise; D: diabetes *mellitus* + beta-glucan + exercise.

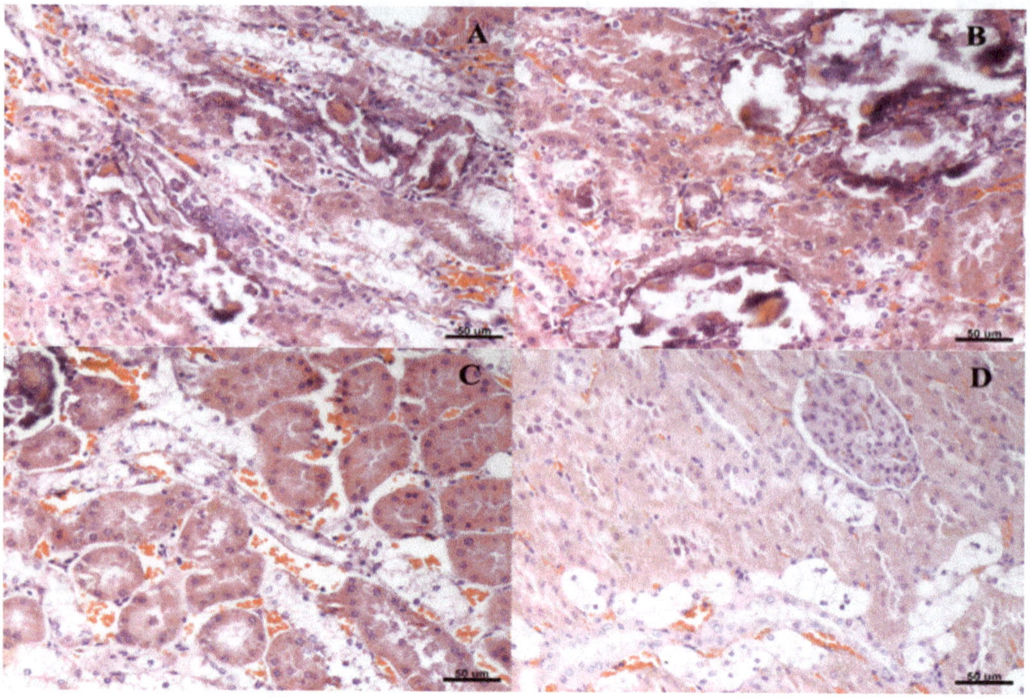

Figure 3. Histological representation (hematoxylin and eosin—20×) of degrees of renal degeneration in type 2 diabetic rats (HFD/STZ) submitted to physical training and/or treated with beta-glucans (30 mg/kg/day). (**A**) diabetes *mellitus*; (**B**) diabetes *mellitus* + beta-glucan; (**C**) diabetes *mellitus* + exercise; (**D**) diabetes *mellitus* + beta-glucan + exercise.

4. Discussion

The main findings of this study were related to improved glycemic control and reduced predisposition to atherosclerosis in animals subjected to both exercise beta-glucan consumption. Moreover, circulating lipoproteins levels, such as total cholesterol, LDL-C, and HDL-C, were improved in animals consuming beta-glucan, independently of physical exercise.

The effects of physical exercise on the improvement of glycemic control in diabetic patients (decrease in HbA1c and fasting glucose) are frequently reported [32–34]. Generally, this effect is due to the increased glucose uptake by skeletal muscle during exercise and increased insulin sensitivity for some hours after physical activity [35]. A beneficial effect in the glycemic control, in our study, was also observed after beta-glucan ingestion, as reported elsewhere in both animal [10] and in human studies [36]. Blood glucose control by beta-glucan consumption is probably due to the fact that these fibers form a gelatinous barrier in the intestinal lumen, hindering the absorption of carbohydrates and lipids by enterocytes [10,37,38]. In this sense, the same mechanism can be used to justify a reduction in circulating levels of total cholesterol, LDL-C and TAG found in groups treated with beta-glucan, with and without exercise. The improvement of the lipid profile, despite the consumption of beta-glucan, was a feature also observed in previous studies from our group [10,17]. The lower lipid absorption in the intestine favors the use of excessive cholesterol to the formation of bile salts in the liver, causing decreased blood concentrations of total cholesterol and LDL-C [39]. This mechanism is generally used to explain the anti-hypercholesterolemic effect of dietary fibers [39].

Among the possible beta-glucan's action, we can highlight the stimulation of intestinal motility, as well as changes in the microbiota and modulation of hormones secretion in the intestine [27,40,41]. Intestinal motility can be stimulated by the increase in the viscosity of the digesta in the lumen, due to the formation of a gelatinous layer [42,43]. In addition, beta-glucan decreases carbohydrates and lipid absorption [42], and consequently decreasing constipation problems [11]. High molecular weight beta-glucans (1,3/1,6) can also serve as a substrate for symbiotic microorganisms present in the intestine, increasing IgA and lysozyme secretion, and, as a consequence, immune resistance [40]. Another mechanism related to the functional effect of beta-glucans is satiety, mediated by gastrointestinal hormones [41]. Beta-glucans modulate the secretion of ghrelin and peptide YY, in order to inhibit hunger, acting indirectly in glycemic and lipidemic control [44].

In this study, we did not observe reduction of circulating lipids in trained animals. This may be related to the training time or duration of exercise sessions. Moura et al. [45] also found similar levels of HDL-C, LDL-C and TAG in diabetic rats (induced by alloxan) and subjected to 44 days of training, compared to sedentary diabetic rats. Another study demonstrated that twelve weeks of aquatic training decreased cholesterol levels and TAG in diabetic Zucker rats [46]. However, in the present study, no significant differences were observed in circulating lipids in animals submitted to physical training, and the atherosclerotic plasma index was reduced when there was an association of exercise and beta-glucan consumption. This additive effect may be related to improvement of the lipid profile provided by the dietary fiber [47], and to the recognized cardiovascular benefits of exercise [48].

Liver and renal lesions observed in all groups are consistent with those observed in type 2 diabetes, where circulating lipid levels promote increased fat deposition both in the liver and kidney [49,50]. However, even with the benefits observed with beta-glucan consumption or exercise, no changes were found in the degree of steatosis in any treatment. Beta-glucan consumption did not significantly alter steatosis either in a recent study of our group that investigated the effects of these fibers in rats submitted to high-fat diet [18]. On the other hand, it was observed that, in Sprague–Dawley rats, hepatic steatosis was reversed after eight weeks of treadmill exercise associated with restrictive diet (low-fat) [51]. Thus, it is possible that, in this study, steatosis was not attenuated because the animals were consuming a high-fat diet throughout the experimental period.

Regarding the effects of exercise, with or without the beta-glucan on the attenuation of renal lesions, it can be considered two mechanisms. The first one involves the reduction in lipotoxicity against moderate exercise [52], since the oxidative stress observed in diabetic patients is one of the factors that predispose to kidney damage [53]. The second one, more likely to explain the results of the present study, is the fact that exercise in moderate intensity promotes improvement in glycemic control, which consequently reduces the generation of advanced glycation-end products (AGE) [54]. Thus, the higher the blood glucose levels, the higher the formation of AGE that attack the kidney tissue and cause diabetic nephropathy [55].

Results of the present research show very promising effects of beta-glucan ingestion for glucose control. Complimentary studies are encouraged, evaluating insulin/leptin levels and inflammatory and cardiovascular parameters as well. The improvement of metabolic parameters in animals that consumed beta-glucans may be related to a decrease in the absorption of nutrients that increase plasma levels of glucose and lipids [37,39]. These changes were not as evident in animals subjected to exercise, possibly due to high-fat diet maintenance for the entire period.

5. Conclusions

Both exercise and beta-glucan consumption alone improved glycemic control in diabetic rats. In the present study, the combination of exercise and beta-glucans improved the atherosclerotic index and decreased renal lesions when compared to the isolated use of the treatments.

Acknowledgments: The authors thank the Coordination of Improvement of Higher Education Personnel (CAPES), the Research Foundation of the State of Minas Gerais (FAPEMIG), the National Council for Research and Technological Development (CNPq), and the Federal University of Lavras (UFLA), Brazil.

Author Contributions: E.F.A., L.J.P. and M.G.Z. conceptualized the study. E.F.A., A.R.V.L., P.N.G. and I.E.N. conducted the experiments. D.R.O. performed histopathologic analysis. M.G.Z. contributed to statistical analysis. E.F.A., F.H.F.A., and L.J.P. were involved in writing and editing the manuscript. All authors participated in the design of the study, study supervision, data interpretation, and revision and approval of the final version of the manuscript.

References

1. Forbes, J.M.; Cooper, M.E. Mechanisms of diabetic complications. *Physiol. Rev.* **2013**, *93*, 137–188. [CrossRef] [PubMed]
2. Chen, L.; Magliano, D.J.; Zimmet, P.Z. The worldwide epidemiology of type 2 diabetes mellitus—Present and future perspectives. *Nat. Rev. Endocrinol.* **2012**, *8*, 228–236. [CrossRef] [PubMed]
3. Kahn, S.E.; Cooper, M.E.; del Prato, S. Pathophysiology and treatment of type 2 diabetes: Perspectives on the past, present, and future. *Lancet (Lond. Engl.)* **2014**, *383*, 1068–1083. [CrossRef]
4. Atkinson, M.A.; Eisenbarth, G.S.; Michels, A.W. Type 1 diabetes. *Lancet* **2014**, *383*, 69–82. [CrossRef]
5. American Diabetes Association. Standards of medical care in diabetes—2015 abridged for primary care providers. *Clin. Diabetes* **2015**, *33*, 97–111.
6. Teixeira-Lemos, E.; Nunes, S.; Teixeira, F.; Reis, F. Regular physical exercise training assists in preventing type 2 diabetes development: Focus on its antioxidant and anti-inflammatory properties. *Cardiovasc. Diabetol.* **2011**, *10*, 12. [CrossRef] [PubMed]
7. Stevens, J.W.; Khunti, K.; Harvey, R.; Johnson, M.; Preston, L.; Woods, H.B.; Davies, M.; Goyder, E. Preventing the progression to type 2 diabetes mellitus in adults at high risk: A systematic review and network meta-analysis of lifestyle, pharmacological and surgical interventions. *Diabetes Res. Clin. Pract.* **2015**, *107*, 320–331. [CrossRef] [PubMed]
8. Thompson, D.; Karpe, F.; Lafontan, M.; Frayn, K. Physical activity and exercise in the regulation of human adipose tissue physiology. *Physiol. Rev.* **2012**, *92*, 157–191. [CrossRef] [PubMed]
9. Samuelsen, A.B.C.; Schrezenmeir, J.; Knutsen, S.H. Effects of orally administered yeast-derived beta-glucans: A review. *Mol. Nutr. Food Res.* **2014**, *58*, 183–193. [CrossRef] [PubMed]
10. De Oliveira Silva, V.; Lobato, R.V.; Andrade, E.F.; de Macedo, C.G.; Napimoga, J.T.C.; Napimoga, M.H.; Messora, M.R.; Murata, R.M.; Pereira, L.J. β-Glucans (*Saccharomyces cereviseae*) Reduce Glucose Levels and Attenuate Alveolar Bone Loss in Diabetic Rats with Periodontal Disease. *PLoS ONE* **2015**, *10*, e0134742.
11. Rahar, S.; Swami, G.; Nagpal, N.; Nagpal, M.A.; Singh, G.S. Preparation, characterization, and biological properties of β-glucans. *J. Adv. Pharm. Technol. Res.* **2011**, *2*, 94–103. [CrossRef] [PubMed]
12. Sonck, E.; Stuyven, E.; Goddeeris, B.; Cox, E. The effect of beta-glucans on porcine leukocytes. *Vet. Immunol. Immunopathol.* **2010**, *135*, 199–207. [CrossRef] [PubMed]
13. Mantovani, M.S.; Bellini, M.F.; Angeli, J.P.F.; Oliveira, R.J.; Silva, A.F.; Ribeiro, L.R. Beta-Glucans in promoting health: Prevention against mutation and cancer. *Mutat. Res.* **2008**, *658*, 154–161. [CrossRef] [PubMed]
14. Andrade, E.F.; Lobato, R.V.; Araújo, T.V.; Zangerônimo, M.G.; Sousa, R.V.; Pereira, L.J. Effect of beta-glucans in the control of blood glucose levels of diabetic patients: A systematic review. *Nutr. Hosp.* **2014**, *31*, 170–177.
15. Akramiene, D.; Kondrotas, A.; Didziapetriene, J.; Kevelaitis, E. Effects of beta-glucans on the immune system. *Medicina (Kaunas)* **2007**, *43*, 597–606. [PubMed]
16. Stier, H.; Ebbeskotte, V.; Gruenwald, J. Immune-modulatory effects of dietary Yeast Beta-1,3/1,6-D-glucan. *Nutr. J.* **2014**, *13*, 38. [CrossRef] [PubMed]
17. Lobato, R.V.; de Silva, V.O.; Andrade, E.F.; Orlando, D.R.; Zangeronimo, M.G.; de Sousa, R.V.; Pereira, L.J. Metabolic effects of β-glucans (*Saccharomyces cerevisae*) per os administration in rats with streptozotocin-induced diabetes. *Nutr. Hosp.* **2015**, *32*, 256–264.
18. De Araújo, T.V.; Andrade, E.F.; Lobato, R.V.; Orlando, D.R.; Gomes, N.F.; de Sousa, R.V.; Zangeronimo, M.G.; Pereira, L.J. Effects of beta-glucans ingestion (*Saccharomyces cerevisiae*) on metabolism of rats receiving high-fat diet. *J. Anim. Physiol. Anim. Nutr. (Berl)* **2016**. [CrossRef] [PubMed]
19. Wang, L.; Duan, G.; Lu, Y.; Pang, S.; Huang, X.; Jiang, Q.; Dang, N. The effect of simvastatin on glucose homeostasis in streptozotocin induced type 2 diabetic rats. *J. Diabetes Res.* **2013**, *2013*, 274986. [CrossRef] [PubMed]
20. Skovsø, S. Modeling type 2 diabetes in rats using high-fat diet and streptozotocin. *J. Diabetes Investig.* **2014**, *5*, 349–358. [CrossRef] [PubMed]
21. Rambo, L.M.; Ribeiro, L.R.; Oliveira, M.S.; Furian, A.F.; Lima, F.D.; Souza, M.A.; Silva, L.F.A.; Retamoso, L.T.; Corte, C.L.D.; Puntel, G.O.; et al. Additive anticonvulsant effects of creatine supplementation and physical exercise against pentylenetetrazol-induced seizures. *Neurochem. Int.* **2009**, *55*, 333–340. [CrossRef] [PubMed]

22. Gobatto, C.A.; de Mello, M.A.; Sibuya, C.Y.; de Azevedo, J.R.; dos Santos, L.A.; Kokubun, E. Maximal lactate steady state in rats submitted to swimming exercise. *Comp. Biochem. Physiol. A Mol. Integr. Physiol.* **2001**, *130*, 21–27. [CrossRef]
23. Andrade, E.F.; Lobato, R.V.; de Araújo, T.V.; Orlando, D.R.; da Costa, D.V.; de Oliveira Silva, V.; Rogatto, G.P.; Zangeronimo, M.G.; Rosa, P.V.; Pereira, L.J. Adaptation to physical training in rats orally supplemented with glycerol. *Can. J. Physiol. Pharmacol.* **2015**, *93*, 63–69. [CrossRef] [PubMed]
24. Amr, A.R.; Abeer, E.E.-K. Hypolipideimic and Hypocholestermic Effect of Pine Nuts in Rats Fed High Fat, Cholesterol-Diet. *World Appl. Sci. J.* **2011**, *15*, 1667–1677.
25. Martinez-flores, H.E.; Kil, Y. Effect of high fiber products on blood lipids and lipoproteins in hamsters. *Nutr. Res.* **2004**, *24*, 85–93. [CrossRef]
26. Hemmati, M.; Zohoori, E.; Mehrpour, O.; Karamian, M.; Asghari, S.; Zarban, A.; Nasouti, R. Anti-atherogenic potential of jujube, saffron and barberry: Anti-diabetic and antioxidant actions. *EXCLI J.* **2015**, *14*, 908–915. [PubMed]
27. Gleissner, C.A.; Galkina, E.; Nadler, J.L.; Ley, K. Mechanisms by which diabetes increases cardiovascular disease. *Drug Discov. Today Dis. Mech.* **2007**, *4*, 131–140. [CrossRef] [PubMed]
28. Lee, M.O. Determination of the surface area of the white rat with its application to the expression of metabolic results. *Am. J. Physiol.* **1929**, *89*, 24–33.
29. Vickers, S.P.; Cheetham, S.; Headland, K.; Dickinson, K.; Grempler, R.; Mayoux, E.; Mark, M.; Klein, T. Combination of the sodium-glucose cotransporter-2 inhibitor empagliflozin with orlistat or sibutramine further improves the body-weight reduction and glucose homeostasis of obese rats fed a cafeteria diet. *Diabetes Metab. Syndr. Obes. Targets Ther.* **2014**, *7*, 265–275. [CrossRef] [PubMed]
30. Andrade, E.F.; Lobato, R.V.; Araújo, T.V.; Orlando, D.R.; Gomes, N.F.; Alvarenga, R.R.; Rogatto, G.P.; Zangeronimo, M.G.; Pereira, L.J. Metabolic effects of glycerol supplementation and aerobic physical training on Wistar rats. *Can. J. Physiol. Pharmacol.* **2014**, *92*, 744–751. [CrossRef] [PubMed]
31. Ferreira, D.F. Sisvar: A computer statistical analysis system. *Ciênc. Agrotec.* **2011**, *35*, 1039–1042.
32. Hall, K.E.; McDonald, M.W.; Grisé, K.N.; Campos, O.A.; Noble, E.G.; Melling, C.W.J. The role of resistance and aerobic exercise training on insulin sensitivity measures in STZ-induced Type 1 diabetic rodents. *Metabolism* **2013**, *62*, 1485–1494. [CrossRef] [PubMed]
33. Ghiasi, R.; Ghadiri Soufi, F.; Somi, M.H.; Mohaddes, G.; Mirzaie Bavil, F.; Naderi, R.; Alipour, M.R. Swim Training Improves HOMA-IR in Type 2 Diabetes Induced by High Fat Diet and Low Dose of Streptozotocin in Male Rats. *Adv. Pharm. Bull.* **2015**, *5*, 379–384. [CrossRef] [PubMed]
34. Silveira, A.P.S.; Bentes, C.M.; Costa, P.B.; Simão, R.; Silva, F.C.; Silva, R.P.; Novaes, J.S. Acute effects of different intensities of resistance training on glycemic fluctuations in patients with type 1 diabetes mellitus. *Res. Sports Med.* **2014**, *22*, 75–87. [CrossRef] [PubMed]
35. Borghouts, L.B.; Keizer, H.A. Exercise and insulin sensitivity: A review. *Int. J. Sports Med.* **2000**, *21*, 1–12. [CrossRef] [PubMed]
36. He, L.; Zhao, J.; Huang, Y.; Li, Y. The difference between oats and beta-glucan extract intake in the management of HbA1c, fasting glucose and insulin sensitivity: A meta-analysis of randomized controlled trials. *Food Funct.* **2016**, *7*, 1413–1428. [CrossRef] [PubMed]
37. Tappy, L.; Gügolz, E.; Würsch, P. Effects of breakfast cereals containing various amounts of beta-glucan fibers on plasma glucose and insulin responses in NIDDM subjects. *Diabetes Care* **1996**, *19*, 831–834. [CrossRef] [PubMed]
38. Choi, J.S.; Kim, H.; Jung, M.H.; Hong, S.; Song, J. Consumption of barley beta-glucan ameliorates fatty liver and insulin resistance in mice fed a high-fat diet. *Mol. Nutr. Food Res.* **2010**, *54*, 1004–1013. [CrossRef] [PubMed]
39. Rideout, T.C.; Harding, S.V.; Jones, P.J.; Fan, M.Z. Guar gum and similar soluble fibers in the regulation of cholesterol metabolism: Current understandings and future research priorities. *Vasc. Health Risk Manag.* **2008**, *4*, 1023–1033. [CrossRef] [PubMed]
40. Raa, J. Immune modulation by non-digestible and non-absorbable beta-1,3/1,6-glucan. *Microb. Ecol. Health Dis.* **2015**, *26*, 27824. [CrossRef] [PubMed]
41. Rebello, C.J.; Burton, J.; Heiman, M.; Greenway, F.L. Gastrointestinal microbiome modulator improves glucose tolerance in overweight and obese subjects: A randomized controlled pilot trial. *J. Diabetes Complicat.* **2015**, *29*, 1272–1276. [CrossRef] [PubMed]

42. Reyna, N.Y.; Cano, C.; Bermúdez, V.J.; Medina, M.T.; Souki, A.J.; Ambard, M.; Nuñez, M.; Ferrer, M.A.; Inglett, G.E. Sweeteners and beta-glucans improve metabolic and anthropometrics variables in well controlled type 2 diabetic patients. *Am. J. Ther.* **2003**, *10*, 438–443. [CrossRef] [PubMed]
43. Battilana, P.; Ornstein, K.; Minehira, K.; Schwarz, J.M.; Acheson, K.; Schneiter, P.; Burri, J.; Jéquier, E.; Tappy, L. Mechanisms of action of beta-glucan in postprandial glucose metabolism in healthy men. *Eur. J. Clin. Nutr.* **2001**, *55*, 327–333. [CrossRef] [PubMed]
44. Vitaglione, P.; Lumaga, R.B.; Stanzione, A.; Scalfi, L.; Fogliano, V. β-Glucan-enriched bread reduces energy intake and modifies plasma ghrelin and peptide YY concentrations in the short term. *Appetite* **2009**, *53*, 338–344. [CrossRef] [PubMed]
45. Moura, L.P.; Puga, G.M.; Beck, W.R.; Teixeira, I.P.; Ghezzi, A.C.; Silva, G.A.; Mello, M.A.R. Exercise and spirulina control non-alcoholic hepatic steatosis and lipid profile in diabetic Wistar rats. *Lipids Health Dis.* **2011**, *10*, 2–7. [CrossRef] [PubMed]
46. De Lemos, E.T.; Pinto, R.; Oliveira, J.; Garrido, P.; Sereno, J.; Mascarenhas-Melo, F.; Páscoa-Pinheiro, J.; Teixeira, F.; Reis, F. Differential effects of acute (extenuating) and chronic (training) exercise on inflammation and oxidative stress status in an animal model of type 2 diabetes mellitus. *Mediat. Inflamm.* **2011**, *2011*, 253061.
47. Bays, H.E.; Evans, J.L.; Maki, K.C.; Evans, M.; Maquet, V.; Cooper, R.; Anderson, J.W. Chitin-glucan fiber effects on oxidized low-density lipoprotein: A randomized controlled trial. *Eur. J. Clin. Nutr.* **2013**, *67*, 2–7. [CrossRef] [PubMed]
48. Roberts, C.K.; Chen, A.K.; Barnard, R.J. Effect of a short-term diet and exercise intervention in youth on atherosclerotic risk factors. *Atherosclerosis* **2007**, *191*, 98–106. [CrossRef] [PubMed]
49. Alsaad, K.O.; Herzenberg, A.M. Distinguishing diabetic nephropathy from other causes of glomerulosclerosis: An update. *J. Clin. Pathol.* **2007**, *60*, 18–26. [CrossRef] [PubMed]
50. Birkenfeld, A.L.; Shulman, G.I. Nonalcoholic fatty liver disease, hepatic insulin resistance, and type 2 Diabetes. *Hepatology* **2014**, *59*, 713–723. [CrossRef] [PubMed]
51. Gauthier, M.-S.; Couturier, K.; Latour, J.-G.; Lavoie, J.-M. Concurrent exercise prevents high-fat-diet-induced macrovesicular hepatic steatosis. *J. Appl. Physiol.* **2003**, *94*, 2127–2134. [CrossRef] [PubMed]
52. Ghosh, S.; Khazaei, M.; Moien-Afshari, F.; Ang, L.S.; Granville, D.J.; Verchere, C.B.; Dunn, S.R.; McCue, P.; Mizisin, A.; Sharma, K.; et al. Moderate exercise attenuates caspase-3 activity, oxidative stress, and inhibits progression of diabetic renal disease in db/db mice. *Am. J. Physiol. Renal Physiol.* **2009**, *296*, 700–708. [CrossRef] [PubMed]
53. Tanaka, Y.; Kume, S.; Araki, S.; Isshiki, K.; Chin-Kanasaki, M.; Sakaguchi, M.; Sugimoto, T.; Koya, D.; Haneda, M.; Kashiwagi, A.; et al. Fenofibrate, a PPARα agonist, has renoprotective effects in mice by enhancing renal lipolysis. *Kidney Int.* **2011**, *79*, 871–882. [CrossRef] [PubMed]
54. Boor, P.; Celec, P.; Behuliak, M.; Grančič, P.; Kebis, A.; Kukan, M.; Pronayová, N.; Liptaj, T.; Ostendorf, T.; Šebeková, K. Regular moderate exercise reduces advanced glycation and ameliorates early diabetic nephropathy in obese Zucker rats. *Metabolism* **2009**, *58*, 1669–1677. [CrossRef] [PubMed]
55. Yamagishi, S.-I.; Matsui, T. Advanced glycation end products, oxidative stress and diabetic nephropathy. *Oxid. Med. Cell. Longev.* **2010**, *3*, 101–108. [CrossRef] [PubMed]

13

Wheat Bran does not Affect Postprandial Plasma Short-Chain Fatty Acids from ^{13}C-inulin Fermentation in Healthy Subjects

Lise Deroover [1], Joran Verspreet [2,3], Anja Luypaerts [1], Greet Vandermeulen [1], Christophe M. Courtin [2,3] and Kristin Verbeke [1,3,*]

1. Translational Research in Gastrointestinal Disorders, KU Leuven, Leuven 3000, Belgium; lise.deroover@kuleuven.be (L.D.); anja.luypaerts@kuleuven.be (A.L.); greet.vandermeulen@kuleuven.be (G.V.)
2. Centre for Food and Microbial Technology, KU Leuven, Leuven 3000, Belgium; joran.verspreet@kuleuven.be (J.V.); christophe.courtin@kuleuven.be (C.M.C.)
3. Leuven Food Science and Nutrition Research Centre, KU Leuven, Leuven 3000, Belgium

* Correspondence: kristin.verbeke@kuleuven.be;

Abstract: Wheat bran (WB) is a constituent of whole grain products with beneficial effects for human health. Within the human colon, such insoluble particles may be colonized by specific microbial teams which can stimulate cross-feeding, leading to a more efficient carbohydrate fermentation and an increased butyrate production. We investigated the extent to which WB fractions with different properties affect the fermentation of other carbohydrates in the colon. Ten healthy subjects performed four test days, during which they consumed a standard breakfast supplemented with 10 g ^{13}C-inulin. A total of 20 g of a WB fraction (unmodified WB, wheat bran with a reduced particle size (WB RPS), or de-starched pericarp-enriched wheat bran (PE WB)) was also added to the breakfast, except for one test day, which served as a control. Blood samples were collected at regular time points for 14 h, in order to measure ^{13}C-labeled short-chain fatty acid (SCFA; acetate, propionate and butyrate) concentrations. Fermentation of ^{13}C-inulin resulted in increased plasma SCFA for about 8 h, suggesting that a sustained increase in plasma SCFA can be achieved by administering a moderate dose of carbohydrates, three times per day. However, the addition of a single dose of a WB fraction did not further increase the ^{13}C-SCFA concentrations in plasma, nor did it stimulate cross-feeding (Wilcoxon signed ranks test).

Keywords: colonic fermentation; short-chain fatty acids; wheat bran; inulin

---

1. Introduction

The short-chain fatty acids (SCFA) acetate, propionate, and butyrate, constitute a major class of bacterial metabolites that are derived from colonic carbohydrate fermentation. They are increasingly considered as signaling molecules with a beneficial impact on gut and systemic health [1,2]. Indeed, besides serving as energy substrates for the colonocytes, SCFA influence the expression of many genes by acting as inhibitors of histone deacetylases, and affect metabolic processes through the activation of G-protein coupled receptors (GPR41 and GPR43, later renamed as free fatty acid receptor (FFAR)-3 and (FFAR)-2). Several studies have indicated that SCFA, and in particular butyrate, improve the intestinal barrier function and reduce inflammation by inhibiting NFκB activation [3,4]. In addition, SCFA that enter the systemic circulation modulate energy homeostasis, and peripheral glucose and lipid metabolism [4–6]. Furthermore, SCFA regulate immune function by affecting T cell differentiation into effector and regulatory T cells (Treg) [7], and colonic Treg cell homeostasis [8].

As a consequence, strategies that target the microbiota to improve health often aim at increasing saccharolytic fermentation. The production of colonic SCFA may be stimulated by modulating the intestinal microbiota and increasing the numbers of acetate and butyrate producing bacteria via administration of probiotics. Many probiotics are selected strains of lactobacilli or bifidobacteria [9], which are known lactate and acetate producers. In addition, there is a growing interest in the use of butyrate producing bacteria, such as *Faecalibacterium prausnitzii* and *Butyrcicoccus pullicaecorum*, as probiotics [10–13].

An alternative strategy for increasing SCFA production is to stimulate the indigenous saccharolytic bacterial population by administration of prebiotics or fermentable dietary fibers [14]. The best studied prebiotic substrates are inulin-type fructans (comprising oligofructose), galacto-oligosaccharides, xylo-oligosaccharides, and arabinoxylanoligosaccharides. In vitro fermentation studies with fecal inocula indicate that the amount and proportion of SCFA produced, depends on the type of fermentable substrate [15]. For example, inulin-type fructans induce a relatively high proportion of acetate, whereas resistant starch favors butyrate production [16].

Here, we applied a third strategy for modulating the entire intestinal ecosystem, which involves the administration of disperse insoluble particles that act as platforms on which the bacteria can adhere, grow, and interact. We hypothesize that these particles facilitate the exchange of microbial nutrients and metabolites, resulting in a more complete carbohydrate fermentation and increased cross-feeding. For example, the production of butyrate requires collaboration between primary degraders, such as bifidobacteria, that produce acetate and lactate, and butyrate producing bacteria, such as *Faecalibacterium* and *Roseburia*, that convert acetate into butyrate [17,18]. This interaction may be facilitated if both species adhere to the dietary platforms. Wheat bran (WB) was selected as an interesting dietary component for this purpose, as bacterial communities attached to WB that was incubated in vitro with human fecal inocula, were found to be dominated by *Clostridium* cluster XIVa bacteria, known as butyrate producers [19]. In addition, WB can be easily technically modified to control its physical properties. In this study, we evaluated the impact of three WB fractions that differed in particle size and tissue composition, on the fermentation of a readily fermentable carbohydrate (^{13}C-inulin) in healthy subjects. Concentrations of ^{13}C-SCFA were measured in plasma as an indication of carbohydrate fermentation and the relative proportions of acetate, propionate, and butyrate, were considered as a marker of cross-feeding.

2. Materials and Methods

2.1. WB Fractions

2.1.1. Unmodified WB

Commercial WB with a particle size of 1690 μm was obtained from Dossche Mills (Deinze, Belgium) and was used without further modification. Its chemical composition (amounts of dietary fiber, starch, protein, lipid, and ash) was analysed as previously described [20–22].

2.1.2. Wheat Bran with Reduced Particle Size (WB RPS)

The unmodified commercial WB mentioned above was milled in a Cyclotec 1093 Sample mill (FOSS, Höganäs, Sweden), as described previously [22], in order to obtain WB particles with an average size of 150 μm.

2.1.3. Destarched Pericarp-Enriched Wheat Bran (PE WB)

PE WB was ascertained from Fugeia N.V. (Leuven, Belgium) and was obtained after an amylase and xylanase treatment of untreated WB, as described by Swennen et al. [23]. Subsequently, the PE WB was reduced in particle size to about 280 μm, using the same method as mentioned above.

2.2. Fermentable Substrate

Highly ^{13}C-enriched inulin with an atom percent (AP) beyond 97% was purchased from Isolife (Wageningen, The Netherlands) and was mixed with unlabeled native inulin (Fibruline instant, Cosucra Groupe Warcoing SA, Warcoing, Belgium; AP 0.98%), to form a homogeneous mixture with an AP of 1.93%.

2.3. Study Population

Ten healthy men and woman, aged between 18 and 65 years, were recruited to participate in the study. All subjects had a body mass index (BMI) between 18 and 27 kg/m^2 and a regular diet defined as three meals per day, on at least five days per week. Exclusion criteria were the use of antibiotics, prebiotics and probiotics, in the month preceding the study and during the study, consumption of a low calorie diet or another special diet in the month prior to the study, the use of medication that could affect the gastrointestinal tract in the two weeks before the start of the study and during the study, abdominal surgery in the past (except for appendectomy), chronic gastrointestinal diseases, blood donation in the three months prior to the study, hemoglobin (Hb) levels below reference values, and for woman, pregnancy or breast feeding. Subjects that had participated in a clinical trial involving radiation exposure in the year prior to the study were also excluded. The study protocol conformed to the Declaration of Helsinki and was approved by the Ethics Committee of the University of Leuven (Belgian Registration Number: B322201423101). All participants signed written informed consent. The study has been registered at ClinicalTrials.gov (clinical trial number: NCT02422537).

2.4. Study Design

Each subject performed four test days, with at least one week in between each test. During the three days prior to each test day, subjects were instructed to consume a low fiber diet, consisting of a maximum of one piece of fruit per day, white bread instead of wholegrain products, and no more than 100 g vegetables per day. They were also asked to avoid alcohol consumption. On the evening prior to the test day, the subjects consumed a completely digestible and non-fermentable meal (lasagna), eventually supplemented with white bread. After an overnight fast, the subjects presented themselves at the laboratory and provided two basal breath samples for the measurement of $^{13}CO_2$ and $^{14}CO_2$. A catheter (BD, Erembodegem, Belgium) was placed into an antecubital vein in the forearm to collect all blood samples during the test day. After collection of a basal blood sample, a standard breakfast was administered to the subjects. The breakfast consisted of 250 g low-fat yoghurt labeled with inulin-^{14}C-carboxylic acid (74 kBq, Perkin Elmer, Boston, MA, USA), a marker for oro-cecal transit time (OCTT), and 10 g of ^{13}C-labeled inulin, which served as a model fermentable substrate. The OCTT was defined as the time that elapses between the intake of the meal, and the arrival in the colon, which is reflected by the appearance of $^{14}CO_2$ in the breath. Depending on the test day, the breakfast was further supplemented with 20 g of one of the three WB fractions, or no supplement on the control test day. The participants were blind to the order of the different WB fractions and control tests, which were randomized using online software [24]. Breath samples were collected every 20 min, up to 14 h after consumption of the breakfast. Blood samples were collected every hour during the first 4 h, every 40 min from 4 h to 10 h, and again every hour from 10 h to 14 h. A light digestible meal was offered to the subjects 4 h and 8 h after consumption of the breakfast. Water was offered *ad libitum* during the whole test day. The course of a test day is represented in Figure 1.

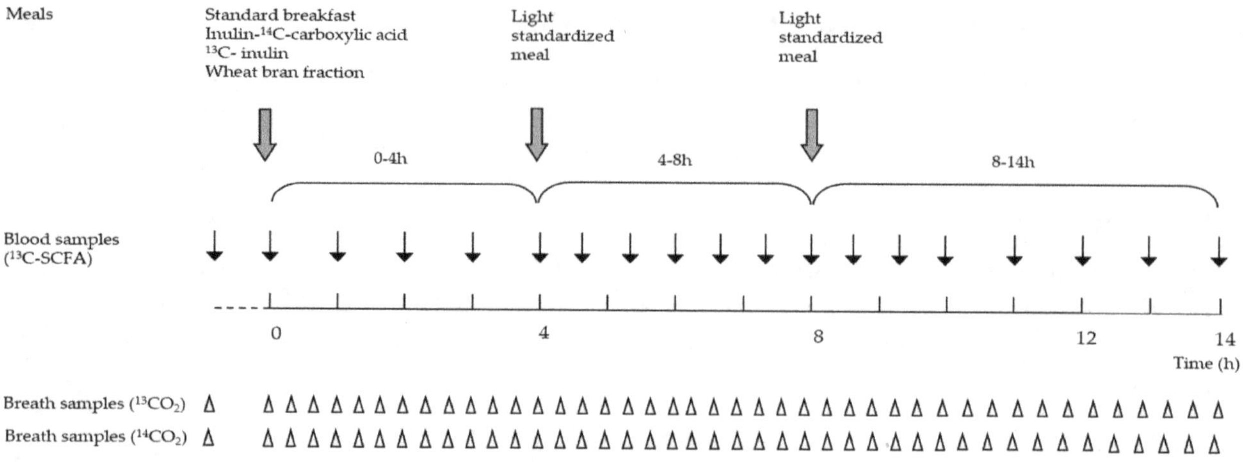

Figure 1. After a standard breakfast, labeled with ^{13}C-inulin, inulin-^{14}C-carboxylic acid and a WB fraction, breath samples were collected for the measurement of $^{13}CO_2$ and $^{14}CO_2$ and blood samples were collected for the analysis of ^{13}C-SCFA concentrations for 14 h. A light standardized meal was administered after 4 h and 8 h. The participants were blind to the order of the different WB fractions and control tests, which were randomized.

2.5. Collection and Analysis of Breath Samples

Subjects deposited breath samples for the analysis of $^{13}CO_2$ by blowing through a straw, into a 12-mL glass tube (Exetainer®, Labco Ltd., Ceredigion, UK), whereas samples for the measurement of $^{14}CO_2$ were collected by blowing through a pipet, into a plastic scintillation vial (Sarstedt, Nümbrecht, Germany) containing 4 mL of a 0.5 M hyamine hydroxide solution (Perkin Elmer, Boston MA, USA). Thymolphtaleine acted as a color indicator, which became discolored when 2 mmol CO_2 was exhaled.

The abundance of $^{13}CO_2$ was measured using isotope ratio mass spectrometry (ABCA, Sercon, Crewe, UK) and the results were expressed as delta over baseline (DOB). $^{14}CO_2$ was measured using β-scintillation counting (Packard Tricarb Liquid Scintillation Spectrometer, model 3375, Packard Instruments, Downers Grove, IL, USA), after addition of 10 mL hionic fluor (Perkin Elmer, Boston MA, USA), and was expressed as disintegrations per minute (DPM) [25]. The arrival time of the breakfast in the colon (OCTT) and the start of the fermentation, were defined as the time at which a significant increase in $^{14}CO_2$ and $^{13}CO_2$, respectively, from the background was observed in the breath. This increase was defined as 2.5 times the standard deviation of all previous points, above the running average of all previous points [26].

2.6. Analysis of Plasma ^{13}C-Abundance

Blood samples were centrifuged at 3000× *g* and 4 °C for 10 min to obtain plasma. The samples were immediately aliquoted and stored at −80 °C until analysis. Plasma samples were deproteinized using Amicon® Ultra-15 filters (Molecular weight cut-off: 30 kDa, Merck, Kenilworth, NJ, USA). Before application of the sample, the filters were rinsed twice using 0.2 N HCl to avoid SCFA contamination. Subsequently, 3 mL plasma was mixed with 3 mL MilliQ® water (Sartorius Arium® 611-VF, Sartorius, Göttingen, Germany) and 150 μL 0.15 N NaOH, and centrifuged at 2000× *g* and 4 °C for 20 min. Following this, the samples were transferred to the cleaned filters and deproteinized by centrifugation at 3000× *g* and 4 °C for 3 h. After addition of 120 μL 1 M NaOH, the filtrate was dried overnight in a vacuum concentrator (RVC 2-18, Christ, Germany) at 50 °C.

Prior to injection, the dried samples were acidified with 100 μL 4 M HCl with trypan blue (0.4%, Sigma, UK), and extracted in 400 μL diethyl ether (Sigma-Aldrich, Steinheim, Germany). The ether layer was pipetted into a crimp neck vial (1.5 mL) and evaporated with nitrogen gas (N_2) to about 50 μL, before injection in the gas chromatograph combustion isotope ratio mass spectrometer (GC-C-IRMS) (Delta plus-XP, Thermo Fisher, Bremen, Germany), equipped with a trace gas chromatograph (Interscience, Breda, The Netherlands) and a combustion interface type 3 (Thermo Fisher). Four µL of the SCFA solution was injected on an AT-Aquawax-DA column (30 m × 0.53 mm, i.d., 1.00 µm, Grace, Lokeren, Belgium), with the injector temperature at 240 °C. Helium 5.0 was used as a carrier gas at a constant flow of 2.5 mL/min. The initial oven temperature was held at 80 °C for 3 min and was increased by 4 °C/min to 140 °C, then further increased by 8 °C/min to 240 °C, and kept at this temperature for 10 min. The separated GC-effluents were combusted and oxidised to NO_x, CO_2, and H_2O in an oxidation furnace (CuO/NiO/Pt) at 940 °C [25]. All oxidised components were passed over the reduction column at 640 °C and the H_2O in the system was eliminated by a Nafion membrane (Thermo Fisher). The delta (δ^{13} Pee Dee Belemnite (PDB)) values were calculated by Isodat 2.0 software (Thermo Fisher) and converted to AP. The measured AP at any time point *t* was subtracted from the abundance measured in the baseline sample at time point 0, to obtain results in atom per cent excess (APE) [25]. The linearity of the system (slope < 0.06) was confirmed to be in the range between 0.8 and 11 volts, with CO_2 as the reference gas (5.0 quality, $\delta = -32.16‰$).

2.7. Analysis of Total SCFA Concentrations in Plasma

The total concentration of acetate, propionate, and butyrate in the plasma was measured using gas chromatography coupled with a flame ionization detector (GC-FID) after preconcentration of the SCFA, using a hollow fiber liquid membrane extraction. Plasma samples were thawed prior to analysis, and prepared and analyzed as described by Zhao et al. [27], with slight modifications. Plasma samples (100 µL) were rapidly spiked with internal standard (12.5 µg 2-ethyl butyric acid and 30 µg 3-methyl-valeric acid), acidified with 20 µL 0.2 N HCl, and diluted to 1.5 mL. A hollow fiber coated with tri-n-octylphoshphine oxide and filled with 10 µL 0.15 N NaOH, was immersed in the diluted plasma and shaken overnight. In this way, protonated SCFA diffuse into the fiber, where they become ionized and remain trapped. After acidification of the fiber content, 0.5 µL of the acidified SCFA solution was injected in a GC (HP 6890 series, Agilent, Wilmington, NC, USA) equipped with a FID and a DB-FAPP capillary column (30 m × 0.53 mm id, 1.00 µm film, Agilent, Wilmington, NC, USA). Helium was used as a carrier gas at a flow rate of 4.2 mL/min. The initial oven temperature was 100 °C for 3 min, raised by 4 °C/min to 140 °C, and held at this temperature for 5 min, before being further increased by 40 °C/min to 235 °C, and finally held at 235 °C for 5 min. The temperature of the FID heater and the injection port were set at 240 °C and 200 °C, respectively. The flow rates of hydrogen, air, and nitrogen as the make-up gas, were 30, 300, and 20 mL/min, respectively.

2.8. Calculations

At each time point, the concentration of ^{13}C-SCFA in plasma is the sum of the concentration that was already present at the baseline, and the concentration that originates from the colon (Equation (1)).

$$\left[{}^{13}\text{C-SCFA}\right] = \left[{}^{13}\text{C-SCFA}\right]_{t_0} + \left[{}^{13}\text{C-SCFA}\right]_{colon} \tag{1}$$

where $\left[{}^{13}\text{C-SCFA}\right]_{t_0}$ is the concentration of ^{13}C-SCFA present in plasma at time point 0 and $\left[{}^{13}\text{C-SCFA}\right]_{colon}$ is the concentration of ^{13}C-SCFA coming from the colon at time point t.

Substitution of the concentration of ^{13}C-SCFA by the product of its total concentration and abundance, results in Equation (2).

$$n_t \times AP_t = n_0 \times AP_{plasma_{t_0}} + n_{colon} \times AP_{colon} \tag{2}$$

In addition, the total concentration of SCFA at each time point t is the sum of the SCFA already present in the plasma, and the SCFA produced in the colon (Equation (3)).

$$n_t = n_0 + n_{colon} \tag{3}$$

Substitution of n_0 by n_t-n_{colon} in Equation (2), allows one to calculate the concentration of SCFA originating from the colon, thus produced from the ^{13}C-inulin at a time point t, according to Equation (4).

$$n_{colon} = n_t \times \frac{\left(AP_t - AP_{plasma_{t_0}}\right)}{\left(AP_{colon} - AP_{plasma_{t_0}}\right)} \tag{4}$$

where n_{colon} is the concentration of SCFA originating from the colon; n_t is the total concentration of SCFA at time point t; AP_t is the AP of ^{13}C-acetate, ^{13}C-propionate, or ^{13}C-butyrate at time point t; AP_{colon} is the AP of the administered inulin; $AP_{plasma_{t_0}}$ is the atom percent of ^{13}C-acetate, ^{13}C-propionate, or ^{13}C-butyrate in the plasma at time point t_0.

The concentrations of ^{13}C-acetate, ^{13}C-propionate, and ^{13}C-butyrate, originating from the colon at each time point, were used to draw concentration versus time curves for each test day. Subsequently, the cumulative concentrations of ^{13}C-acetate, ^{13}C-propionate, and ^{13}C-butyrate (area under the curve (AUC)) were calculated using the trapezoidal rule and were expressed in μmol·h/L.

The starting point of the fermentation was ascertained by calculating the mean time at which ^{13}C-acetate, ^{13}C-propionate, and ^{13}C-butyrate concentrations in plasma increased. The end of the fermentation was the mean time at which ^{13}C-acetate, ^{13}C-propionate, and ^{13}C-butyrate concentrations returned to the baseline. The duration of the fermentation was the difference between the end and start points of the fermentation.

2.9. Statistical Analysis

Statistical analysis was performed using SPSS software, version 23.0 (IBM, Brussels, Belgium). Because of the small sample size, non-parametric tests were used (Wilcoxon signed ranks test).

3. Results

3.1. Characterisation of the WB Fractions

Untreated WB had an average particle size of 1690 μm and was composed of 50% dietary fiber (arabinoxylan, cellulose, β-glucan, lignin and fructan), 17% starch, 20% protein, 6% lipids, and 7% ash (Figure 2a). WB RPS did not differ in tissue composition from the unmodified WB (Figure 2a). In contrast, PE WB was composed of 71% dietary fiber (mainly insoluble), 2% starch, 18% protein, 6% lipids, and 7% ash (Figure 2b).

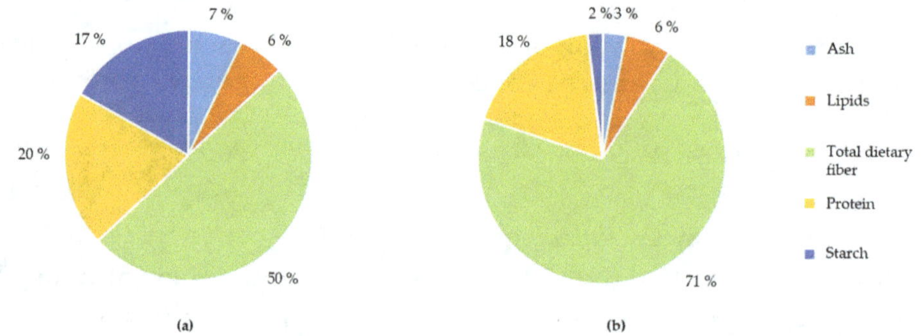

Figure 2. Unmodified wheat bran (WB) and wheat bran with reduced particle size (WB RPS) (**a**) contain less total dietary fiber and more starch compared to destarched pericarp-enriched wheat bran (PE WB) (**b**).

3.2. Study Population

From the 58 subjects that responded to the advertisement, 15 subjects underwent screening, which included an assessment of height and body weight, plasma Hb levels, medical history, and dietary habits (Figure 3). Five volunteers withdrew from the study before the start because of a lack of time (n = 3), pregnancy (n = 1), or because they did not meet the inclusion criteria (n = 1). Ten subjects (4M/6F, aged 25 ± 4 years, BMI 23.7 ± 2.0 kg/m^2) completed the four test days according to the study protocol.

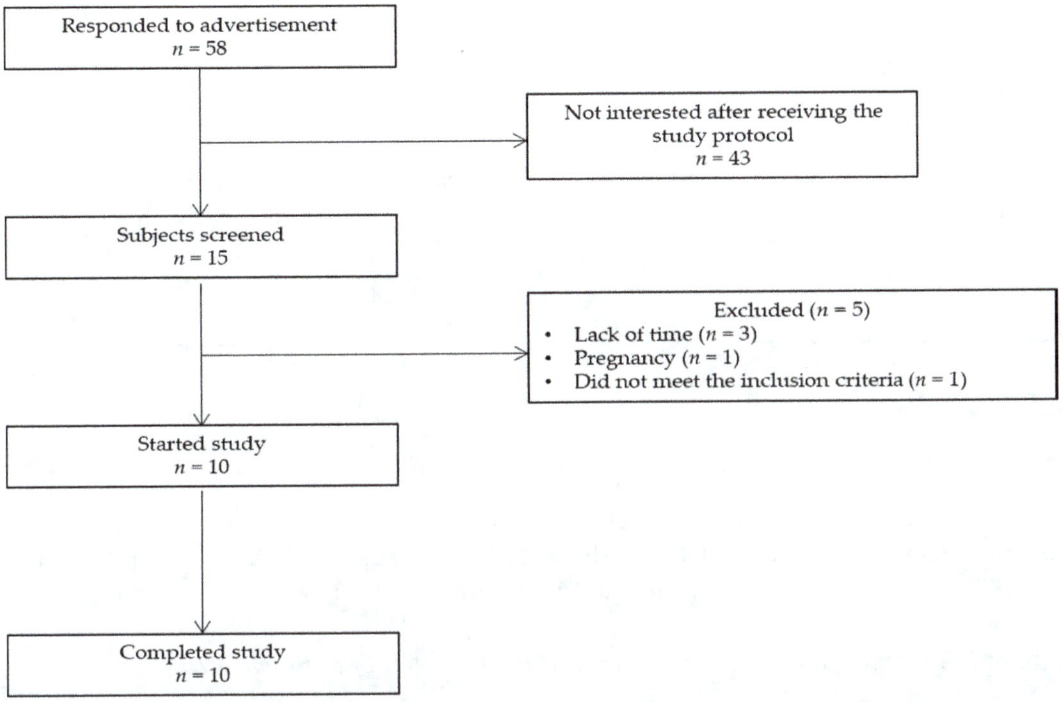

Figure 3. Flow chart depicting the passage of subjects through the study.

3.3. Estimation of the OCTT and the Start of the Fermentation Using Breath and Plasma Samples

The start of the fermentation was defined as the time point at which $^{13}CO_2$ started to increase in the breath, or as the mean time point at which the concentration of ^{13}C-acetate, ^{13}C-propionate, and ^{13}C-butyrate started to increase in the plasma. An increase in breath $^{14}CO_2$, which was generated from bacterial fermentation of ^{14}C-labeled inulin carboxylic acid, was used as a marker for the OCTT. Figure 4a,b compare the OCTT to the start of fermentation, based on breath $^{13}CO_2$ excretion and plasma ^{13}C-SCFA concentrations, respectively. The increase in breath $^{13}CO_2$ and in plasma ^{13}C-SCFA occurred slightly before the increase in breath $^{14}CO_2$, suggesting that fermentation of ^{13}C-inulin had already started in the terminal ileum.

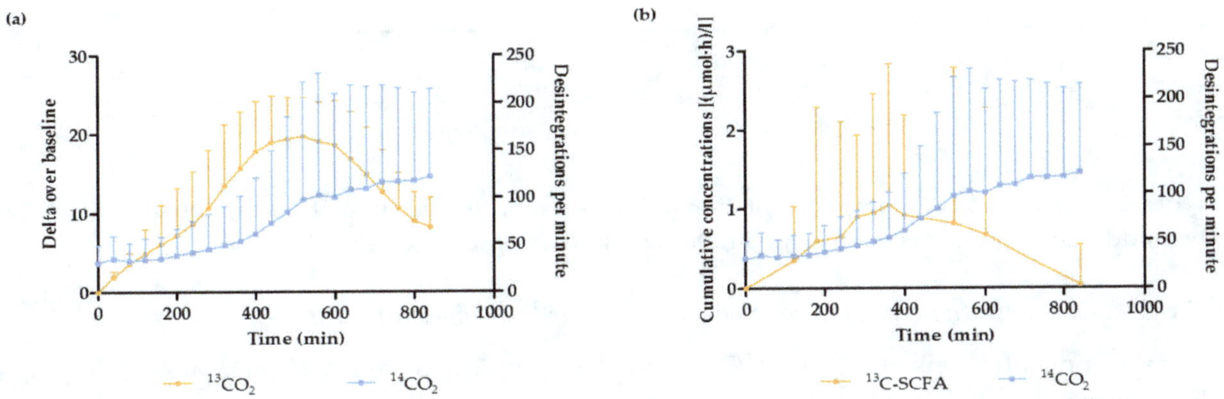

Figure 4. Both ^{13}C-excretion in breath (**a**) and plasma ^{13}C-SCFA concentrations (**b**) start to increase before the increase in breath $^{14}CO_2$ (n = 40).

On average, the fermentation started 208.5 ± 29 min and 219 ± 24.2 min after consumption of the breakfast, based on the breath samples and the plasma samples, respectively. The start of the fermentation was not affected by the addition of any of the WB fractions, when compared to the control (Wilcoxon signed ranks test; Breath samples: $p_{WB} = 0.073$, $p_{WBRPS} = 0.125$, $p_{PEWB} = 0.619$; Plasma samples: $p_{WB} = 0.123$, $p_{WBRPS} = 0.482$, $p_{PEWB} = 0.066$) (Figure 5a,b).

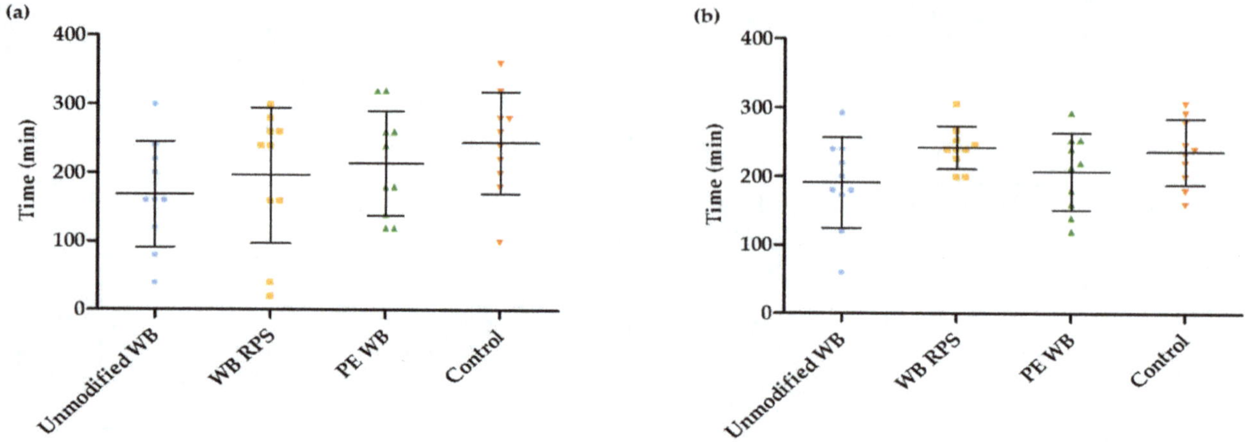

Figure 5. Wheat bran (WB) supplementation did not affect the start of the fermentation based on the $^{13}CO_2$-breath excretion (**a**) nor ^{13}C-labeled short-chain fatty acids (SCFA) concentrations in plasma (**b**) (n = 10). The middle line represents the mean with the standard deviation (whiskers).

3.4. Estimation of the Duration of the Fermentation in the Presence of Different WB Fractions

The duration of the fermentation was considered as a measure for the efficiency of fermentation with shorter duration, indicating a more efficient fermentation. On average, fermentation continued for 486 ± 40.9 min. However, the duration of the fermentation was not different when unmodified WB, WB RPS, and PE WB were administered to the subjects, compared to the control condition (Wilcoxon signed rank test; $p_{WB} = 0.201$, $p_{\ WBRPS} = 0.236$, $p_{PEWB} = 0.878$) (Figure 6).

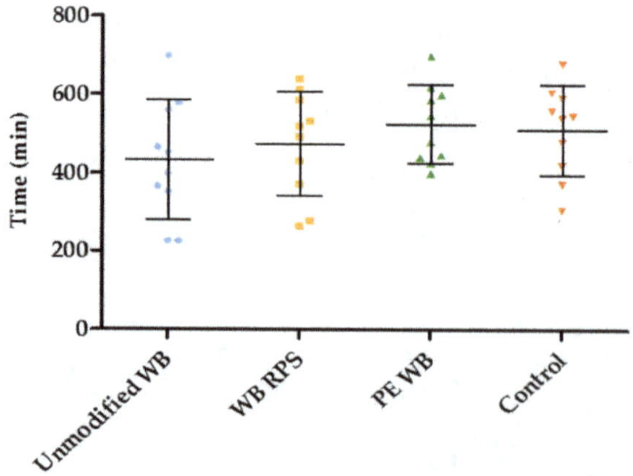

Figure 6. Wheat bran (WB) supplementation did not modify the duration of the fermentation (n = 10). The middle line represents the mean with the standard deviation (whiskers).

3.5. ^{13}C-SCFA Concentrations in Plasma Produced from the ^{13}C-Labeled Inulin

Average concentrations of plasma ^{13}C-acetate, ^{13}C-propionate, and ^{13}C-butyrate originating from the colon, were presented as a function of time (Figure 7).

Influx of ^{13}C-acetate, ^{13}C-propionate, and ^{13}C-butyrate from the colon, reached a maximum value 360 ± 119 min after consuming the breakfast. Mean cumulative ^{13}C-SCFA concentrations

($n = 40$) amounted to 18.5 ± 3.88 μmol·h·L^{-1} for acetate, 0.59 ± 0.17 μmol·h·L^{-1} for propionate, and 0.99 ± 0.3 μmol·h·L^{-1} for butyrate. However, cumulative ^{13}C-SCFA plasma concentrations were not different in the presence of any WB fraction, when compared to the control condition (Wilcoxon signed ranks test; Acetate: $p_{WB} = 0.114$, $p_{WBRPS} = 0.878$, $p_{PEWB} = 0.721$; Propionate: $p_{WB} = 0.169$, $p_{WBRPS} = 0.646$, $p_{PEWB} = 0.139$; Butyrate: $p_{WB} = 0.169$, $p_{WBRPS} = 0.721$, $p_{PEWB} = 0.646$; Total SCFA: $p_{WB} = 0.074$, $p_{WBRPS} = 0.799$, $p_{PEWB} = 0.646$) (Figure 8).

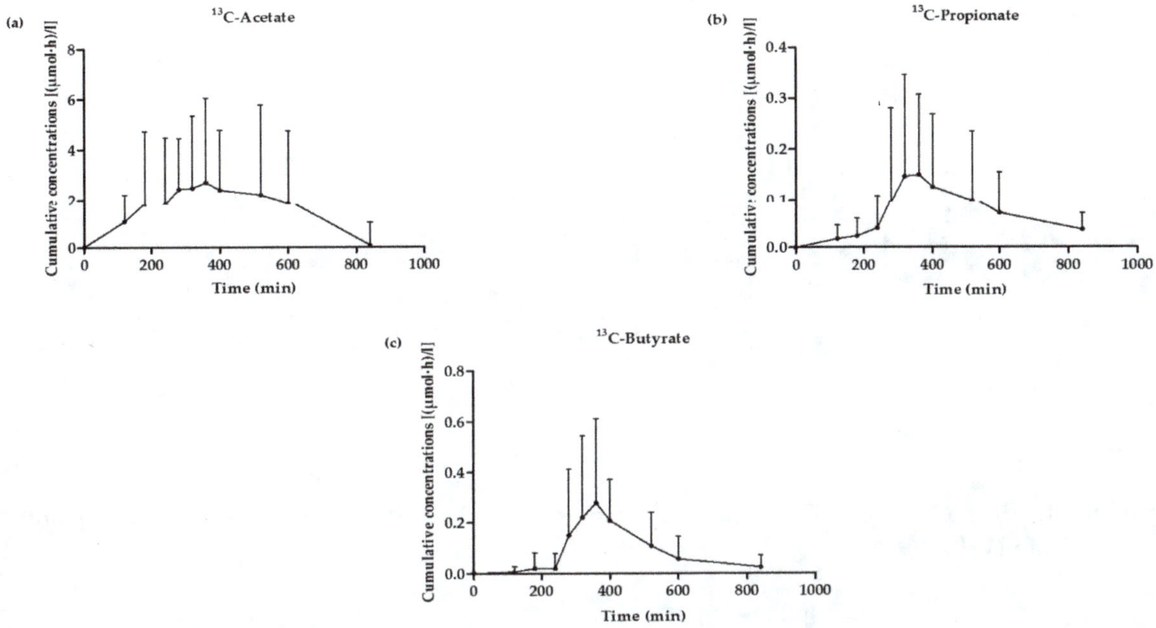

Figure 7. Average plasma concentrations of ^{13}C-acetate (**a**), ^{13}C-propionate (**b**) and ^{13}C-butyrate (**c**) originating from the colon as a function of time ($n = 40$).

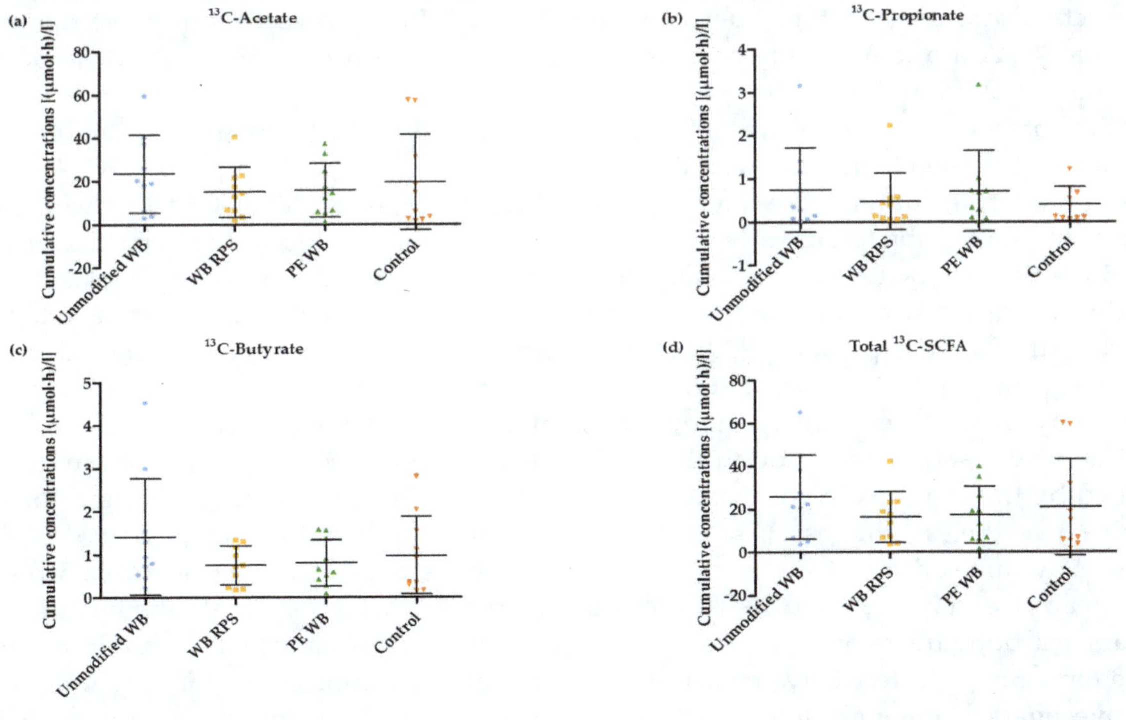

Figure 8. Wheat bran (WB) supplementation did not affect the cumulative ^{13}C-acetate (**a**), ^{13}C-propionate (**b**), ^{13}C-butyrate (**c**), total ^{13}C-SCFA (**d**) concentrations in plasma ($n = 10$). The middle line represents the mean with the standard deviation (whiskers).

3.6. Relative Proportion of Acetate, Propionate, and Butyrate after WB Supplementation

Stimulation of cross-feeding between colonic bacteria was evaluated by calculating the relative proportion of acetate, propionate, and butyrate for the different conditions. However, none of the WB fractions significantly influenced the relative proportion of acetate, propionate, and butyrate in the plasma, when compared to the control (Wilcoxon signed rank test; Acetate: $p_{WB} = 0.721$, $p_{WBRPS} = 0.959$, $p_{PEWB} = 0.575$; Propionate: $p_{WB} = 0.959$, $p_{WBRPS} = 0.445$, $p_{PEWB} = 0.959$; Butyrate: $p_{WB} = 0.575$, $p_{WBRPS} = 0.799$, $p_{PEWB} = 0.799$ (Figure 9).

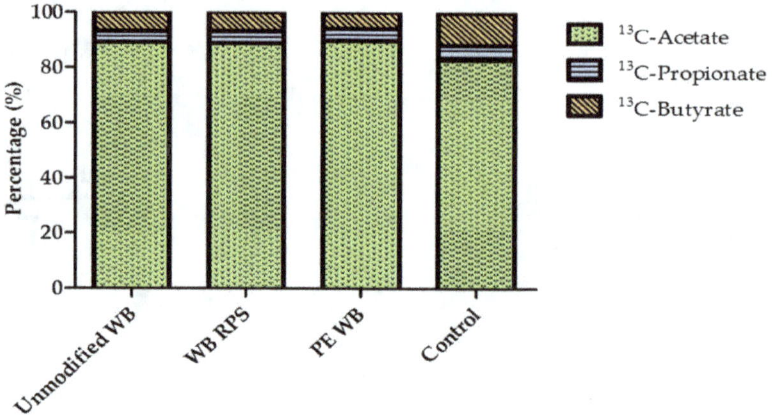

Figure 9. The proportions of ^{13}C-acetate, ^{13}C-propionate, and ^{13}C-butyrate in plasma were not affected by wheat bran (WB) (n = 10).

4. Discussion

Colonic production of SCFA from undigested carbohydrates has been increasingly recognized as a key process that contributes to both local gut and systemic health. The extent to which colonic-derived SCFA reach the systemic circulation may be an important parameter that determines the systemic health effects induced by dietary fiber consumption [25]. In the present study, we demonstrated that plasma SCFA are temporarily increased after consumption of a moderate dose of an easily fermentable carbohydrate.

The fact that we used uniformly stable isotope labeled inulin which, upon fermentation, resulted in the formation of labeled SCFA, allowed us to selectively quantify in plasma those SCFA originating from the inulin fermentation in the colon and to exclude confounders, like SCFA that were present in the colon at the start of the test days, SCFA that might have been produced due to partial fermentation of the WB fractions, or SCFA that have been endogenously produced. For example, plasma acetate is also produced from fatty acid oxidation and amino acid metabolism [28], and during ketogenesis in the mitochondria of the hepatocytes [29]. Colonic fermentation of ^{13}C-inulin contributed to increased plasma ^{13}C-SCFA concentrations for about 8 h, with maximal concentrations 6 h after consumption of the carbohydrate. It needs to be mentioned that the peak SCFA concentrations depend on the transit time of the substrates through the gastrointestinal tract, which is, apart from host factors, determined by the composition and caloric load of the breakfast meal and may vary with another test meal. Nevertheless, the results suggest that sustained increased plasma levels of SCFA might be obtained by three administrations of a considerable dose of an easily fermentable carbohydrate, evenly spread over a 24-h period. Furthermore, experiments which evaluate the health benefits of fermentable carbohydrates or prebiotics that are attributed to systemic SCFA, should preferably be performed in a time window between 6 and 10 h after administration of the carbohydrate.

To investigate whether insoluble particles could stimulate the fermentation of other carbohydrates in the colon, we used WB fractions that differed in tissue composition and particle size. Although reduction of particle size does not alter the composition of the WB fraction, it clearly modifies the physical properties of the WB. Destruction of cell walls during milling increases the specific surface area and the accessibility of intracellular cell components to degrading enzymes and, in this way, augments the fermentability of the WB fractions. In contrast, PE WB has been stripped of any fermentable material and mainly contains highly cross-linked dietary fiber that is hardly fermentable. We hypothesized that PE WB might facilitate fermentation by providing a platform on which bacteria can adhere, resulting in a more efficient exchange of microbial nutrients and metabolites between different types of bacteria; so-called cross-feeding. RPS WB may act in the same way, but has the additional advantage of being partly fermentable. If we would compare PE WB with a dinner table to which the bacteria draw up, WB RPS would be a dinner table filled with nutrients. Hence, we expected WB RPS to be more efficient in stimulating carbohydrate fermentation and cross-feeding.

Several factors may explain why WB did not stimulate the fermentation of inulin. First, inulin is an easily and rapidly fermentable substrate for colonic bacteria. It is possible that the fermentation proceeds so efficiently in baseline conditions that no room is left for improvement by the additional administration of WB platforms. Future studies may be performed with less rapidly fermentable carbohydrates, such as arabinoxylanoligosaccharides (AXOS). These oligosaccharides consist of a xylose backbone that is substituted with arabinose residues. By varying the degree of polymerization (DP) and the degree of substitution (DS), the rate of fermentation can be modulated. Unfortunately, ^{13}C-labeled AXOS derivatives are not commercially available. Second, the appearance of $^{13}CO_2$ in the breath and of ^{13}C-SCFA in the plasma, consistently occurred before arrival of the test meal in the colon, indicated by the appearance of $^{14}CO_2$ in the breath, suggesting that the fermentation of inulin had already started in the terminal ileum, where the bacterial density rapidly increases [30]. We used native inulin, which is a mixture of oligo- and polysaccharides, with a DP varying from 3 to 70 and an average DP of 25. The presence of short fructo-oligosaccharides most likely explains the early fermentation, as fermentation of short oligosaccharides proceeds more easily than that of longer chains [31]. Indeed, studies that use the increase in breath hydrogen excretion after administration of inulin as a marker of OCTT [26,32,33], generally use Raftiline HP® (Beneo, Mannheim, Germany) as the substrate, which only contains the long chains of inulin. This, at least in part, physical disconnection between the site of fermentation (terminal ileum) and main location of bacteria (colon), might hamper stimulation of the carbohydrate fermentation by bacteria adhered to the WB fractions.

Finally, repeated administration, rather than a single dose of WB, might have been more efficient for inducing a more efficient bacterial ecosystem. Nevertheless, in vitro incubation of human fecal samples with insoluble WB, showed that within 24 h (no earlier time point was tested) WB was already colonized by subsets of bacteria, suggesting a rapid colonization of insoluble particles [19]. Few studies have evaluated the impact of insoluble particles on SCFA production in vivo. Administration of resistant starch (RS) to pigs for two weeks resulted in increased cecal concentrations of butyrate, whereas combined administration of RS and WB resulted in increased butyrate concentrations in the more distal parts of the colon and in feces, suggesting that the addition of WB distally shifted fermentation [34]. These results could not be explained by partial fermentation of WB, as WB alone did not significantly increase butyrate concentrations. Also in humans, a diet supplemented with WB and RS for three weeks resulted in higher fecal proportions of butyrate and lower propionate proportions than WB alone, whereas fecal SCFA concentrations after the WB diet were not different from the values recorded during the control diet [35]. These observations support our hypothesis of improved carbohydrate fermentation due to the colonization of WB particles. However, alternative mechanisms also need to be considered. Increased fecal SCFA may also be due to the fact that WB accelerates whole gut transit time [36]. Indeed, both in vitro fermentation studies and human studies, indicate that SCFA production is increased with short transit time, and that longer transit times are associated with a shift from carbohydrate to protein fermentation [37–39]. It is important to note that fecal SCFA concentrations are the net result of production and absorption, and are difficult to relate to plasma SCFA.

Finally, we observed large inter- and intra-individual variations in plasma SCFA concentrations, which may have hampered detection of subtle changes in plasma SCFA due to WB intervention. Such large variations have also been reported in previous studies measuring SCFA [40–42] and may be due to variability in intestinal microbiota composition, colonic SCFA absorption and metabolism, and SCFA metabolism in the liver.

5. Conclusions

In this study, we showed that fermentation of a readily fermentable substrate results in increased plasma SCFA for about 8 h, suggesting that a sustained increase in plasma SCFA concentrations can be achieved when a moderate dose of fermentable carbohydrate is administered three times per day. Nevertheless, the addition of a single dose of different WB fractions did not further increase either the fermentation of the readily fermentable inulin, or cross-feeding between gut bacteria.

Acknowledgments: This research was conducted in the framework of an SBO-IWT project entitled "BRANDING: Cereal bran-based dispersions for gut health" and is supported by the "Vlaams Agentschap Innoveren en Ondernemen" (Vlaio, former IWT or "Agentschap voor Innovatie door Wetenschap en Technologie").

Author Contributions: L.D. and K.V. conceived and designed the experiments and wrote the paper; L.D., A.L. and G.V. performed the experiments and analyzed the data; J.V. and C.M.C. provided the wheat bran fractions and contributed to the revision of the manuscript.

References

1. Den Besten, G.; van Eunen, K.; Groen, A.K.; Venema, K.; Reijngoud, D.J.; Bakker, B.M. The role of short-chain fatty acids in the interplay between diet, gut microbiota, and host energy metabolism. *J. Lipid Res.* **2013**, *54*, 2325–2340. [CrossRef] [PubMed]
2. Macfarlane, G.T.; Macfarlane, S. Bacteria, colonic fermentation, and gastrointestinal health. *J. AOAC Int.* **2012**, *95*, 50–60. [CrossRef] [PubMed]
3. Hamer, H.M.; Jonkers, D.; Venema, K.; Vanhoutvin, S.; Troost, F.J.; Brummer, R.J. Review article: The role of butyrate on colonic function. *Aliment. Pharmacol. Ther.* **2008**, *27*, 104–119. [CrossRef] [PubMed]
4. Macfarlane, G.T.; Macfarlane, S. Fermentation in the human large intestine: Its physiologic consequences and the potential contribution of prebiotics. *J. Clin. Gastroenterol.* **2011**, *45*, S120–S127. [CrossRef] [PubMed]
5. Canfora, E.E.; Jocken, J.W.; Blaak, E.E. Short-chain fatty acids in control of body weight and insulin sensitivity. *Nat. Rev. Endocrinol.* **2015**, *11*, 577–591. [CrossRef] [PubMed]
6. Hong, Y.H.; Nishimura, Y.; Hishikawa, D.; Tsuzuki, H.; Miyahara, H.; Gotoh, C.; Choi, K.C.; Feng, D.D.; Chen, C.; Lee, H.G.; et al. Acetate and propionate short chain fatty acids stimulate adipogenesis via GPCR43. *Endocrinology* **2005**, *146*, 5092–5099. [CrossRef] [PubMed]
7. Park, J.; Kim, M.; Kang, S.G.; Jannasch, A.H.; Cooper, B.; Patterson, J.; Kim, C.H. Short-chain fatty acids induce both effector and regulatory T cells by suppression of histone deacetylases and regulation of the mtor-s6k pathway. *Mucosal. Immunol.* **2015**, *8*, 80–93. [CrossRef] [PubMed]
8. Smith, P.M.; Howitt, M.R.; Panikov, N.; Michaud, M.; Gallini, C.A.; Bohlooly, Y.M.; Glickman, J.N.; Garrett, W.S. The microbial metabolites, short-chain fatty acids, regulate colonic Treg cell homeostasis. *Science* **2013**, *341*, 569–573. [CrossRef] [PubMed]
9. Floch, M.H.; Hong-Curtiss, J. Probiotics and functional foods in gastrointestinal disorders. *Curr. Treat. Opt. Gastroenterol.* **2002**, *5*, 311–321. [CrossRef]
10. Marteau, P. Butyrate-producing bacteria as pharmabiotics for inflammatory bowel disease. *Gut* **2013**, *62*, 1673. [CrossRef] [PubMed]
11. Eeckhaut, V.; Ducatelle, R.; Sas, B.; Vermeire, S.; Van Immerseel, F. Progress towards butyrate-producing pharmabiotics: Butyricicoccus pullicaecorum capsule and efficacy in TNBS models in comparison with therapeutics. *Gut* **2014**, *63*, 367. [CrossRef] [PubMed]
12. Eeckhaut, V.; Machiels, K.; Perrier, C.; Romero, C.; Maes, S.; Flahou, B.; Steppe, M.; Haesebrouck, F.; Sas, B.; Ducatelle, R.; et al. Butyricicoccus pullicaecorum in inflammatory bowel disease. *Gut* **2013**, *62*, 1745–1752. [CrossRef] [PubMed]

13. Miquel, S.; Martin, R.; Rossi, O.; Bermudez-Humaran, L.G.; Chatel, J.M.; Sokol, H.; Thomas, M.; Wells, J.M.; Langella, P. Faecalibacterium prausnitzii and human intestinal health. *Curr. Opin. Microbiol.* **2013**, *16*, 255–261. [CrossRef] [PubMed]
14. Gibson, G.; Scott, K.; Rastal, R.A.; Kieran, M.T.; Hotchkiss, A.; Dubert-Ferrandon, A.; Gareau, M.; Eileen, M.F.; Saulnier, D.; Loh, G.; et al. Dietary prebiotics: Current status and new definition. *Food Sci. Technol. Bull.* **2010**, *7*, 1–19. [CrossRef]
15. Velázquez, M.; Davies, C.; Marett, R.; Slavin, J.L.; Feirtag, J.M. Effect of oligosaccharides and fibre substitutes on short-chain fatty acid production by human faecal microflora. *Anaerobe* **2000**, *6*, 87–92. [CrossRef]
16. Brouns, F.; Kettlitz, B.; Arrigoni, E. Resistant starch and "the butyrate revolution". *Trends Food Sci. Technol.* **2002**, *13*, 251–261. [CrossRef]
17. Moens, F.; Weckx, S.; De Vuyst, L. Bifidobacterial inulin-type fructan degradation capacity determines cross-feeding interactions between bifidobacteria and faecalibacterium prausnitzii. *Int. J. Food Microbiol.* **2016**, *231*, 76–85. [CrossRef] [PubMed]
18. Riviere, A.; Gagnon, M.; Weckx, S.; Roy, D.; De Vuyst, L. Mutual cross-feeding interactions between bifidobacterium longum subsp. Longum NCC2705 and eubacterium rectale ATCC 33656 explain the bifidogenic and butyrogenic effects of arabinoxylan oligosaccharides. *Appl. Environ. Microbiol.* **2015**, *81*, 7767–7781. [CrossRef] [PubMed]
19. Leitch, E.C.; Walker, A.W.; Duncan, S.H.; Holtrop, G.; Flint, H.J. Selective colonization of insoluble substrates by human faecal bacteria. *Environ. Microbiol.* **2007**, *9*, 667–679. [CrossRef] [PubMed]
20. Courtin, C.M.; Van den Broeck, H.; Delcour, J.A. Determination of reducing end sugar residues in oligo- and polysaccharides by gas-liquid chromatography. *J. Chromatogr. A* **2000**, *866*, 97–104. [CrossRef]
21. Gerits, L.R.; Pareyt, B.; Delcour, J.A. Single run hplc separation coupled to evaporative light scattering detection unravels wheat flour endogenous lipid redistribution during bread dough making. *LWT-Food Sci. Technol.* **2013**, *53*, 426–433. [CrossRef]
22. Jacobs, P.J.; Hemdane, S.; Dornez, E.; Delcour, J.A.; Courtin, C.M. Study of hydration properties of wheat bran as a function of particle size. *Food Chem.* **2015**, *179*, 296–304. [CrossRef] [PubMed]
23. Swennen, K.; Courtin, C.M.; Lindemans, G.C.J.E.; Delcour, J.A. Large-scale production and characterisation of wheat bran arabinoxylooligosaccharides. *J. Sci. Food Agric.* **2006**, *86*, 1722–1731. [CrossRef]
24. Urbaniak, G.U.; Plous, S. Research Randomizer. Available online: http://www.randomizer.org (accessed on 10 January 2015).
25. Boets, E.; Deroover, L.; Houben, E.; Vermeulen, K.; Gomand, S.V.; Delcour, J.A.; Verbeke, K. Quantification of in vivo colonic short chain fatty acid production from inulin. *Nutrients* **2015**, *7*, 8916–8929. [CrossRef] [PubMed]
26. Verbeke, K.; de Preter, V.; Geboes, K.; Daems, T.; van den Mooter, G.; Evenepoel, P.; Rutgeerts, P. In vivo evaluation of a colonic delivery system using isotope techniques. *Aliment. Pharmacol. Ther.* **2005**, *21*, 187–194. [CrossRef] [PubMed]
27. Zhao, G.; Liu, J.F.; Nyman, M.; Jonsson, J.A. Determination of short-chain fatty acids in serum by hollow fiber supported liquid membrane extraction coupled with gas chromatography. *J. Chromatogr. B Anal. Technol. Biomed. Life Sci.* **2007**, *846*, 202–208. [CrossRef] [PubMed]
28. Layden, B.T.; Angueira, A.R.; Brodsky, M.; Durai, V.; Lowe, W.L., Jr. Short chain fatty acids and their receptors: New metabolic targets. *Transl. Res.* **2013**, *161*, 131–140. [CrossRef] [PubMed]
29. Yamashita, H.; Kaneyuki, T.; Tagawa, K. Production of acetate in the liver and its utilization in peripheral tissues. *Biochim. Biophys. Acta* **2001**, *1532*, 79–87. [CrossRef]
30. Sartor, R.B. Microbial influences in inflammatory bowel diseases. *Gastroenterology* **2008**, *134*, 577–594. [CrossRef] [PubMed]
31. Van der Meulen, R.; Makras, L.; Verbrugghe, K.; Adriany, T.; De Vuyst, L. In vitro kinetic analysis of oligofructose consumption by *Bacteroides* and *Bifidobacterium* spp. Indicates different degradation mechanisms. *Appl. Environ. Microbiol.* **2006**, *72*, 1006–1012. [CrossRef] [PubMed]
32. Geboes, K.P.; Luypaerts, A.; Rutgeerts, P.; Verbeke, K. Inulin is an ideal substrate for a hydrogen breath test to measure the orocaecal transit time. *Aliment. Pharmacol. Ther.* **2003**, *18*, 721–729. [CrossRef] [PubMed]
33. Schneider, A.R.; Jepp, K.; Murczynski, L.; Biniek, U.; Stein, J. The inulin hydrogen breath test accurately reflects orocaecal transit time. *Eur. J. Clin. Investig.* **2007**, *37*, 802–807. [CrossRef] [PubMed]

34. Govers, M.J.; Gannon, N.J.; Dunshea, F.R.; Gibson, P.R.; Muir, J.G. Wheat bran affects the site of fermentation of resistant starch and luminal indexes related to colon cancer risk: A study in pigs. *Gut* **1999**, *45*, 840–847. [CrossRef] [PubMed]
35. Muir, J.G.; Yeow, E.G.; Keogh, J.; Pizzey, C.; Bird, A.R.; Sharpe, K.; O'Dea, K.; Macrae, F.A. Combining wheat bran with resistant starch has more beneficial effects on fecal indexes than does wheat bran alone. *Am. J. Clin. Nutr.* **2004**, *79*, 1020–1028. [PubMed]
36. De Vries, J.; Miller, P.E.; Verbeke, K. Effects of cereal fiber on bowel function: A systematic review of intervention trials. *World J. Gastroenterol.* **2015**, *21*, 8952–8963. [CrossRef] [PubMed]
37. Lewis, S.J.; Heaton, K.W. Increasing butyrate concentration in the distal colon by accelerating intestinal transit. *Gut* **1997**, *41*, 245–251. [CrossRef] [PubMed]
38. Macfarlane, G.T.; Macfarlane, S.; Gibson, G.R. Validation of a three-stage compound continuous culture system for investigating the effect of retention time on the ecology and metabolism of bacteria in the human colon. *Microb. Ecol.* **1998**, *35*, 180–187. [CrossRef] [PubMed]
39. Roager, H.M.; Hansen, L.B.; Bahl, M.I.; Frandsen, H.L.; Carvalho, V.; Gobel, R.J.; Dalgaard, M.D.; Plichta, D.R.; Sparholt, M.H.; Vestergaard, H.; et al. Colonic transit time is related to bacterial metabolism and mucosal turnover in the gut. *Nat. Microbiol.* **2016**, *1*, 16093. [CrossRef] [PubMed]
40. Bloemen, J.G.; Venema, K.; van de Poll, M.C.; Olde Damink, S.W.; Buurman, W.A.; Dejong, C.H. Short chain fatty acids exchange across the gut and liver in humans measured at surgery. *Clin. Nutr.* **2009**, *28*, 657–661. [CrossRef] [PubMed]
41. Boets, E.; Gomand, S.V.; Deroover, L.; Preston, T.; Vermeulen, K.; De Preter, V.; Hamer, H.; Van den Mooter, G.; De Vuyst, L.; Courtin, C.M.; et al. Systemic availability and metabolism of colonic-derived short-chain fatty acids in healthy subjects—A stable isotope study. *J. Physiol.* **2017**, *595*, 541–555. [CrossRef] [PubMed]
42. Peters, S.G.; Pomare, E.W.; Fisher, C.A. Portal and peripheral blood short chain fatty acid concentrations after caecal lactulose instillation at surgery. *Gut* **1992**, *33*, 1249–1252. [CrossRef] [PubMed]

14

Role of Fiber in Symptomatic Uncomplicated Diverticular Disease

Marilia Carabotti [1,2,*], Bruno Annibale [1], Carola Severi [2] and Edith Lahner [1]

1 Medical-Surgical Department of Clinical Sciences and Translational Medicine, University Sapienza, Via di Grottarossa 1035, 00189 Rome, Italy; bruno.annibale@uniroma1.it (B.A.); edith.lahner@uniroma1.it (E.L.)

2 Department of Internal Medicine and Medical Specialties, University Sapienza, Viale del Policlinico 155, 00161 Rome, Italy; carola.severi@uniroma1.it

* Correspondence: mariliacarabotti@gmail.com;

Abstract: Symptomatic uncomplicated diverticular disease (SUDD) is a syndrome characterized by recurrent abdominal symptoms in patients with colonic diverticula. There is some evidence that a high-fiber diet or supplemental fibers may reduce symptoms in SUDD patients and a high-fiber diet is commonly suggested for these patients. This systematic review aims to update the evidence on the efficacy of fiber treatment in SUDD, in terms of a reduction in symptoms and the prevention of acute diverticulitis. According to PRISMA, we identified studies on SUDD patients treated with fibers (PubMed and Scopus). The quality of these studies was evaluated by the Jadad scale. The main outcome measures were a reduction of abdominal symptoms and the prevention of acute diverticulitis. Nineteen studies were included, nine with dietary fiber and 10 with supplemental fiber, with a high heterogeneity concerning the quantity and quality of fibers employed. Single studies suggest that fibers, both dietary and supplemental, could be beneficial in SUDD, even if the quality is very low, with just one study yielding an optimal score. The presence of substantial methodological limitations, the heterogeneity of the therapeutic regimens employed, and the lack of ad hoc designed studies, did not permit a summary of the outcome measure. Thus, the benefit of dietary or supplemental fiber in SUDD patients still needs to be established.

Keywords: diverticular disease; dietary fiber; supplemental fiber; symptomatic uncomplicated diverticular disease

---

1. Introduction

Colonic diverticula are common in Western countries, affecting up to 60% of subjects over 70 years of age [1]. In about 80% of patients, colonic diverticula remain asymptomatic (diverticulosis), while approximately 20% of patients may develop abdominal symptoms (symptomatic uncomplicated diverticular disease, SUDD) and, eventually, complications such as bouts of diverticulitis or bleeding [2]. SUDD has been defined as a syndrome which is characterized by recurrent abdominal symptoms (i.e., abdominal pain and bloating resembling or overlapping those present in irritable bowel syndrome), attributed to diverticula in the absence of macroscopically evident alterations, other than the presence of diverticula [3,4]. The impact of these complaints is variable, and the severity and frequency of symptoms may range from mild and rare episodes, to a severe, chronic, recurrent disorder, impacting daily activities and the quality of life of patients [5,6]. About 4% of patients develop acute diverticulitis, an inflammatory process that may result in complications in about 15% of patients, with the development of abscesses, perforation, fistula, obstruction, or peritonitis [7]. A recurrence of diverticulitis after the first episode has been reported to occur in 15%–30% of patients [8,9].

The main goals of managing SUDD are both the reduction of abdominal symptoms and the prevention of acute diverticulitis. Even if recommendations for the treatment of SUDD have been issued by the medical societies of various countries [3,10–13], a standard therapeutic approach still remains to be defined. Fibers have been suggested for the treatment of SUDD patients, but the therapeutic benefit is not yet fully understood. Fibers might confer benefits by increasing fecal mass and regularizing bowel movements, as well as acting as prebiotics in the colon, favoring health-promoting species of the intestinal microbiota [14]. Fibers are defined as the edible parts of plants or the analogous carbohydrates that are resistant to digestion and absorption in the human small intestine, with complete or partial fermentation in the colon [15]. Fiber intake may be achieved by consuming fruits, vegetables, and cereal grains (dietary fibers), and/or by diet supplementation with specific commercial preparations containing fibers (supplemental fibers).

A previous systematic review assessed whether a high-fiber diet can improve symptoms or prevent complications of diverticular disease. Few studies were identified, and the authors concluded that evidence for a therapeutic benefit of a high-fiber diet in the treatment of diverticular disease is poor [16].

This systematic review aims to update the evidence on the efficacy of treatment with fiber in SUDD, in terms of the reduction of symptoms and the prevention of acute diverticulitis.

2. Methods

2.1. Study Selection

The search was conducted according to the PRISMA (Preferred Reporting Items for Systematic Reviews and Meta-Analyses) guidelines [17]. The electronic databases PubMed MEDLINE (U.S. National Library of Medicine, Bethesda, MD, USA) and Scopus were systematically searched according to the following search strategy, using the following MesH terms:

((("diverticulum" [MeSH Terms] OR "diverticulum" [All Fields] OR "diverticulosis" [All Fields]) OR diverticular [All Fields] OR ("diverticulum" [MeSH Terms] OR "diverticulum" [All Fields] OR "diverticula" [All Fields]) OR ("diverticulitis" [MeSH Terms] OR "diverticulitis" [All Fields])) AND (("colon" [MeSH Terms] OR "colon" [All Fields]) OR ("colon" [MeSH Terms] OR "colon" [All Fields] OR "colonic" [All Fields]) OR ("colon, sigmoid" [MeSH Terms] OR ("colon" [All Fields] AND "sigmoid" [All Fields]) OR "sigmoid colon" [All Fields] OR "sigmoid" [All Fields])) AND (("dietary fiber" [MeSH Terms] OR ("dietary" [All Fields] AND "fiber" [All Fields]) OR "dietary fiber" [All Fields] OR "fiber" [All Fields]) OR fibre [All Fields] OR ("diet" [MeSH Terms] OR "diet" [All Fields] OR "dietary" [All Fields]) OR insoluble [All Fields] OR soluble [All Fields] OR ("fruit" [MeSH Terms] OR "fruit" [All Fields]) OR ("vegetables" [MeSH Terms] OR "vegetables" [All Fields] OR "vegetable" [All Fields]) OR ("(1-6)-alpha-glucomannan" [Supplement *] OR "(1-6)-alpha-glucomannan" [All Fields] OR "glucomannan" [All Fields]) OR ("starch" [MeSH Terms] OR "starch" [All Fields]) OR fructooligosaccharides [All Fields] OR bran [All Fields] OR ("inulin" [MeSH Terms] OR "inulin" [All Fields]) OR ("psyllium" [MeSH Terms] OR "psyllium" [All Fields]))) AND ("humans" [MeSH Terms] AND (English [lang] OR French [lang] OR German [lang] OR Italian [lang] OR Spanish [lang]) AND "adult" [MeSH Terms]) AND ("therapy" [Subheading] OR "therapy" [All Fields] OR "treatment" [All Fields] OR "therapeutics" [MeSH Terms] OR "therapeutics" [All Fields]) AND ("humans" [MeSH Terms] AND (English [lang] OR French [lang] OR German [lang] OR Italian [lang] OR Spanish [lang]) AND "adult" [MeSH Terms]).

The search strategy excluded reviews, meta-analyses, case reports, and animal studies. The following study types were included: randomized controlled trials (blinded and/or placebo-controlled), open randomized clinical trials, and non-randomized open studies. Pediatric subjects were excluded from this review. No publication data restriction was imposed. Reports published in English, German, French, Italian, and Spanish were considered.

Clinical studies published up to 7 October 2016 were considered for inclusion in this review, if they described in adults (>18 years) with SUDD, the efficacy of fiber treatment with respect to the baseline (i) on reduction or remission of abdominal symptoms; and/or (ii) on prevention of acute diverticulitis.

Potentially relevant articles were independently screened for eligibility in an un-blinded standardized manner by the two reviewers (M.C., E.L.), initially by abstract, and then by full text when necessary, in order to determine whether they met the inclusion criteria. Reviews, letters, books, and/or editorials were excluded on the basis of the abstract and/or title; in other cases, the judgement of inclusion/exclusion was based on an evaluation of the full-text. Disagreement between reviewers was resolved by discussion. The reference lists of the identified articles, as well as of the identified relevant reviews, were manually searched for additional studies that may have been overlooked using a computer-assisted search strategy.

2.2. Data Extraction

We developed a data extraction sheet, pilot-tested it on three randomly-selected included studies, and refined it accordingly. One review author (M.C.) extracted the data from the included studies and the second author (E.L.) checked the extracted data. Disagreements were resolved by discussion between the two review authors. The following information was extracted from each included paper: (1) author and year of publication; (2) characteristics of fibers; (3) characteristics of study participants (number, mean age, and gender); (4) diagnosis of SUDD; (5) study type and treatment arms; (6) type of intervention; (7) follow-up; (8) outcome measure (reduction of abdominal symptoms; occurrence of acute diverticulitis); (9) efficacy of intervention; (10) adverse effects of fiber arms; (11) single or multiple centers.

The diagnosis of SUDD was considered appropriate when patients with colonic diverticula had recurrent abdominal symptoms such as abdominal pain, which were eventually associated with bloating or bowel habit alteration [3]. Studies which did not completely fulfill this definition were not excluded a priori, but the specific clinical settings were singularly extracted and described in detail.

For the purpose of this paper, dietary fibers were defined as the intake of food fibers in fruits, vegetables, and cereal grains. A high-fiber diet has been defined as at least a 30 g daily intake of dietary fibers [18]. When indicated, the amount of daily fiber intake was extracted from each paper. Supplemental fibers were defined as diet supplementation with specific commercial preparations containing one or more types of fiber.

2.3. Statistical Analysis

Originally, a meta-analysis was planned in order to provide a numerical estimate of the overall effect of interest, for which the outcome measure (effect size) comprised the proportion of patients who showed a positive response to fiber treatment with respect to the baseline, or with respect to controls, defined as the reduction of abdominal symptoms and prevention of acute diverticulitis. Due to the heterogeneity of the retrieved studies and their low quality, a meta-analysis was not considered applicable. The efficacy of the interventions reported in the retrieved studies was described in a qualitative manner.

2.4. Quality Assessment

The two reviewers evaluated the quality of all of the included studies, using the Jadad scale for randomized controlled trials [19]. This scale awards a maximum of five points to each study. The considered categories are randomization, blinding of outcome assessment, description of withdrawals and dropouts, and description and appropriateness of randomization and blinding. A study can be awarded a maximum of one point for each category (Table S1). Discrepancies in the quality assessment were discussed and resolved by the two reviewers.

3. Results

3.1. Search Results

The electronic search study identified a total of 374 records from electronic databases, 351 of which were unique (Figure 1).

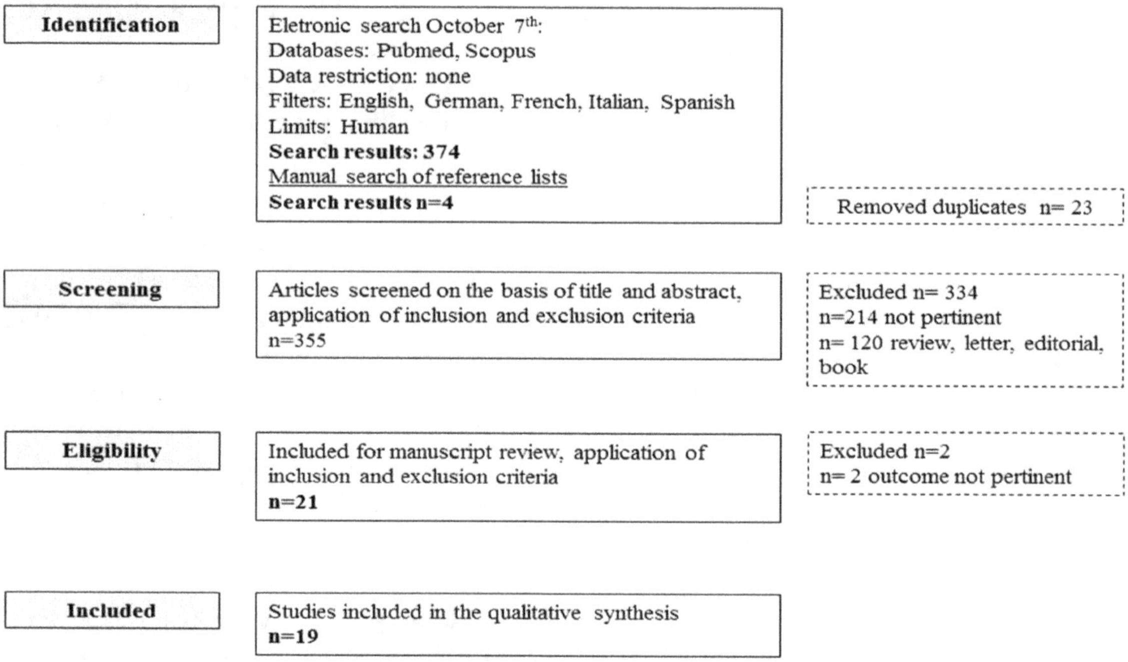

Figure 1. Flow-chart of study selection.

Manual searching of a reference list of potentially relevant papers contributed another four articles. The articles were screened on the basis of the title and abstract and, after application of the inclusion and exclusion criteria, 21 articles were retrieved for a full-paper evaluation. Of these 21 papers, 19 met the eligibility criteria and were subjected to data extraction. Two studies were excluded because the outcome was not pertinent to the present study purpose, since it only evaluated constipated patients [20,21]. Thus, 19 articles were included for qualitative synthesis (Table 1).

Table 1. Type of fibers and dosage used in the included studies.

Author, Year (Reference)	Type of Fibers and Dosage
	Dietary
Lahner E., 2012 [22]	Dietary fiber (at least 30 gr/day)
Annibale B., 2011 [23]	Dietary fiber (at least 30 gr/day)
Colecchia A., 2007 [24]	Dietary fiber (at least 20 gr/day)
Smits B.J., 1990 [25]	Dietary fiber (30–40 gr/day)
Leahy A.L., 1985 [26]	Dietary fiber (>25 gr/day)
Hyland J.M.P., 1980 [27]	Dietary fiber (37.9 gr/day)
Brodribb A.J.M., 1977 [28]	Bran crispbread (6.7 gr/day) Wheat crispbread (0.6 gr/day)
Plumley P.F., 1973 [29]	High-fiber crispbread (96 gr/day total unavailable fraction)
Painter N.S., 1972 [30]	High-residue, low sugar diet with unprocessed bran (12–14 gr/day)

Table 1. *Cont.*

Author, Year (Reference)	Type of Fibers and Dosage
	Supplemental
Lanas A., 2013 [31]	Plantago ovata (7 gr/day)
Latella G., 2003 [32]	Glucomannan (4 gr/day)
Papi C., 1995 [33]	Glucomannan (2 gr/day)
Papi C., 1992 [34]	Glucomannan (2 gr/day)
Thorburn H.A., 1992 [35]	Ispaghula husk (7 gr/day)
Ornstein M.H., 1981 [36]	Bran (6.99 g/day) Ispaghula (9.04 gr/day)
Eastwood M.A., 1978 [37]	Bran (20 g/day) Isphaghula (2 sachets/day)
Hodgson W.J.B., 1977 [38]	Methylcellulose (1000 mg/day)
Brodribb A.J.M., 1976 [39]	Wheat bran (24 gr/day)
Taylor I., 1976 [40]	High roughage diet with bran supplement Bran (18 gr/day)

3.2. Quality Assessment

Details of the quality assessment of the included studies are given in Supplementary Table S1 (see Supplementary material). Of the 19 studies included, six achieved 0 points [26,27,35,36,39,40], three achieved 1 point [25,29,30], two achieved 2 points [28,38], seven achieved 3 points [22–24,31,33,34,36], and only one achieved 5 points [33], according to Jadad scale.

3.3. Characteristics of Included Studies

The main characteristics of the 19 included studies are summarized in Table 2. Considering the high heterogeneity of the fibers used, studies are grouped on the basis of dietary (nine articles) or supplemental fibers (ten articles).

Table 2. Main characteristics of the 19 selected studies on fibers in symptomatic uncomplicated diverticular disease (SUDD).

Author, Year (Reference)	N/F/Mean Age	Diagnosis of SUDD	Study Type/Arms	Single Center Yes/No
Dietary				
Lahner E., 2012 [22]	44/35/66	App	Open RCT/2	No
Annibale B., 2011 [23]	50/32/65	App	Open RCT/3	No
Colecchia A., 2007 [24]	307/189/62	App	Open RCT/2	No
Smits B.J., 1990 [25]	43/28/59	App	Open RCT/2	Yes
Leahy A.L., 1985 [26]	56/-/-	App	Retrospective study/2	Yes
Hyland J.M.P., 1980 [27]	100/73/67	NcApp [1]	Retrospective study/1	Yes
Brodribb A.J.M., 1977 [28]	18/9/60	App	Double-blind RCT	Yes
Plumley P.F., 1973 [29]	48/-/71	NcApp [2]	Prospective interventional, partly cross-over study/2	Yes
Painter N.S., 1972 [30]	70/25/60	App	Prospective interventional study, not controlled/1	Yes
Supplemental				
Lanas A., 2013 [31]	165/59/54	NcApp [3]	Open RCT/2	No
Latella G., 2003 [32]	968/501/63	App	Open RCT/2	No
Papi C., 1995 [33]	168/100/62	App	Double-blind placebo controlled/2	No
Papi C., 1992 [34]	217/112/65	App	Open RCT/2	No
Thorburn H.A., 1992 [35]	10/4/66	NcApp [4]	Open/1	Yes
Ornstein M.H., 1981 [36]	58/36/64	App	Double-blind, cross-over, RCT/3	No
Eastwood M.A., 1978 [37]	31/-/60	NcApp [5]	Prospective, not randomized/3	Yes
Hodgson W.J.B., 1977 [38]	30/18/60	App	Double-blind, cross-over RCT/2	Yes
Brodribb A.J.M., 1976 [39]	40/-/-	App	Prospective, not controlled/1	Yes
Taylor I., 1976 [40]	20/-/-	NcApp [6]	Cross-over RCT	Yes

App: appropriate; NcApp: not completely appropriate; F: female gender; N: number of patients; RCT: randomized controlled trial; [1] an unspecified number of pts with acute diverticulitis were included; [2] 4 pts with diverticulosis were included; [3] pts with a recent episode of colonic diverticulitis, current in remission were included, [4] 3 pts with diverticulosis were included; [5] an unspecified number of pts with diverticulosis were included; [6] 8 pts with acute diverticulitis were included.

In thirteen studies, SUDD was appropriately diagnosed [22–26,28,30,32–34,36,38,39], while in six studies, the diagnosis was not completely appropriated [27,29,35,37,40] (see Table 2). The latter studies include three in which SUDD patients with diverticulosis were included [29,35,37], and in the other two studies, SUDD patients with acute diverticulitis were included [27–40]. In one study, patients who had reported a recent episode of colonic diverticulitis, but were currently in remission, were included [31].

3.4. Dietary Fiber

Articles concerning dietary fibers were performed over a period of 40 years, from 1972 to 2012, and only three of them were published in the last 10 years [22–24]. Six of these were single center studies and three were multicenter studies [22–24]. Six studies were conducted in the United Kingdom [25–30] and three were completed in Italy [22–24].

An overall number of 736 patients with SUDD were investigated, for which the female gender was slightly prevalent (n = 391), but in two articles [26–29], the gender of the patients was lacking. Patients had a mean age of 64 years, ranging from 59 to 71 years. In one study, the age of patients was lacking [26].

With regard to the study type, four were randomized controlled open trials [22–25], two were retrospective studies [26,27], one was a double-blind RCT [28], one was a prospective partly cross-over study [29], and the remaining one was an un-controlled study [30].

With regard to the fibers used, in the majority of the studies, patients were treated with dietary fibers [22–27], in two articles crispbread was used [28,29], and in the last study, a high residue, low sugar with unprocessed bran was utilized [30]. In addition, the amount of dietary fiber utilized was variable, ranging from 20 [24] to 96 gr/day [29]. In five studies, a high-fiber diet was employed [22,23,25,27,29], but in the other studies, the dosage of fiber seemed to be lower than 30 gr daily [24,26,28,30]. Unfortunately, it was not possible to assess the proportion of soluble or insoluble fibers for each dietary regimen, since its exact composition was not reported.

The follow-up protocol was very variable between studies, ranging from three [25–28] to 65 months [27]. Also, the interventions were variable between studies: in four studies, the dietary fiber was a control arm and was compared in two articles to symbiotic preparations [22,23], in another it was compared to rifaximin [24], and in the last it was compared to lactulose [25]. In one study, a high-fiber diet was compared to one which was not high in fiber [26], and in two studies, high-fiber crispbread was compared to lower fiber crispbread [28,29]. One study used a high-fiber diet without a control arm [27], and the other study used a high-residue, low sugar diet with unprocessed bran [30]. With regard to the outcome measures, seven articles assessed the reduction of abdominal symptoms [22,23,25,27–30], and two assessed the reduction of symptoms and/or complications.

Two of the most recent open RCT studies compared a high-fiber diet with the combined treatment of a high-fiber diet and a symbiotic preparation [22,23]. In the first study, both treatments significantly reduced abdominal pain [22], whereas in the second, the high-fiber diet alone did not improve abdominal symptoms, compared to the baseline [23]. Another open RCT study compared a high-fiber diet with the combination of a high-fiber diet and rifaximin, and showed that both treatments significantly improved abdominal symptoms, compared to the baseline [24]. The occurrence of diverticulitis was reduced during the administration of a high-fiber diet in comparison to one which was not high in fiber, at a follow-up of 65 months [26]. Another study showed a similar frequency of diverticulitis occurrence in both treatment arms, for both dietary fiber and dietary fiber plus rifaximin, after 24 months [24]. Table 3 summarizes the type of intervention, follow-up protocols, the outcome measure, and the efficacy of each intervention included in the selected studies.

Table 3. Intervention and follow-up protocol in the selected studies of dietary fiber treatment in symptomatic uncomplicated diverticular disease (SUDD).

Author, Year (Reference)	Intervention	FU (Months)	Outcome Measure	Efficacy of Intervention	Adverse Effects
Lahner E., 2012 [22]	T1: High-fiber diet T2: Symbiotic preparation + high-fiber diet	6	Reduction of abdominal symptoms	T1 and T2: decrease of abdominal pain <24 h and >24 h in T1 and T2 ($p < 0.05$); T1 and T2: decrease of intensity of abdominal pain <24 h and bloating ($p < 0.05$)	None
Annibale B., 2011 [23]	T1: High-fiber diet T2: Symbiotic (1 sachet bid) + high-fiber diet for 14 days/months T3: Symbiotic (2 sachets bid) + high-fiber diet for 14 day/months	6	Reduction of abdominal symptoms	T1: no significant efficacy; T2 and T3: decrease of bloating VAS ($p < 0.05$), and abdominal pain >24 h ($p = 0.016$)	T3: 1 pt diarrhea
Colecchia A., 2007 [24]	T1: Dietary fiber T2: Dietary fiber + Rifaximin 400 mg bid for 7 days/months	24	Reduction of abdominal symptoms and diverticulitis	T1 and T2: significant reduction of symptomatic score compared to baseline; T1 has similar frequency of diverticulitis of T2 (4 pts in T1 vs. 2 pts in T2; $p = 1$)	Nausea, headache and weakness, T1: 3 pts, T2: 4 pts (p = ns)
Smits B.J., 1990 [25]	T1: High-fiber diet T2: Lactulose 15 mL bid	3	Reduction of abdominal symptoms	T1 and T2: reduction of abdominal pain frequency (T1: $p = 0.022$ and T2 $p = 0.0015$) and severity (T1: $p = 0.028$ and T2 $p = 0.009$) in comparison to baseline	T1: none, T2 :4 pts drops out for abdominal pain, nausea, vomiting
Leahy A.L., 1985 [26]	T1: High-fiber diet T2: Non High-fiber diet	65	Occurrence of symptoms and diverticulitis	T1 reported fewer symptoms and surgery or complications in comparison to T2 (19.3% vs. 44% and 6.4% vs. 32%; $p < 0.05$)	Not reported
Hyland J.M.P., 1980 [27]	T1: High dietary fiber	60	Reduction of abdominal symptoms	T1: 91% (91/100) were symptoms free at 5 years	Not reported
Brodribb A.J.M., 1977 [28]	T1: Bran crispbread T2: Wheat crispbread	3	Reduction of symptoms	T1 reduction of total symptom score in comparison to T2 (from 34.3 to 8.1 and from 42.0 to 35.1 respectively $p < 0.002$)	Not reported
Plumley P.F., 1973 [29]	T1: High fiber crispbread T2: Standard crispbread for at least 2 months	21	Reduction of abdominal symptoms	T1: 29/42 (69%) pts with pain were controlled satisfactory. Only 14 pts took part in the cross over trial (taking T2), but no results are available	Not reported
Painter N.S., 1972 [30]	T1: High-residue, low sugar diet with unprocessed bran	22	Reduction of abdominal symptoms	T1: 88.6% of symptoms relieved or resolved	8 pts did not tolerate bran diet

FU: follow-up; pts: patients; T1: treatment arm 1; T2: treatment arm 2; T3: treatment arm 3.

Due to the poor quality of the studies and the heterogeneity of the study design (mean Jadad score 1.5 ± 1.2 points), a meta-analysis could not be performed to provide a pooled estimate of the outcome measure. With regard to adverse effects, data were not reported in four studies [26–29], no adverse effect was observed in two studies [22–25], and in three studies, some minor effects were reported [23,24,30].

3.5. Supplemental Fiber

These studies were performed over a range of 37 years, from 1976 to 2013, and just one article was published in the last 10 years. Five studies were single center in nature [35,37–40] and five were multicenter studies [31–34,36]. Five studies were conducted in the United Kingdom [35–37,39,40], three in Italy [32–34], one in Spain [31], and one in the USA [38]. The ten included studies investigated an overall total number of 1707 patients, of which 830 were female, but in three studies, the gender of the patients was lacking [37–39]. Patients had a median age of 62 years, ranging from 54 to 66 years, but in two studies, the age of patients was lacking [39,40].

With regard to the study type, three were open randomized controlled trials [31,32,34], two were double blind-cross over studies [36,38], one was a double-blind randomized placebo controlled study [33], two were open un-controlled studies [35,39], and the last was a cross-over RCT [40].

With regard to the type of supplementation, patients were treated with glucomannan [32,34], ispaghula [35–37], bran [36–38,40], plantago ovata [31], and methylcellulose [38]. None of the studies achieved a high dosage of fiber intake with the prescribed supplementation regimen. Because the fiber intake of the diet was not reported, it may be that the total amount of the daily fiber intake is higher than that reported. With regard to fiber solubility, soluble fibers were used in five studies [31–35], both insoluble and soluble fibers were used in two studies [36,37], and in three studies, insoluble fibers were used [38–40].

With regard to the follow-up protocol, the studies were variable, ranging from one to 12 months. Five studies observed patients for a period of less than six months [35–38,40]. In addition, the interventions were very variable: in four studies, fibers were administrated together with a drug (rifaximin) and compared with the efficacy of the fiber alone [32–34]; in two studies, the efficacy of ispaghula and bran was respectively compared to a placebo [36] or lactulose [37], or were administrated as a unique arm of treatment in open un-controlled studies [35,39]. In another study, the efficacy of bran was compared to a high roughage diet or bulk laxative [40], or methylcellulose was compared to a placebo [38]. With regard to the outcome measures, the majority of studies evaluated the reduction of abdominal symptoms [33,35–40], two evaluated the reduction of symptoms and the occurrence of diverticulitis [32,34], and another study only considered the recurrence of diverticulitis [31]. In three open RCTs, the efficacy of glucomannan (2 or 4 gr/day) was compared to glucomannan, together with cyclic rifaximin, analysing the improvement of abdominal symptoms in SUDD patients [32–34]. In all three studies, a significant reduction of abdominal symptoms in the treatment arm with just glucomannan was achieved. In two of these three studies, the glucomannan treatment arm had a similar occurrence of diverticulitis to the antibiotic arm [33,34], while in the Latella study, the glucomannan arm treatment reported more complications ($p < 0.05$) [32]. Table 4 summarizes the type of intervention, follow-up protocols, outcome measures, and efficacy of interventions.

Table 4. Intervention and follow-up protocol in the selected studies of supplemental fiber treatment in symptomatic uncomplicated diverticular disease (SUDD).

Author, Year (Reference)	Intervention	FU (Months)	Outcome Measure	Efficacy of Intervention	Adverse Effects
Lanas A., 2013 [31]	T1: Plantago ovata 3.5 gr bid T2: Plantago ovata 3.5 gr bid + Rifaximin 400 mg bid for 7 days/months	12	Recurrence of diverticulitis	T1: recurrences in 17/88 pts (19.3%) T2: recurrences in 8/77 (10.4%) T1 had a significant higher risk of recurrence $p = 0.025$; OR 3.2 (95% CI: 1.16–8.82)	T1: 13/88 (14.8%) T2: 17/77 (22.1%) ($p = 0.225$)
Latella G., 2003 [32]	T1: Glucomannan 4 gr/day T2: Glucomannan 4 gr/day + Rifaximin 400 mg bid for 7 days/months	12	Reduction of abdominal symptoms and occurrence of diverticulitis	T1 and T2: significant reduction of global symptomatic score in comparison to baseline; T2 had more asymptomatic pts in comparison to T1: 29.2% vs. 56.5% pts at 12 months ($p < 0.001$); T1 reported more diverticulitis in comparison to T2: 11 pts vs. 6 pts ($p < 0.05$).	Nausea, headache, and asthenia: T1: 5 (1.34%) T2: 10 (1.68%) ($p = 0.7932$)
Papi C., 1995 [33]	T1: Glucomannan 2 gr/die + placebo T2: Glucomannan 2 gr/die + Rifaximin 400 mg bid for 7 days/month	12	Reduction of abdominal symptoms	T1 and T2: reduction of global symptom score in comparison to baseline; T2 had more asymptomatic pts in comparison to T1: 68.9% vs. 39.5% pts at 12 month ($p = 0.001$); No differences in preventing diverticulitis.	None
Papi C., 1992 [34]	T1: Glucomannan 2 gr/die T2: Glucomannan 2 gr/die + Rifaximin 400 mg bid for 7 days/months	12	Reduction of abdominal symptoms and occurrence of diverticulitis	T1 and T2: reduction of global symptom score in comparison to baseline. T2 had a marked reduction of score in comparison to T1 (47.6% vs. 63.9%: $p < 0.001$); No differences in preventing diverticulitis (T1: 3 vs. T2: 0, $p = 0.2467$)	Not reported
Thorburn H.A., 1992 [35]	T1: Ispaghula husk	1	Reduction of abdominal symptoms	Improvement of abdominal pain in 71.4% (5/7); Bowel habit improves in 66.6% (6/9)	Not reported
Ornstein M.H., 1981 [36]	T1: Bran (6.99 gr/day) T2: Ispaghula (9.04 gr/day) T3: Placebo (2.34 gr/die)	4	Reduction of abdominal symptoms	No change in pain. T1 and T2: improvement of straining ($p < 0.01$)	T2: 2 pts diarrhea T3: 1 pt constipation
Eastwood M.A., 1978 [37]	T1: Bran (20 gr/die) T2: Ispaghula (2 sachets/day) T3: Lactuose (20–40 mL/day)	1	Reduction of abdominal symptoms	T1, T2 and T3 alleviated symptoms	Not reported
Hodgson W.J.B., 1977 [38]	T1: Methylcellulose 500 mg bid T2: Placebo	3	Reduction of abdominal symptoms	Symptoms score decrease significantly in T1 (from 19 ± 6, to 13 ± 4 $p < 0.01$) but not in T2 (from 21 ± 7 to 17 ± 9, $p = ns$)	Not reported
Brodribb A.J.M., 1976 [39]	T1:Wheat bran 24 gr/die	6	Reduction of abdominal symptoms	60% of symptoms were abolished and 28% relieved	Not reported
Taylor I., 1976 [40]	T1: High roughage diet with bran supplement T2: Bulk laxative plus antispasmodic T3: Bran tablets (18 gr/day)	2	Reduction of abdominal symptoms	T3 was most effective in reduce symptoms. Asymptomatics pts were: T1 = 20%; T2 = 40%; T3 = 60%	Not reported

FU: follow-up; pts: patients; T1: treatment arm 1; T2: treatment arm 2; T3: treatment arm 3.

Also, due to the poor quality of the studies and their heterogeneity (mean Jadad score 1.9 ± 1.8 points), a meta-analysis could not be performed.

On the basis of the heterogeneity of these papers, it was not possible to perform a sub-analysis assessing the differences between dietary and supplemental fibers, the effects of high- or low fiber diet/supplementation, or the differences between soluble and insoluble fibers.

With regard to adverse effects, data were not reported in six studies [34,35,37–40], some minor adverse effects were reported in the fiber arm in three studies [31,32,36], and in another study, the only double-blind randomized placebo controlled report, no adverse effects were observed [33].

4. Discussion

Dietary fibers are defined as the edible parts of plants or the analogous carbohydrates that are resistant to digestion and absorption in the human small intestine, with complete or partial fermentation in the colon [15]. Dietary fibers include non-starch polysaccharides, resistant oligosaccharides, and other carbohydrates, such as resistant starch and dextrins, and lignin [41,42]. Non-starch polysaccharides can be further subdivided into soluble and insoluble fibers: soluble fibers dissolve in water-forming viscous gels, bypass the digestion of the small intestine, and are easily fermented by the gut microbiota (i.e., pectins, gums, inulin-type fructans, and some hemicelluloses). In contrast, insoluble fibers are not water soluble, they do not form gels due to their water insolubility, and fermentation is severely limited (i.e., lignin, cellulose, and some hemicelluloses). The Academy of Nutrition and Dietetics declared that the adequate intake of fiber is 14 gr total per 1000 kcal, or 25 gr for adult women and 38 gr for adult men [18]. In Western countries, the daily fiber intake can change from region to region, and may change over the years. The mean intake of dietary fiber in the United States is 17 gr/day, with only 5% of the general population meeting the adequate intake [18]. In contrast, in a recent study evaluating the changes in food consumption and nutrient intake in a Mediterranean cohort, it has been observed that fiber intake has a baseline of 24.3 ± 9.4 gr/day; after 10 years, it was observed that fiber intake increased by 1.8 gr/day, thus augmenting over time [43]. Even if the health benefits of dietary fibers have long been appreciated, especially for their effect on cardiovascular diseases, type II diabetes, glycemic control, and gastrointestinal conditions [14], these data underline that dietary habits in Western countries may be far from the recommended adequate intake.

With regard to the risk of developing colonic diverticula, it has been proposed that "fiber deficiency", caused by the spreading of refined carbohydrates in the Western diet, may play an important role. However, little evidence is available to substantiate this hypothesis [44,45], and more recently, this concept has been reviewed. A colonoscopy-based, cross-sectional study on the dietary risk factors for diverticulosis found that a high fiber diet was even associated with a higher prevalence of colonic diverticula [46]. The association with dietary fiber intake was dose-dependent and stronger when limited to cases with multiple diverticula. Although it has been suggested that a high-fiber diet does not protect against the development of colonic diverticulosis, it may reduce the abdominal symptoms related to diverticular disease.

Patients with SUDD may complain of chronic recurrent abdominal symptoms, and fibers might confer benefits by increasing fecal mass and promoting the regularity of bowel movements. Another beneficial effect of fibers in the treatment of SUDD may be ascribed to their capability to act as prebiotics in the colon, by favoring health-promoting species of the intestinal microbiota, especially bifidobacteria and lactobacilli [14].

Diverticular disease is a complex, multifactorial disorder, in which the gut microbiota could play a key role. Recently, Barbara et al. reported that patients with diverticular disease showed depletion of microbiota members with anti-inflammatory properties, including Clostridium cluster IV, Clostridium cluster IX, Fusobacterium, and Lactobacillaceae, with microbiota changes being correlated with mucosal immune activation [47]. The gut microbiota, indeed, shifts rapidly in response to dietary changes, particularly with fiber intake [48]. For this reason, high-fiber intake represents a promising treatment option in diverticular disease. In this condition, a high-fiber diet based on fruits, vegetables, and cereal grains may be difficult to achieve and should be supported with an adequate dietary counseling, and in a subset of patients, the use of supplemental fibers might be useful.

The beneficial effect on potential microbiota changes achieved with dietary fibers, based on different amounts of soluble and insoluble fibers, or the supplementation of commercial fibers of the same type, may be different and not necessarily comparable. However, it was not possible to perform a sub-analysis assessing the differences between dietary or supplemental fibers, or between high- or low-fiber diet/supplementation. Unfortunately, on the basis of these studies, it was not possible to assess differences between the effect of soluble or insoluble fibers, even if the relative amount might have influenced the outcome of treatment. In patients with irritable bowel syndrome, a condition that might be considered similar to SUDD, the effect of fibers appears to be limited to the soluble type [49].

In clinical practice, a high-fiber diet or fiber supplementation are commonly used in patients affected by diverticular disease, even if most recommendations are based on poor evidence. A previous systematic review, performed in 2012, was restricted to the use of a high-fiber diet in diverticular disease and only included controlled studies in the English language, reporting that high-quality evidence for a high-fiber diet in the treatment of this condition is scarce [16].

The present systematic review represents an attempt to provide an updated measure of evidence on the efficacy of dietary and supplemental fibers in SUDD, in terms of the reduction of abdominal symptoms and the prevention of acute diverticulitis.

The research was updated until October 2016, considering randomized controlled trials (blinded and/or placebo-controlled), open randomized clinical trials, non-randomized open studies, and also taking into consideration papers in German, French, Italian, and Spanish. The selected studies, all of which came from Western countries with just one study from the USA, presented a high heterogeneity concerning the quantity and quality of the fibers employed, notwithstanding dietary and supplemental fibers, which were evaluated separately. However, the quality of the studies was very low, with just one study yielding an optimal score [33]. Based on the available studies, it was not possible to draw conclusions regarding the efficacy of fiber treatment in SUDD patients, neither in terms of the reduction of abdominal symptoms, nor for the prevention of acute diverticulitis.

5. Conclusions

Single low quality studies suggest that fibers, both dietary and supplemental, could be beneficial in the treatment of SUDD. The presence of substantial methodological limitations, the heterogeneity of therapeutic regimens employed, and the lack of ad hoc designed studies, do not permit a summary of the outcome measures. Up to now, high-quality evidence on the efficacy of fiber treatment for the reduction of symptoms in SUDD and for the prevention of acute diverticulitis, is lacking. Thus, further, well-designed studies, specifically focusing on the efficacy of fibers in SUDD, dietary or supplemental, are needed.

Acknowledgments: This study was in part supported by a Grant of University Sapienza, Roma 2014.

Author Contributions: Marilia Carabotti performed the data extraction and collection, and wrote the manuscript. Edith Lahner performed the data extraction, collection, and contributed to final revision of the manuscript. Carola Severi contributed to the critical revision of the manuscript. Bruno Annibale contributed to the conception and design of the study and to the final revision of the manuscript. All authors approved the final draft submitted.

References

1. Parra-Blanco, A. Colonic diverticular disease: Pathophysiology and clinical picture. *Digestion* **2006**, *73* (Suppl. 1), 47–57. [CrossRef] [PubMed]
2. Stollman, N.; Raskin, J.B. Diverticular disease of the colon. *Lancet* **2004**, *363*, 631–639. [CrossRef]

3. Cuomo, R.; Barbara, G.; Pace, F.; Annese, V.; Bassotti, G.; Binda, G.A.; Casetti, T.; Colecchia, A.; Festi, D.; Fiocca, R.; et al. Italian consensus conference for colonic diverticulosis and diverticular disease. *United Eur. Gastroenterol. J.* **2014**, *2*, 413–442. [CrossRef] [PubMed]
4. Annibale, B.; Lahner, E.; Maconi, G.; Usai, P.; Marchi, S.; Bassotti, G.; Barbara, G.; Cuomo, R. Clinical features of symptomatic uncomplicated diverticular disease: A multicenter Italian survey. *Int. J. Colorectal Dis.* **2012**, *27*, 1151–1159. [CrossRef] [PubMed]
5. Bolster, L.T.; Papagrigoriadis, S. Diverticular disease has an impact on quality of life-results of a preliminary study. *Colorectal Dis.* **2003**, *5*, 320–323. [CrossRef] [PubMed]
6. Comparato, G.; Fanigliulo, L.; Aragona, G.; Cavestro, G.M.; Cavallaro, L.G.; Leandro, G.; Pilotto, A.; Nervi, G.; Soliani, P.; Sianesi, M.; et al. Quality of life in uncomplicated symptomatic diverticular disease: Is it another good reason for treatment? *Dig. Dis.* **2007**, *25*, 252–259. [CrossRef] [PubMed]
7. Shahedi, K.; Fuller, G.; Bolus, R.; Cohen, E.; Vu, M.; Shah, R.; Agarwal, N.; Kaneshiro, M.; Atia, M.; Sheen, V.; et al. Long-term risk of acute diverticulitis among patients with incidental diverticulosis found during colonoscopy. *Clin. Gastroenterol. Hepatol.* **2013**, *11*, 1609–1613. [CrossRef] [PubMed]
8. Anaya, D.A.; Flum, D.R. Risk of emergency colectomy and colostomy in patients with diverticular disease. *Arch. Surg.* **2005**, *140*, 681–685. [CrossRef] [PubMed]
9. Broderick-Villa, G.; Burchette, R.J.; Collins, J.C.; Abbas, M.A.; Haigh, P.I. Hospitalization for acute diverticulitis does not mandate routine elective colectomy. *Arch. Surg.* **2005**, *140*, 576–581. [CrossRef] [PubMed]
10. Binda, G.A.; Cuomo, R.; Laghi, A.; Nascimbeni, R.; Serventi, A.; Bellini, D.; Gervaz, P.; Annibale, B.; Italian society of colon and rectal surgery. Practice parameters for the treatment of colonic diverticular disease: Italian society of colon and rectal surgery (SICCR) guidelines. *Tech. Coloproctol.* **2015**, *19*, 615–626. [CrossRef] [PubMed]
11. Andersen, J.C.; Bundgaard, L.; Elbrønd, H.; Laurberg, S.; Walker, L.R.; Støvring, J.; Danish Surgical Society. Danish national guidelines for treatment of diverticular disease. *Dan. Med. J.* **2012**, *59*, C4453. [PubMed]
12. Pietrzak, A.; Bartnik, W.; Szczepkowski, M.; Krokowicz, P.; Dziki, A.; Reguła, J.; Wallner, G. Polish interdisciplinary consensus on diagnostics and treatment of colonic diverticulosis (2015). *Pol. Przegl. Chir.* **2015**, *87*, 203–220. [CrossRef] [PubMed]
13. Strate, L.L.; Peery, A.F.; Neumann, I. American gastroenterological association institute technical review on the management of acute diverticulitis. *Gastroenterology* **2015**, *149*, 1950–1976. [CrossRef] [PubMed]
14. Slavin, J. Fiber and prebiotics: Mechanisms and health benefits. *Nutrients* **2013**, *5*, 1417–1435. [CrossRef] [PubMed]
15. The Definition of Dietary Fiber. Available online: http://www.aaccnet.org/initiatives/definitions/documents/dietaryfiber/dfdef.pdf (accessed on 16 February 2017).
16. Ünlü, C.; Daniels, L.; Vrouenraets, B.C.; Boermeester, M.A. A systematic review of high-fibre dietary therapy in diverticular disease. *Int. J. Colorectal Dis.* **2012**, *27*, 419–427. [CrossRef] [PubMed]
17. Moher, D.; Liberati, A.; Tetzlaff, J.; Altman, D.G.; PRISMA Group. Preferred reporting items for systematic reviews and meta-analyses: The PRISMA statement. *PLoS Med.* **2009**, *6*, e1000097. [CrossRef] [PubMed]
18. Dahl, W.J.; Stewart, M.L. Position of the academy of nutrition and dietetics: Health implications of dietary fiber. *J. Acad. Nutr. Diet.* **2015**, *115*, 1861–1870. [CrossRef] [PubMed]
19. Jadad, A.R.; Moore, R.A.; Carroll, D.; Jenkinson, C.; Reynolds, D.J.; Gavaghan, D.J.; McQuay, H.J. Assessing the quality of reports of randomized clinical trials: Is blinding necessary? *Control Clin. Trials* **1996**, *17*, 1–12. [CrossRef]
20. Coste, T.; Rautureau, J.; Paraf, A. Treatment of constipation and colonic diverticulosis by bran. *Med. Chir. Dig.* **1978**, *7*, 631–634. [PubMed]
21. Ewerth, S.; Ahlberg, J.; Holmström, B.; Persson, U.; Udén, R. Influence on symptoms and transit-time of Vi-SiblinR in diverticular disease. *Acta Chir. Scand. Suppl.* **1980**, *500*, 49–50. [PubMed]
22. Lahner, E.; Esposito, G.; Zullo, A.; Hassan, C.; Cannaviello, C.; Di Paolo, M.C.; Pallotta, L.; Garbagna, N.; Grossi, E.; Annibale, B. High-fibre diet and *Lactobacillus paracasei* B21060 in symptomatic uncomplicated diverticular disease. *World J. Gastroenterol.* **2012**, *18*, 5918–5924. [CrossRef] [PubMed]
23. Annibale, B.; Maconi, G.; Lahner, E.; De Giorgi, F.; Cuomo, R. Efficacy of *Lactobacillus paracasei* sub. *paracasei* F19 on abdominal symptoms in patients with symptomatic uncomplicated diverticular disease: A pilot study. *Minerva Gastroenterol. Dietol.* **2011**, *57*, 13–22. [PubMed]

24. Colecchia, A.; Vestito, A.; Pasqui, F.; Mazzella, G.; Roda, E.; Pistoia, F.; Brandimarte, G.; Festi, D. Efficacy of long term cyclic administration of the poorly absorbed antibiotic Rifaximin in symptomatic, uncomplicated colonic diverticular disease. *World J. Gastroenterol.* **2007**, *13*, 264–269. [CrossRef] [PubMed]
25. Smits, B.J.; Whitehead, A.M.; Prescott, P. Lactulose in the treatment of symptomatic diverticular disease: A comparative study with high-fibre diet. *Br. J. Clin. Pract.* **1990**, *4*, 314–318.
26. Leahy, A.L.; Ellis, R.M.; Quill, D.S.; Peel, A.L. High fibre diet in symptomatic diverticular disease of the colon. *Ann. R. Coll. Surg. Engl.* **1985**, *67*, 173–174. [PubMed]
27. Hyland, J.M.; Taylor, I. Does a high fibre diet prevent the complications of diverticular disease? *Br. J. Surg.* **1980**, *67*, 77–79. [CrossRef] [PubMed]
28. Brodribb, A.J. Treatment of symptomatic diverticular disease with a high-fibre diet. *Lancet* **1977**, *1*, 664–666. [CrossRef]
29. Plumley, P.F.; Francis, B. Dietary management of diverticular disease. *J. Am. Diet. Assoc.* **1973**, *63*, 527–530. [PubMed]
30. Painter, N.S.; Almeida, A.Z.; Colebourne, K.W. Unprocessed bran in treatment of diverticular disease of the colon. *Br. Med. J.* **1972**, *2*, 137–140. [CrossRef] [PubMed]
31. Lanas, A.; Ponce, J.; Bignamini, A.; Mearin, F. One year intermittent rifaximin plus fibre supplementation vs. fibre supplementation alone to prevent diverticulitis recurrence: A proof-of-concept study. *Dig. Liver Dis.* **2013**, *45*, 104–109. [CrossRef] [PubMed]
32. Latella, G.; Pimpo, M.T.; Sottili, S.; Zippi, M.; Viscido, A.; Chiaramonte, M.; Frieri, G. Rifaximin improves symptoms of acquired uncomplicated diverticular disease of the colon. *Int. J. Colorectal Dis.* **2003**, *18*, 55–62. [CrossRef] [PubMed]
33. Papi, C.; Ciaco, A.; Koch, M.; Capurso, L. Efficacy of rifaximin in the treatment of symptomatic diverticular disease of the colon. A multicentre double-blind placebo-controlled trial. *Aliment. Pharmacol. Ther.* **1995**, *9*, 33–39. [CrossRef] [PubMed]
34. Papi, C.; Ciaco, A.; Koch, M.; Capurso, L. Efficacy of rifaximin on symptoms of uncomplicated diverticular disease of the colon. A pilot multicentre open trial. Diverticular Disease Study Group. *Ital. J. Gastroenterol.* **1992**, *24*, 452–456. [PubMed]
35. Thorburn, H.A.; Carter, K.B.; Goldberg, J.A.; Finlay, I.G. Does ispaghula husk stimulate the entire colon in diverticular disease? *Gut* **1992**, *33*, 352–356. [CrossRef] [PubMed]
36. Ornstein, M.H.; Littlewood, E.R.; Baird, I.M.; Fowler, J.; North, W.R.; Cox, A.G. Are fibre supplements really necessary in diverticular disease of the colon? A controlled clinical trial. *Br. Med. J.* **1981**, *282*, 1353–1356. [CrossRef]
37. Eastwood, M.A.; Smith, A.N.; Brydon, W.G.; Pritchard, J. Comparison of bran, ispaghula, and lactulose on colon function in diverticular disease. *Gut* **1978**, *19*, 1144–1147. [CrossRef] [PubMed]
38. Hodgson, W.J. The placebo effect. Is it important in diverticular disease? *Am. J. Gastroenterol.* **1977**, *67*, 157–162. [PubMed]
39. Brodribb, A.J.; Humphreys, D.M. Diverticular disease: Threee studies. Part II—Treatment with bran. *Br. Med. J.* **1976**, *1*, 425–428. [CrossRef] [PubMed]
40. Taylor, I.; Duthie, H.L. Bran tablets and diverticular disease. *Br. Med. J.* **1976**, *1*, 988–990. [CrossRef] [PubMed]
41. Hamaker, B.R.; Tuncil, Y.E. A perspective on the complexity of dietary fiber structures and their potential effect on the gut microbiota. *J. Mol. Biol.* **2014**, *426*, 3838–3850. [CrossRef] [PubMed]
42. Jones, J.M. CODEX-aligned dietary fiber definitions help to bridge the 'fiber gap'. *Nutr. J.* **2014**, *13*, 34. [CrossRef] [PubMed]
43. De la Fuente-Arrillaga, C.; Zazpe, I.; Santiago, S.; Bes-Rastrollo, M.; Ruiz-Canela, M.; Gea, A.; Martinez-Gonzalez, M.A. Beneficial changes in food consumption and nutrient intake after 10 years of follow-up in a Mediterranean cohort: The SUN project. *BMC Public Health* **2016**, *16*, 203. [CrossRef] [PubMed]
44. Painter, N.S.; Burkitt, D.P. Diverticular disease of the colon: A deficiency disease of Western civilization. *Br. Med. J.* **1971**, *2*, 450–454. [CrossRef] [PubMed]
45. Korzenik, J.R. Case closed? Diverticulitis: Epidemiology and fiber. *J. Clin. Gastroenterol.* **2006**, *40* (Suppl. 3), S112–S116. [CrossRef] [PubMed]

46. Peery, A.F.; Barrett, P.R.; Park, D.; Rogers, A.J.; Galanko, J.A.; Martin, C.F.; Sandler, R.S. A high-fiber diet does not protect against asymptomatic diverticulosis. *Gastroenterology* **2012**, *142*, 266–272. [CrossRef] [PubMed]
47. Barbara, G.; Scaioli, E.; Barbaro, M.R.; Biagi, E.; Laghi, L.; Cremon, C.; Marasco, G.; Colecchia, A.; Picone, G.; Salfi, N.; et al. Gut microbiota, metabolome and immune signatures in patients with uncomplicated diverticular disease. *Gut* **2016**. [CrossRef] [PubMed]
48. David, L.A.; Maurice, C.F.; Carmody, R.N.; Gootenberg, D.B.; Button, J.E.; Wolfe, B.E.; Ling, A.V.; Devlin, A.S.; Varma, Y.; Fischbach, M.A.; et al. Diet rapidly and reproducibly alters the human gut microbiome. *Nature* **2014**, *505*, 559–563. [CrossRef] [PubMed]
49. Moayyedi, P.; Quigley, E.M.; Lacy, B.E.; Lembo, A.J.; Saito, Y.A.; Schiller, L.R.; Soffer, E.E.; Spiegel, B.M.; Ford, A.C. The effect of fiber supplementation on irritable bowel syndrome: A systematic review and meta-analysis. *Am. J. Gastroenterol.* **2014**, *109*, 1367–1374. [CrossRef] [PubMed]

15

Intake and Dietary Food Sources of Fibre in Spain: Differences with Regard to the Prevalence of Excess Body Weight and Abdominal Obesity in Adults of the ANIBES Study

Liliana G. González-Rodríguez [1,2], José Miguel Perea Sánchez [1,2], Javier Aranceta-Bartrina [3,4], Ángel Gil [4,5], Marcela González-Gross [4,6], Lluis Serra-Majem [4,7], Gregorio Varela-Moreiras [8,9] and Rosa M. Ortega [2,10,*]

1 Department of Nutrition and Dietetics, Faculty of Health Sciences, University Alfonso X El Sabio, Madrid 28691, Spain; liligoro@uax.es (L.G.G.-R.); josepesa@uax.es (J.M.P.S.)
2 VALORNUT Research Group, Department of Nutrition, Faculty of Pharmacy, Complutense University, Madrid 28040, Spain
3 Department of Preventive Medicine and Public Health, University of Navarra, Pamplona, Navarra 31008, Spain; jaranceta@unav.es
4 Biomedical Research Networking Center for Physiopathology of Obesity and Nutrition (CIBEROBN), Carlos III Health Institute, Madrid 28029, Spain; agil@ugr.es (A.G.); marcela.gonzalez.gross@upm.es (M.G.-G.); lluis.serra@ulpgc.es (L.S.-M.)
5 Department of Biochemistry and Molecular Biology II and Institute of Nutrition and Food Sciences, University of Granada, Granada 18100, Spain
6 ImFINE Research Group, Department of Health and Human Performance, Technical University of Madrid, Madrid 28040, Spain
7 Research Institute of Biomedical and Health Sciences, University of Las Palmas de Gran Canaria, Faculty of Health Sciences, c/Doctor Pasteur s/n Trasera del Hospital, Las Palmas de Gran Canaria, 35016 Las Palmas, Spain
8 Department of Pharmaceutical and Health Sciences, Faculty of Pharmacy, CEU San Pablo University, Madrid 28668, Spain; gvarela@ceu.es
9 Spanish Nutrition Foundation (FEN), Madrid 28010, Spain
10 Department of Nutrition, Faculty of Pharmacy, Madrid Complutense University, Madrid 28040, Spain
* Correspondence: rortega@ucm.es;

Abstract: The aim was to study the intake and food sources of fibre in a representative sample of Spanish adults and to analyse its association with excess body weight and abdominal obesity. A sample of 1655 adults (18–64 years) from the ANIBES ("Anthropometric data, macronutrients and micronutrients intake, practice of physical activity, socioeconomic data and lifestyles") cross-sectional study was analysed. Fibre intake and dietary food sources were determined by using a three-day dietary record. Misreporters were identified using the protocol of the European Food Safety Authority. Mean (standard deviation) fibre intake was 12.59 (5.66) g/day in the whole sample and 15.88 (6.29) g/day in the plausible reporters. Mean fibre intake, both in the whole sample and the plausible reporters, was below the adequate intake established by European Food Safety Authority (EFSA) and the Institute of Medicine of the United States (IOM). Main fibre dietary food sources were grains, followed by vegetables, fruits, and pulses. In the whole sample, considering sex, and after adjusting for age and physical activity, mean (standard error) fibre intake (adjusted by energy intake) was higher in subjects who had normal weight (NW) 13.40 (0.184) g/day, without abdominal obesity 13.56 (0.192) g/day or without excess body weight and/or abdominal obesity 13.56 (0.207) g/day compared to those who were overweight (OW) 12.31 (0.195) g/day, $p < 0.001$ or obese (OB) 11.83 (0.266) g/day, $p < 0.001$, with abdominal obesity 12.09 (0.157) g/day, $p < 0.001$ or with excess body weight and/or abdominal obesity 12.22 (0.148) g/day, $p < 0.001$. There were no significant differences in relation with the fibre intake according to the body mass index (BMI), presence or absence of abdominal obesity or excess body weight and/or abdominal obesity in the plausible reporters. Fibre from afternoon snacks was higher in subjects with NW (6.92%) and without abdominal obesity (6.97%) or without excess body weight and/or abdominal obesity (7.20%), than those with OW (5.30%), $p < 0.05$ or OB (4.79%), $p < 0.05$, with abdominal obesity (5.18%), $p < 0.01$, or with excess body weight and/or abdominal obesity (5.21%), $p < 0.01$, in the whole sample. Conversely, these differences were not observed in the plausible reporters. The present study demonstrates an insufficient fibre intake both in the whole sample and in the plausible reporters and confirms its association with excess body weight and abdominal obesity only when the whole sample was considered.

Keywords: fibre; food sources; obesity; abdominal obesity; misreporting; adults; Spain; ANIBES

---

1. Introduction

In recent decades, there has been a significant increase in the prevalence of overweight (OW) and obesity (OB) in children and adults, in both developed and developing countries [1]. Excess body weight increases the risk of developing various diseases, such as cardiovascular disease, type 2 diabetes, some types of cancers, musculoskeletal disorders, and neurodegenerative diseases, which have an important health and social impact [1–3].

Diet and physical activity are the main factors that influence the development of OW and OB [1,4]. In this respect, several studies have shown that the intake of dietary fibre may have a positive effect on body weight control; however, the available results are inconsistent [5–8]. There are several possible mechanisms to explain the anti-obesogenic effect of dietary fibre. Among the most documented mechanisms is the one that refers to the benefits of the fibre capacity (mainly soluble fibre) to form viscous gels that delay the gastric emptying, which helps, on the one hand, to increase the satiety sensation and consequently reduces energy intake [9] and, secondly, to control the postprandial glycaemia by delaying the intestinal absorption [10]. Another possible mechanism is associated with short-chain fatty acid produced during fermentation of fibre in the gastrointestinal tract [11] since it has been shown that this can contribute to regulating the secretion of some gastrointestinal hormones, such as glucagon-like peptide-1 (GLP-1), involved in satiety, and ghrelin, involved in appetite control [12,13], and to increase the oxidation of fatty acids and energy expenditure and to regulate glucose metabolism [11].

In addition, there are few recent studies regarding the intake of fibre in a representative Spanish adults sample and none of these studies have analysed the relation between the fibre intake, fibre from different meals of the day and food sources and the problematic of excess body weight and abdominal obesity [14,15]. Additionally, it is the first Spanish study that takes into account the dietary misreporting of the participants.

Therefore, the aim of the present work was to study the intake and dietary food sources of fibre in a representative sample of the Spanish adults from the ANIBES ("Anthropometric data, macronutrients and micronutrients intake, practice of physical activity, socioeconomic data and lifestyles") study and to analyse the differences in fibre intake between people with different body weight and with or without abdominal obesity. The present work shows the analysed data for the total sample and plausible reporters of the study.

2. Materials and Methods

2.1. Study Design and Sampling Procedure

The complete design, protocol, and methodology of the ANIBES study have been already described in detail elsewhere [16,17]. In summary, the ANIBES study was carried out to analyse anthropometric data, physical activity, intake of food and beverages, and dietary habits in the Spanish population (9–75 years old, $n = 2009$). The participants were randomly selected from the Northeast, East, Southwest, North-Central, Barcelona, Madrid, Balearic, and Canary Islands areas of Spain, including rural, semi-urban and urban populations [16,17]. The present study is focused on 1655 adults (779 men and 858 women) with ages ranging 18–64.

The following exclusion criteria were applied:

- Those individuals living in an institutional setting (e.g., colleges, nursing homes, hospitals, and others);
- Individuals following a therapeutic diet owing to recent surgery or taking any medical prescriptions;
- Potential participants with a transitory illness (i.e., flu, gastroenteritis) at the time of the fieldwork; and
- Individuals employed in areas related to consumer science, marketing, or the media [16,17].

The fieldwork for the ANIBES study was carried out from mid-September 2013 to mid-November 2013. The final protocol was approved by the Ethical Committee for Clinical Research of the Region of Madrid (Spain) (code FEN 2013/31, May 2013). All participants were informed of the protocol and risks and benefits of their participation in the study and a written informed consent was obtained from all the study's participants.

2.2. Anthropometric Data

Weight, height, and waist circumference (WC) were measured by trained interviewers following standardized procedures [18]. Weight was measured once with a Seca® model 804 weighing scale (Medizinische Messsysteme und Waagen seit 1840, Hamburg, Germany; range: 70–205 cm, precision: 1 mm). Height was assessed in triplicate using a Seca® model 206 stadiometer (Medizinische Messsysteme und Waagen seit 1840, Hamburg, Germany; range: 0.1–150 kg, precision: 100 g). WC was measured in triplicate using a Seca® 201 tape measure (Seca, Hamburg, Germany; range: 0–150 cm, precision: 1 mm).

Excess body weight was assessed using the body mass index (BMI) and abdominal obesity by the waist to height ratio (WHtR). BMI was calculated as weight (kg)/height (m)^2 and WHtR as WC (cm)/height (cm). Participants were classified into the following categories using the BMI: underweight (UW) (BMI <18.5 kg/m^2), normal weight (NW) (BMI 18.5–24.9 kg/m^2), OW (BMI 25–29.9 kg/m^2), and OB (BMI $\geq$30 kg/m^2), based on the World Health Organization classification [19], and using the WHtR respondents were classified into two categories: "non-abdominal obesity" (WHtR <0.5) and those with "abdominal obesity" (WHtR $\geq$0.5) [20–23]. BMI and WHtR were combined into one category called "excess body weight and/or abdominal obesity" (BMI $\geq$25 kg/m^2 and/or WHtR $\geq$0.5) for subsequent analysis [19,21–23].

2.3. Physical Activity

To obtain physical activity data of the studied participants, a detailed interview using the International Physical Activity Questionnaire (IPAQ) for adults was performed [24]. In addition, different physical activity measurements were obtained with an accelerometer ActiGraph (model GT3x and GT3x+; ActiGraph, Pensacola, FL, USA) in a subsample of 167 adults. Individuals were asked to wear the ActiGraph on a belt above the right hip, for three consecutive full days. This previous information was used to validate the physical activity questionnaire administered to the whole sample.

There were calculated the following indicators of physical activity in the participants of the present study:

- Total physical activity expressed as minutes of activity per week;
- Time spent in vigorous physical activity expressed as minutes of activity per week.

Subjects were classified into two levels of physical activity based on two questions of the IPAQ [24]:

"Sedentary activity level" as those subjects who have performed less than 30 min per day of physical activity of daily life and less than 2 h per week of structured physical exercise.

"Active activity level" as those subjects who have performed at least 30 min per day of physical activity of daily life or have performed at least 2 h per week of structured physical exercise.

2.4. Food and Beverage Record

Study participants were provided with a tablet device (Samsung Galaxy Tab 2 7.0, Samsung Electronics, Suwon, South Korea) and trained in how to record information by taking photos of all food and beverages consumed during the three days of the study, both at home and outside the home. Photos had to be taken before beginning to eat and drink, and again after finishing, so as to record the actual intake. Additionally, a brief description of meals (including the type of food), recipes, brands, and the use of dietary supplements were recorded using the device.

Energy and fibre intake were calculated from food consumption records using VD-FEN 2.1 software (Dietary Evaluation Programme, Spanish Nutrition Foundation, Madrid, Spain) which was newly developed for the ANIBES study by the Spanish Nutrition Foundation and is based mainly on Spanish food composition tables [25], with several expansions and updates. Data obtained from food manufacturers and nutritional information provided on food labels were also included. A food photographic atlas was also used to assist in assigning gram weights to serving sizes [26].

The present study was focused on the intake of fibre expressed in grams per day (g/day) raw (before the energy intake adjustment) and after the energy intake adjustment by the residual methods [27,28] and the intake of fibre expressed in grams per 1000 kcal per day. The mean intake of fibre of the studied participants was compared with the adequate intake set out by European Food Safety Authority (EFSA): 25 g/day in adults [29], and by the Institute of Medicine of the United States (IOM): 38 g/day for men and 25 g/day for women of 19–50 years and 30 g/day for men and 21 g/day for women of 51–70 years (14 g/1000 kcal/day) [30].

Once fibre intake has been established, the percentage of fibre from each one of the meal times (breakfast, mid-morning snack, lunch, afternoon snack, and dinner) was calculated.

The contribution of each food to total fibre intake has been calculated by adding the amount of fibre provided by each specific food and dividing by the total intake of fibre, all multiplied by 100 [31].

2.5. Evaluation of Misreporting

The assessment of dietary intake based on self-reported or self-recorded data by the study subjects is often prone to bias. One of the main sources of error is misreporting, including both under- and over-reporting, which are often influenced by age, sex, and other individual characteristics, including BMI [32]. The magnitude of misreporting of the intake of food may lead to biased interpretation of the results. In the present study the protocol of the EFSA was used to identify misreporters [33,34]. This method is based mainly on the Goldberg [35] and Black [36,37] work. This method evaluates the reported energy intake (EIrep) against the presumed energy requirements. EIrep is expressed as a multiple of the mean basal metabolic rate estimated (BMRest) (from formulas), and it is compared with the presumed energy expenditure of the studied population. Then the ratio EIrep:BMRest is referred to as the physical activity levels (PAL) [33,34]. The PAL is established for adults ($\geq$18 years) in three levels: low, 1.4; moderate, 1.6; and vigorous, 1.8. Additionally, the protocol indicates that analyses should be performed at two levels, group and individual. The group level determines the overall bias to the reported energy intake, and the individual level shows the rate of under and over reporters. The BMRest was calculated using the Schöfield equations [38]. Misreporting cut-offs at group and individual levels for the ANIBES study has been described in a previous paper [39]. Subjects were classified into two categories:

"Plausible reporters" as those subjects with estimated values of the ratio EIrep:BMRest ranging between calculated lower cut-off and upper cut-off values for the studied population allocated to the different category of physical activity [33,34].

"Misreporters" as those subjects with estimated values of EIrep:BMRest below the calculated lower cut-off value (under-reporters) and those subjects with estimated values of EIrep:BMRest above the upper calculated cut -off value (over-reporters) [33,34].

In the present study, the results are showed in the total sample (before the exclusion of the non-plausible reporters) and in the plausible reporters.

2.6. Statistical Analysis

Descriptive data were presented as mean and standard deviation (SD), median and interquartile range (IQR) (both without any adjustment), and frequencies (%) stratified by sex, BMI, presence of abdominal obesity, and excess body weight and/or abdominal obesity. The normality of the data and equality of the variances were tested using the Kolmogorov–Smirnov and Levene's test, respectively.

The statistical differences of the studied quantitative variables by sex were assessed using Student's *t*-test when data were normally distributed, and using the Mann–Whitney test, otherwise. A two-way ANOVA test was used to assess the differences within the studied variables using sex and the variables of BMI, abdominal obesity or excess body weight and/or abdominal obesity. Two-way ANOVA main effects for BMI, abdominal obesity, and excess body weight and/or abdominal obesity were obtained. The Bonferroni post hoc test for comparison for more than two groups was used. A two-way ANCOVA test was used to assess the differences within the studied variables using the previous ANOVA model taking into account the age and the physical activity (PA) of the participants as covariates to control their influence on the dependent variable. Two-way ANCOVA main effects and interactions were analysed and they are only reported in the text as estimated marginal means and the standard error (SE) when a significant inverse trend, significant changes, or an interaction with sex were observed. The level of significance was set at $p < 0.05$. All calculations were performed using IBM SPSS version 22.0 (IBM Corp., Armonk, NY, USA).

3. Results

3.1. Study Population

A sample of 1655 adults (48.2% men and 51.8% women) with ages ranging from 18 to 64 years was studied. In total, 26.16% ($n = 433$) (36.4% men and 63.5% women) of the studied adults were classified as plausible reporters. Table 1 shows the anthropometric and physical activity data of the whole sample and of the plausible reporters. The combined prevalence of OW and OB in the whole sample was 55.70% and 32.80% in the plausible reporters. The prevalence of abdominal obesity was 58.40% and 39.3% and the presence of excess body weight and/or abdominal obesity was 63.93% and 42.7% in the whole sample and in the plausible reporters, respectively. A 44.40% of the whole sample and 44.3% of the plausible reporters were sedentary.

3.2. Fibre Intake and Dietary Food Sources in the Whole Sample and in the Plausible Reporters and by Sex

Mean dietary fibre intake (raw) was 12.59 (SD 5.66) g/day, and adjusted by energy was 12.59 (SD 4.91) g/day, while the intake of fibre expressed as grams per 1000 kcal per day was 7.05 (SD 2.81) in the whole sample (Table 2). Fibre intake (raw) was significantly lower in women than in men, but when it was adjusted by energy intake or when was expressed as grams per 1000 kcal per day, it was significantly lower in men than in women in the whole sample (Table 2). Meanwhile, in the group of plausible reporters, the mean dietary fibre (raw) was 15.88 (SD 6.29) g/day, and it was also significantly lower in women than in men, however, there were no statistically significant differences in relation with the fibre intake adjusted by the energy intake or expressed as g/1000 kcal/day (Table 2). Lunch and dinner contributed the highest proportions of fibre to the total daily intake in the whole sample and in the plausible reporters (75.85% and 70.59%, respectively). It is noteworthy that the fibre from breakfast was quite low in the whole sample (13.04%) as well as in the plausible reporters (14.27%). The proportion of fibre from breakfast and afternoon snacks was higher in women and from dinner in men in the whole sample. No significant differences were observed regarding the fibre from the different meals in the plausible reporters (Table 2).

The main food sources of fibre in the whole studied population and in the plausible reporters were grains (39.13% and 39.14%), vegetables (24.17% and 20.99%), fruits (16.60% and 18.51%), pulses (9.28% and 9.14%), ready-to-eat-meals (4.50% and 4.99%), sauces and condiments (2.18% and 1.97%), appetizers (1.53% and 2.30%), sugars and sweets (0.67% and 1.15%), non-alcoholic beverages (0.49% and 0.53%), dairy products (0.39% and 0.28%), and supplements and meal replacers (0.14% and 0.09%, respectively).

3.3. Fibre Intake and Dietary Food Sources in the Whole Sample and in the Plausible Reporters by Body Mass Index Classification

Considering the whole sample, the fibre intake (raw) was higher in subjects who had NW compared to those who had OW or OB, taking into account sex and after adjusting for the age and PA (Table 3). When the interaction of sex by BMI was analysed, it was noted that the intake of fibre (raw) was slightly different according to sex. Men who presented NW 14.83 (SE 0.327) g/day had a higher intake compared to those who had OW 12.45 (SE 0.304) g/day ($p < 0.001$) or OB 11.67 (SE 0.413) g/day ($p < 0.001$). While women who were UW 14.52 (SE 1.077) g/day had a higher intake than those with OW 11.48 (SE 0.335) g/day ($p < 0.05$) or OB 11.33 (SE 0.455) g/day ($p < 0.05$).

Fibre intake adjusted by energy intake (considering sex) was similar for the different groups of BMI in the whole sample (Table 3). However, after adjusting for the age and the PA, it was observed that subjects with NW 13.29 (SE 0.183) g/day had a higher intake than subjects with OW 12.26 (SE 0.194) g/day ($p < 0.001$) or OB 11.79 (SE 0.265) g/day ($p < 0.001$). Analysing the interaction of sex at different levels of BMI, these differences were observed only in men. Thus, men who presented NW 13.46 (SE 0.279) g/day had a higher intake in comparison with those who had OW 11.81 (SE 0.260) g/day ($p < 0.001$) or OB 11.33 (SE 0.353) g/day ($p < 0.001$).

The intake of fibre per 1000 kcal per day (considering sex) was similar for the different groups of BMI in the whole sample (Table 3). However, after adjusting for the age and the PA, it was observed that subjects with NW 7.35 (SE 0.104) g/1000 kcal/day had a higher intake than subjects with OW 6.92 (SE 0.110) g/1000 kcal/day ($p < 0.05$) or OB 6.68 (SE 0.151) g/1000 kcal/day ($p < 0.01$).

No significant differences were observed regarding the fibre intake (raw, adjusted by the energy intake and expressed as grams per 1000 kcal/day) according with the BMI in the plausible reporters, considering sex and after adjusting for the age and the PA (Table 3).

The proportion of fibre from the lunch was higher in individuals with OW than those with NW taking into account sex, but this difference disappeared when an adjustment for age and PA was performed. Fibre from the afternoon snack was higher in individuals with NW than those with OW or OB (taking into account sex and even after adjusting for age and PA) (Table 3). While fibre from dinner was lower (after adjusting for the age and PA) in individuals who had OW 27.50% (SE 0.581) compared to those with OB 30.27% (SE 0.795) ($p < 0.05$). However, the proportion of fibre from the different meals was similar according the BMI in the plausible reporters (Table 3).

Regarding the fibre food sources according to the BMI in the whole sample, we observed that fibre from breakfast cereals and cereal bars was higher in individuals with NW than those with OW and fibre from vegetables was higher in individuals with OB than those with NW, but these differences disappeared when an adjustment for age and PA was performed (Table S1). Fibre from fruits (taking into account sex and after adjusting for the age and PA) was significantly higher in individuals with NW 18.36% (SE 0.574%) compared to subjects with OW 15.16% (SE 0.605%) ($p < 0.01$). In analysing the interaction of sex, it was observed that only in men, the fibre from fruits was higher in those with NW 18.50% (SE 0.881%) than those with OW 14.01% (SE 0.819%) ($p < 0.001$) or OB 12.92% (SE 1.094%) ($p < 0.001$).

After excluding misreporters, we observed that fibre from grains and flours was higher in subjects with NW than those subjects with OW, but this difference disappeared when an adjustment for age and PA was performed (Table S2). Fibre from pasta (taking into account sex and after adjusting for age and PA) was significantly higher individuals with UW 10.83 (SE 2.231%) compared to subjects with NW 4.72% (0.383%) ($p < 0.05$) or OW 4.59% (0.580%) ($p < 0.05$). In analysing the interaction of sex, it was observed that only in men, the fibre from pasta was higher in those with UW 17.98% (SE 4.207%) than in those with NW 4.71% (SE 0.616%) ($p < 0.05$) or OW 4.62% (SE 0.835%) ($p < 0.05$).

3.4. Fibre Intake and Dietary Food Sources in the Whole Sample and in the Plausible Reporters by the Presence of Abdominal Obesity Determined by the Waist to Height Ratio

Having into account the whole sample, fibre intake (raw) was higher in subjects without abdominal obesity (taking into account sex and even after adjusting for the age and PA) than those with abdominal obesity (Table 4). In analysing the interaction of sex was found that fibre intake in both men and women without abdominal obesity was higher 15.14 (SE 0.337) g/day and 12.76 (SE 0.276) g/day than those subjects with abdominal obesity 12.04 (SE 0.244) g/day ($p < 0.001$) and 11.47 (SE 0.264) g/day ($p < 0.01$), respectively.

Fibre intake (adjusted by energy intake) considering the sex of the participants was similar independently of the presence or absence of abdominal obesity in the whole sample (Table 4). However, after adjusting for the age and PA, subjects without abdominal obesity 13.43 (SE 0.191) g/day had significantly higher intake than subjects with abdominal obesity 12.05 (SE 0.157) g/day ($p < 0.001$). In analysing the interaction of sex was found that fibre intake in both men and women without abdominal obesity was higher 13.63 (SE 0.288) g/day and 13.24 (SE 0.236) g/day that those with abdominal obesity 11.57 (SE 0.208) g/day ($p < 0.001$) and 12.52 (SE 0.226) g/day ($p < 0.05$), respectively.

The intake of fibre per 1000 kcal per day (considering sex) was similar regardless the presence or absence of abdominal obesity in the whole sample (Table 4). However, after adjusting for the age and the PA, it was observed that the subjects without abdominal obesity 7.44 (SE 0.109) g/1000 kcal/day had a higher intake than subjects with abdominal obesity 6.79 (SE 0.089) g/1000 kcal/day ($p < 0.001$). An interaction of sex was found and it was observed that fibre intake only in men without abdominal obesity was higher 7.36 (SE 0.164) g/1000 kcal/day than in those men with abdominal obesity 6.40 (SE 0.119) g/1000 kcal/day ($p < 0.001$).

Nevertheless, no significant differences were observed regarding the fibre intake (raw, adjusted by the energy intake and expressed as grams per 1000 kcal/day) according with the presence or absence of abdominal obesity, considering sex and after adjusting for the age and the PA in the plausible reporters (Table 4).

Fibre from the mid-morning snack was higher in subjects without abdominal obesity than in subjects with abdominal obesity in the whole sample, but this difference disappeared when an adjustment for age and PA was performed (Table 4).

Considering sex and after adjusting for age and PA, the proportion of fibre from lunch was higher in subjects with abdominal obesity than those without abdominal obesity. In contrast, fibre from the afternoon snack was higher in individuals without abdominal obesity unlike those with abdominal obesity (Table 4). The proportion of fibre from the different meals was similar according the presence or absence of abdominal obesity in the plausible reporters (Table 4).

Concerning the fibre food sources according to the presence or absence of abdominal obesity in the whole sample, we observed that fibre from grains, breakfast cereals, and cereal bars, ready-to-eat meals, and sauces and condiments was higher in individuals without abdominal obesity than those with abdominal obesity and fibre from vegetables was higher in individuals with abdominal obesity than those subjects without abdominal obesity, but all of these differences disappeared when an adjustment for age and PA was performed (Table S3). We only found that fibre from bread (taking into account sex and after adjusting for the age and PA) was higher in subjects with abdominal obesity than those who did not have this problem (Table S3). Similarly, after adjusting for the age and the PA, it was observed that the fibre from pasta was higher in individuals with abdominal obesity 6.73% (SE 0.272%) unlike those participants without abdominal obesity 5.68% (SE 0.332%) ($p < 0.05$). In contrast, the fibre from fruits (taking into account sex and after adjusting for the age and PA) was higher in subjects without abdominal obesity 18.46% (SE 0.600%) than in subjects with abdominal obesity 15.46% (SE 0.491%) ($p < 0.001$). However, when the interaction with sex was analysed (Table S3), the previous result only was observed in men without abdominal obesity 19.15% (SE 0.902%) compared to those with abdominal obesity 13.78% (SE 0.654%) ($p < 0.001$). In relation to the group of sugars and sweets and specifically chocolates, individuals without abdominal obesity had a higher intake than subjects with abdominal obesity (Table S3).

In the plausible reporters, we observed that fibre from pasta was higher in subjects without abdominal obesity than those with abdominal obesity, but this difference disappeared when an adjustment for age and PA was performed (Table S4). Fibre from ready-to-eat-meals (taking into account sex and after adjusting for age and PA) was significantly higher in individuals with abdominal obesity 6.39% (SE 0.585%) compared to subjects without abdominal obesity 4.02% (0.484%) ($p < 0.01$).

3.5. Fibre Intake and Dietary Food Sources in the Whole Sample and in the Plausible Reporters by the Presence of Excess Body Weight and/or Abdominal Obesity Using the Body Mass Index and Waist to Height Ratio

Fibre intake (raw) was higher in individuals without excess body weight and/or abdominal obesity in the whole sample (taking into account sex and after adjusting for the age and PA) (Table 5). An interaction of sex was found and it was observed that fibre intake in both men and women without excess body weight and/or abdominal obesity was higher 15.22 (SE 0.371) g/day and 12.81 (SE 0.291) g/day than in those who had excess body weight and/or abdominal obesity 12.28 (SE 0.232) g/day ($p < 0.001$) and 11.55 (SE 0.252) g/day ($p < 0.01$), respectively.

Fibre intake (adjusted by energy intake) considering sex was similar according to the presence or absence of excess body weight and/or abdominal obesity in the whole sample (Table 5). However, after adjusting for the age and PA, it was found that subjects without excess body weight and/or abdominal obesity 13.43 (SE 0.206) g/day had significantly higher intake than subjects with excess body weight and/or abdominal obesity 12.18 (SE 0.148) g/day ($p < 0.001$). An interaction of sex was found and it was observed that fibre intake only in men without excess body weight and/or abdominal obesity was higher 13.68 (SE 0.317) g/day than in those men with excess body weight and/or abdominal obesity 11.74 (SE 0.198) g/day ($p < 0.001$).

The intake of fibre per 1000 kcal per day (considering sex) was similar regardless the presence or absence of excess body weight and/or abdominal obesity in the whole sample (Table 5). However, after adjusting for the age and the PA, it was observed that the subjects without excess body weight and/or abdominal obesity 7.43 (SE 0.117) g/1000 kcal/day had a higher intake than subjects with excess body weight and/or abdominal obesity 6.86 (SE 0.084) g/1000 kcal/day ($p < 0.001$). An interaction of sex was found and it was observed that fibre intake only in men without excess body weight and/or abdominal obesity was higher 7.36 (SE 0.180) g/1000 kcal/day than in those men with excess body weight and/or abdominal obesity 6.48 (SE 0.113) g/1000 kcal/day ($p < 0.001$).

No significant differences were observed regarding the fibre intake (raw, adjusted by the energy intake and expressed as grams per 1000 kcal/day) according with the presence or absence of excess body weight and/or abdominal obesity in the plausible reporters, considering sex and after adjusting for the age and the PA (Table 5).

Considering the sex and after adjusting for the age and the PA, the proportion of fibre from lunch was higher in subjects with excess body weight and/or abdominal obesity than those who did not have excess body weight and/or abdominal obesity. In contrast, the fibre from the afternoon snack was higher in individuals who had no excess body weight and/or abdominal obesity, unlike those with excess body weight and/or abdominal obesity (Table 5). The proportion of fibre from the different meals was similar according the presence or absence of excessive body weight and/or abdominal obesity in the plausible reporters (Table 5).

Table 1. Anthropometric and physical activity data in the whole sample and in plausible reporters of the ANIBES study of the Spanish adult population (18–64 years).

Personal, Anthropometric and Physical Activity Data	Statistical Data	Whole Sample	Plausible Reporters
n		1655	433
Age (years)	Mean (SD)	39.97 (12.19)	38.53 (11.67)
	P50 (IQR)	39.00 (20.00)	37.00 (17.00)
Weight (kg)	Mean (SD)	74.18 (16.47)	65.71 (13.06)
	P50 (IQR)	72.10 (21.80)	63.80 (17.2)
Height (cm)	Mean (SD)	167.67 (9.35)	165.98 (9.56)
	P50 (IQR)	167.00 (14.00)	165.00 (14.00)
Body mass index (kg/m^2)	Mean (SD)	26.31 (5.14)	23.78 (3.88)
	P50 (IQR)	25.60 (6.20)	23.10 (5.00)
Underweight	%	1.80	4.60
Normal	%	42.50	62.60
Overweight	%	35.80	25.20
Obesity	%	19.90	7.60
Waist circumference (cm)	Mean (SD)	88.06 (14.50)	81.42 (11.70)
	P50 (IQR)	86.83 (19.74)	79.73 (16.17)
Waist to height ratio	Mean (SD)	0.52 (0.08)	0.49 (0.07)
	P50 (IQR)	0.51 (0.11)	0.48 (0.09)
Non-abdominal obesity	%	41.60	60.70
Abdominal obesity	%	58.40	39.30
Non-excess body weight and/or abdominal obesity	%	36.07	57.30
Excess body weight and abdominal obesity	%	63.93	42.70
Physical activity (minutes/week)	Mean (SD)	856.60 (637.72)	889.22 (640.23)
	P50 (IQR)	735.00 (920.00)	800.00 (960.00)
Vigorous activity (minutes/week)	Mean (SD)	149.20 (264.15)	168.68 (275.13)
	P50 (IQR)	0 (180.00)	0 (260)
Sedentary activity level	%	44.40	44.30
Active activity level	%	55.60	55.70

SD: standard deviation; P50: 50th percentile; IQR: interquartile range; Abdominal obesity: waist to height ratio ≥ 0.5; Excess body weight and/or abdominal obesity: body mass index ≥ 25 kg/m^2 and/or waist to height ratio ≥ 0.5.

Table 2. Fibre intake in the whole sample and in plausible reporters of the ANIBES study of the Spanish adult population (18–64 years) by sex.

Whole Sample	Statistical Data	Total (n = 1655)	Men (n = 798)	Women (n = 857)	p
Energy (kcal/day)	Mean (SD)	1815.58 (511.96)	1966.22 (543.22)	1675.31 (436.85)	***
	P50 (IQR)	1758.00 (683)	1919.00 (770)	1648.00 (598)	
Total fibre (g/day) (raw)	Mean (SD)	12.59 (5.66)	13.09 (6.09)	12.13 (5.20)	**
	P50 (IQR)	11.63 (6.98)	12.15 (7.27)	11.27 (6.68)	
Total fibre (g/day) (adjusted by energy intake)	Mean (SD)	12.59 (4.91)	12.26 (5.14)	12.91 (4.67)	***
	P50 (IQR)	11.75 (6.01)	11.32 (5.79)	12.25 (6.00)	
Fibre per 1000 kcal/day	Mean (SD)	7.05 (2.81)	6.71 (2.66)	7.37 (2.91)	***
	P50 (IQR)	6.55 (3.53)	6.25 (3.24)	6.99 (3.78)	
Fibre from breakfast (%)	Mean (SD)	13.04 (11.59)	12.15 (11.68)	13.88 (11.44)	***
	P50 (IQR)	10.84 (15.02)	9.73 (15.68)	11.78 (14.48)	
Fibre from mid-morning snack (%)	Mean (SD)	5.16 (8.19)	4.99 (8.21)	5.31 (8.18)	NS
	P50 (IQR)	7.51 (11.69)	0.00 (8.01)	0.87 (8.20)	
Fibre from lunch (%)	Mean (SD)	47.46 (16.60)	48.00 (16.83)	46.96 (16.37)	NS
	P50 (IQR)	47.10 (22.74)	47.61 (23.11)	46.17 (22.50)	
Fibre from afternoon snack (%)	Mean (SD)	5.92 (8.67)	5.48 (8.94)	6.34 (8.39)	***
	P50 (IQR)	1.52 (9.66)	0 (8.55)	3.13 (10.62)	
Fibre from dinner (%)	Mean (SD)	28.39 (14.05)	29.35 (14.43)	27.49 (13.64)	*
	P50 (IQR)	27.03 (18.67)	27.82 (19.40)	26.53 (18.49)	
Plausible Reporters	**Statistical data**	**Total (n = 433)**	**Men (n = 158)**	**Women (n = 275)**	p
Energy (kcal/day)	Mean (SD)	2352 (425)	2712 (358)	2145 (306)	***
	P50 (IQR)	2297 (625)	2640 (490)	2095 (403)	
Total fibre (g/day) (raw)	Mean (SD)	15.88 (6.29)	17.97 (7.19)	14.68 (5.36)	***
	P50 (IQR)	14.89 (7.38)	16.63 (8.26)	14.10 (7.40)	
Total fibre (g/day) (adjusted by energy intake)	Mean (SD)	15.88 (5.81)	15.93 (6.87)	15.85 (5.12)	NS
	P50 (IQR)	14.78 (7.69)	14.26 (8.38)	14.94 (7.46)	
Fibre per 1000 kcal/day	Mean (SD)	6.79 (2.44)	6.64 (2.52)	6.87 (2.38)	NS
	P50 (IQR)	6.31 (3.36)	6.07 (3.03)	6.47 (3.46)	
Fibre from breakfast (%)	Mean (SD)	14.27 (11.39)	13.68 (10.89)	14.61 (11.66)	NS
	P50 (IQR)	12.04 (13.54)	11.75 (13.88)	12.45 (12.90)	
Fibre from mid-morning snack (%)	Mean (SD)	6.32 (8.35)	5.99 (7.91)	6.50 (8.60)	NS
	P50 (IQR)	3.38 (9.32)	2.53 (9.44)	3.78 (9.28)	
Fibre from lunch (%)	Mean (SD)	42.98 (14.84)	44.05 (15.06)	42.37 (14.70)	NS
	P50 (IQR)	42.22 (20.90)	43.32 (21.27)	41.05 (22.17)	
Fibre from afternoon snack (%)	Mean (SD)	8.81 (9.66)	8.16 (9.76)	9.19 (9.60)	NS
	P50 (IQR)	6.15 (13.72)	5.05 (12.22)	6.46 (13.25)	
Fibre from dinner (%)	Mean (SD)	27.61 (12.52)	28.12 (12.11)	27.32 (12.76)	NS
	P50 (IQR)	26.01 (17.25)	27.04 (16.31)	25.79 (18.58)	

SD: standard deviation; P50: 50th percentile; IQR: interquartile range; p: denotes statistical mean differences by sex. * $p < 0.05$. ** $p < 0.01$. *** $p < 0.001$. NS: non-significant.

Table 3. Fibre intake in the whole sample and in the plausible reporters of the ANIBES study of the Spanish adult population (18–64 years) by body mass index.

Whole Sample	Statistical Data	Underweight (n = 30)	Normal Weight (n = 704)	Overweight (n = 592)	Obesity (n = 329)	Two-Way ANOVA	Two-Way ANCOVA
Energy intake (kcal/day)	Mean (SD)	1930.90 (592.45)	1872.51 (526.97)	1773.45 (502.33) $_b$	1759.05 (475.65) $_b$	S ** BMI ***	S ** BMI ***
	P50 (IQR)	1857.00 (2114.00)	1827.00 (4018.00)	1712.50 (2843.00)	1676.00 (3109.00)		
Total fibre intake (g/day) (raw)	Mean (SD)	12.86 (6.35)	13.05 (5.98)	12.27 (5.40) $_b$	12.19 (5.33) $_b$	BMI ** I *	BMI *** I *
	P50 (IQR)	11.20 (22.98)	11.82 (40.66)	11.46 (34.16)	11.46 (35.71)		
Total fibre (g/day) (adjusted by energy) intake)	Mean (SD)	12.22 (4.56)	12.73 (5.13)	12.50 (4.71)	12.50 (4.83)	NS	BMI *** I *
	P50 (IQR)	11.19 (7.68)	11.86 (6.19)	11.90 (6.07)	11.57 (5.81)		
Fibre per 1000 kcal/day	Mean (SD)	6.58 (2.39)	7.06 (2.78)	7.05 (2.79)	7.08 (2.97)	S *	S * BMI **
	P50 (IQR)	6.15 (9.10)	6.56 (18.82)	6.64 (18.35)	6.42 (23.84)		
Fibre from breakfast (%)	Mean (SD)	10.51 (11.89)	13.25 (11.56)	13.16 (11.79)	12.65 (11.30)	NS	NS
	P50 (IQR)	7.34 (41.49)	11.01 (69.25)	10.94 (61.66)	10.37 (64.58)		
Fibre from mid-morning snack (%)	Mean (SD)	6.29 (9.91)	5.32 (8.00)	5.19 (8.48)	4.64 (7.93)	NS	NS
	P50 (IQR)	0.29 (35.40)	1.08 (58.11)	0 (58.29)	0 (63.99)		
Fibre from lunch (%)	Mean (SD)	47.19 (15.69)	45.83 (16.24	48.99 (16.87) $_b$	48.25 (16.71)	BMI **	NS
	P50 (IQR)	46.20 (57.35)	44.81 (93.52)	48.96 (88.61)	48.18 (97.88)		
Fibre from afternoon snack (%)	Mean (SD)	7.43 (5.93)	6.92 (9.11)	5.30 (8.49) $_b$	4.79 (7.99) $_b$	BMI **	BMI *
	P50 (IQR)	6.80 (19.78)	3.25 (52.26)	0.0 (66.44)	0.0 (60.28)		
Fibre from dinner (%)	Mean (SD)	28.58 (12.39)	28.66 (13.96)	27.35 (14.06)	29.65 (14.32)	NS	BMI *
	P50 (IQR)	29.00 (66.69)	27.95 (79.03)	25.80 (91.30)	27.64 (76.37)		
Plausible Reporters	**Statistical Data**	**Underweight (n = 20)**	**Normal Weight (n = 271)**	**Overweight (n = 109)**	**Obesity (n = 33)**	**Two-Way ANOVA**	**Two-Way ANCOVA**
Energy intake (kcal/day)	Mean (SD)	2153 (466)	2307 (425)	2443 (394) $_{a,b}$	2539 (395) $_{a,b}$	BMI **	S *** BMI ***
	P50 (IQR)	2070 (799)	2244 (619)	2405 (616)	2413 (459)		
Total fibre intake (g/day) (raw)	Mean (SD)	14.12 (6.35)	15.58 (6.35)	16.69 (5.86)	16.75 (6.97)	NS	NS
	P50 (IQR)	11.96 (10.08)	14.62 (7.13)	16.45 (8.34)	15.82 (6.45)		
Total fibre (g/day) (adjusted by energy) intake)	Mean (SD)	15.25 (4.93)	15.83 (5.81)	16.17 (5.84)	15.69 (6.41)	NS	NS
	P50 (IQR)	14.24 (8.93)	14.89 (7.09)	15.48 (8.71)	14.31 (7.62)		
Fibre per 1000 kcal/day	Mean (SD)	6.44 (2.19)	6.78 (2.44)	6.93 (2.46)	6.59 (2.48)	NS	NS
	P50 (IQR)	6.15 (4.26)	6.38 (3.12)	6.53 (3.96)	6.08 (3.26)		
Fibre from breakfast (%)	Mean (SD)	11.81 (13.33)	14.47 (11.63)	14.12 (10.64)	14.69 (10.81)	NS	NS
	P50 (IQR)	8.03 (19.27)	12.23 (14.34)	13.08 (12.56)	13.45 (14.12)		
Fibre from mid-morning snack (%)	Mean (SD)	9.07 (11.13)	6.47 (8.57)	6.10 (7.86)	4.14 (5.30)	NS	NS
	P50 (IQR)	6.05 (16.17)	3.78 (9.31)	2.64 (9.42)	1.71 (7.15)		
Fibre from lunch (%)	Mean (SD)	42.40 (15.06)	42.61 (15.11)	43.72 (14.52)	43.97 (14.00)	NS	NS
	P50 (IQR)	42.29 (29.63)	40.16 (20.22)	45.93 (21.66)	43.65 (22.68)		
Fibre from afternoon snack (%)	Mean (SD)	8.12 (6.06)	8.60 (9.28)	9.58 (11.37)	8.43 (8.50)	NS	NS
	P50 (IQR)	6.66 (10.27)	6.15 (13.48)	5.27 (14.07)	7.79 (12.94)		
Fibre from dinner (%)	Mean (SD)	28.61 (12.83)	27.85 (12.69)	26.48 (11.89)	28.77 (13.26)	NS	NS
	P50 (IQR)	26.64 (16.05)	26.68 (17.34)	25.48 (16.86)	26.58 (18.43)		

SD: standard deviation; P50: 50th percentile; IQR: interquartile range; Two-way ANOVA was performed taking into account sex (S) and body mass index (BMI); Two-way ANCOVA was performed taking into account S and BMI and age and physical activity as covariates; Two-way ANOVA significant differences between BMI classification: a: regarding underweight, b: regarding normal weight, c: regarding overweight; I: Interaction; * $p < 0.05$, ** $p < 0.01$, *** $p < 0.001$; NS: non-significant.

Table 4. Fibre intake in the whole sample and in plausible reporters of the ANIBES Study Spanish adult population (18–64 years) by the presence or absence of abdominal obesity using the waist to height ratio.

Whole Sample	Statistical Data	Non-Abdominal Obesity (n = 689)	Abdominal Obesity (n = 966)	Two-Way ANOVA	Two-Way ANCOVA
Energy intake (kcal/day)	Mean (SD)	1886.03 (543.28)	1765.33 (482.43)	S *** WHtR ***	S *** WHtR ***
	P50 (IQR)	1832.00 (701.00)	1705.00 (653.00)		
Total fibre intake (g/day) (raw)	Mean (SD)	12.96 (5.97)	12.33 (5.43)	S *** WHtR ** I **	S *** WHtR *** I **
	P50 (IQR)	11.94 (7.34)	11.46(6.52)		
Total fibre (g/day) (adjusted by energy intake)	Mean (SD)	12.58 (5.06)	12.61 (4.81)	I *	WHtR *** I **
	P50 (IQR)	11.71 (6.06)	11.81 (5.83)		
Fibre per 1000 kcal/day	Mean (SD)	6.97 (2.80)	7.11 (2.82)	S ***	S *** WHtR *** I *
	P50 (IQR)	6.46 (3.54)	6.59 (3.49)		
Fibre from breakfast (%)	Mean (SD)	13.15 (11.81)	12.97 (11.43)	S **	S *
	P50 (IQR)	10.75 (15.44)	10.87 (15.04)		
Fibre from mid-morning snack (%)	Mean (SD)	5.70 (8.59)	4.77 (7.88)	WHtR *	NS
	P50 (IQR)	1.44 (8.23)	0 (7.80)		
Fibre from lunch (%)	Mean (SD)	45.35 (16.26)	48.97 (16.67)	WHtR ***	WHtR **
	P50 (IQR)	44.29 (23.29)	48.81(22.57)		
Fibre from afternoon snack (%)	Mean (SD)	6.97 (8.96)	5.18 (8.38)	WHtR ***	WHtR **
	P50 (IQR)	3.31 (11.75)	0 (8.03)		
Fibre from dinner (%)	Mean (SD)	28.81 (14.26)	28.09 (13.91)	S **	S *
	P50 (IQR)	27.96 (18.71)	26.64 (18.59)		
Plausible Reporters	**Statistical Data**	**Non-Abdominal Obesity (n = 263)**	**Abdominal Obesity (n = 170)**	**Two-Way ANOVA**	**Two-Way ANCOVA**
Energy intake (kcal/day)	Mean (SD)	2319.06 (446.79)	2401.78 (384.418)	S ***	S ***
	P50 (IQR)	2244.00 (641.00)	2366.50 (558)		
Total fibre intake (g/day) (raw)	Mean (SD)	15.36 (6.28)	16.67 (6.23)	S ***	S ***
	P50 (IQR)	14.47 (7.36)	16.32 (7.67)		
Total fibre (g/day) (adjusted by energy intake)	Mean (SD)	15.54 (5.57)	16.39 (6.13)	NS	NS
	P50 (IQR)	14.65 (7.01)	15.27 (8.23)		
Fibre per 1000 kcal/day	Mean (SD)	6.63 (2.31)	7.03 (2.59)	NS	NS
	P50 (IQR)	6.22 (3.21)	6.52 (3.59)		
Fibre from breakfast (%)	Mean (SD)	14.36 (11.94)	14.12 (10.49)	NS	NS
	P50 (IQR)	11.89 (14.42)	13.16 (12.53)		
Fibre from mid-morning snack (%)	Mean (SD)	6.88 (9.00)	5.43 (7.14)	NS	NS
	P50 (IQR)	4.11 (10.44)	2.60 (8.64)		
Fibre from lunch (%)	Mean (SD)	41.97 (14.99)	44.54 (14.50)	NS	NS
	P50 (IQR)	39.91 (19.86)	45.79 (23.04)		
Fibre from afternoon snack (%)	Mean (SD)	8.57 (9.10)	9.18 (10.48)	NS	NS
	P50 (IQR)	6.28 (13.48)	6.03 (13.92)		
Fibre from dinner (%)	Mean (SD)	28.19 (12.64)	26.70 (12.31)	NS	NS
	P50 (IQR)	26.87 (17.32)	25.50 (16.84)		

SD: standard deviation; P50: 50th percentile; IQR: interquartile range; Two-way ANOVA was performed taking into account sex (S) and the waist to height ratio (WHtR); Two-way ANCOVA was performed taking into account S and the WHtR and the age and physical activity as covariates. I: interaction. * $p < 0.05$. ** $p < 0.01$. *** $p < 0.001$. NS: non-significant.

Table 5. Fibre intake in the whole sample and in plausible reporters of the ANIBES study of the Spanish adult population (18–64 years) by the presence or absence of excess body weight and/or abdominal obesity using the body mass index and the waist to height ratio.

Whole Sample	Statistical Data	Non-Excess Body Weight and/or Abdominal Obesity (n = 597)	Excess Body Weight and/or Abdominal Obesity (n = 1058)	Two-Way ANOVA	Two-Way ANCOVA
Energy intake (kcal/day)	Mean (SD)	1892.54 (539.47)	1772.15 (490.72)	S *** BMI_WHtR ***	S *** BMI_WHtR ***
	P50 (IQR)	1848.00 (686.00)	1707.00 (669.00)		
Total fibre intake (g/day) (raw)	Mean (SD)	13.00 (5.96)	12.36 (5.49)	S *** BMI_WHtR** I**	S *** BMI_WHtR *** I**
	P50 (IQR)	11.94 (7.25)	11.47 (6.54)		
Total fibre (g/day) (adjusted by energy intake)	Mean (SD)	12.58 (5.09)	12.60 (4.81)	I *	BMI_WHtR *** I **
	P50 (IQR)	11.71 (6.14)	11.79 (5.86)		
Fibre per 1000 kcal/day	Mean (SD)	6.97 (2.78)	7.1 (2.84)	S ***	S *** BMI_WHtR ** I *
	P50 (IQR)	6.47 (3.56)	6.59 (3.5)		
Fibre from breakfast (%)	Mean (SD)	13.21 (11.85)	12.96 (11.45)	S * I *	S * I *
	P50 (IQR)	10.76 (15.27)	10.85 (15.07)		
Fibre from mid-morning snack (%)	Mean (SD)	5.66 (8.31)	4.88 (8.13)	NS	NS
	P50 (IQR)	1.46 (8.31)	0 (7.76)		
Fibre from lunch (%)	Mean (SD)	45.17 (16.17)	48.76 (16.71)	BMI_WHtR ***	BMI_WHtR **
	P50 (IQR)	44.13 (22.98)	48.64 (22.37)		
Fibre from afternoon snack (%)	Mean (SD)	7.20 (9.09)	5.21 (8.35)	BMI_WHtR ***	BMI_WHtR **
	P50 (IQR)	3.61 (12.03)	0 (8.03)		
Fibre from dinner (%)	Mean (SD)	28.76 (13.84)	28.19 (14.18)	S **	S *
	P50 (IQR)	27.91 (18.71)	26.79 (18.62)		
Plausible Reporters	**Statistical Data**	**Non-Excess Body Weight and/or Abdominal Obesity (n = 248)**	**Excess Body Weight and/or Abdominal Obesity (n = 185)**	**Two-Way ANOVA**	**Two-Way ANCOVA**
Energy intake (kcal/day)	Mean (SD)	2296 (434)	2426 (402)	S ***	S *** BMI_WHtR **
	P50 (IQR)	2223 (623)	2385 (601)		
Total fibre intake (g/day) (raw)	Mean (SD)	15.16 (6.09)	16.85 (6.43)	S ***	S ***
	P50 (IQR)	14.42 (7.27)	16.36 (7.87)		
Total fibre (g/day) (adjusted by energy intake)	Mean (SD)	15.47 (5.47)	16.43 (6.20)	NS	NS
	P50 (IQR)	14.62 (6.84)	15.33 (8.33)		
Fibre per 1000 kcal/day	Mean (SD)	6.62 (2.31)	7.02 (2.58)	NS	NS
	P50 (IQR)	6.22 (3.10)	6.53 (3.71)		
Fibre from breakfast (%)	Mean (SD)	14.34 (12.12)	14.19 (10.35)	NS	NS
	P50 (IQR)	11.47 (14.64)	13.31 (12.24)		
Fibre from mid-morning snack (%)	Mean (SD)	6.98 (9.08)	5.43 (7.17)	NS	NS
	P50 (IQR)	4.22 (10.74)	2.63 (8.70)		
Fibre from lunch (%)	Mean (SD)	41.93 (14.99)	44.40 (14.56)	NS	NS
	P50 (IQR)	39.75 (20.10)	45.69 (22.85)		
Fibre from afternoon snack (%)	Mean (SD)	8.71 (9.22)	8.96 (10.25)	NS	NS
	P50 (IQR)	6.37 (13.86)	5.98 (13.44)		
Fibre from dinner (%)	Mean (SD)	28.05 (12.81)	27.02 (12.13)	NS	NS
	P50 (IQR)	26.71 (17.24)	25.64 (17.04)		

SD: standard deviation; P50: 50th percentile; IQR: interquartile range; Two-way ANOVA was performed taking into account sex (S) and the body mass index and/or waist to height ratio (BMI-WHtR); Two-way ANCOVA was performed taking into account S and the BMI-WHtR and the age and physical activity as covariates. I: interaction. * $p < 0.05$. ** $p < 0.01$. *** $p < 0.001$. NS: non-significant.

Relating to the fibre food sources, according to the presence or absence of excess body weight and/or abdominal obesity in the whole sample, we found that fibre from grains, breakfast cereals, and cereal bars, chocolates, ready-to-eat meals, sauces, and condiments, was higher in individuals without excess body weight and/or abdominal obesity than those with excess body weight and/or abdominal obesity, and fibre from vegetables was higher in individuals with excess body weight and/or abdominal obesity than those subjects without excess body weight and/or abdominal obesity, but all these differences disappeared when an adjustment for age and PA was performed (Table S5). Fibre from bread (taking into account sex and after adjusting for the age and PA) was higher in subjects who had excess body weight and/or abdominal obesity than in those who did not have this problematic (Table S5). Similarly, after adjusting for the age and the PA, it was observed that the fibre from the pasta was higher in individuals with excess body weight and/or abdominal obesity 6.65% (SE 0.256%) as opposed to those without it 5.63% (SE 0.358%) ($p < 0.05$). In contrast, fibre from fruits (taking into account sex and after adjusting for the age and PA) was higher in subjects without excess body weight and/or abdominal obesity 19.06% (SE 0.644%) than in subjects with excess body weight and/or abdominal obesity 15.45% (SE 0.462%) ($p < 0.001$). However, when analysing the interaction with sex (Table S5), this result was only observed in men without excess body weight and/or abdominal obesity 20.12% (SE 0.990%) compared to those with excess body weight and/or abdominal obesity 13.87% (SE 0.619%) ($p < 0.001$).

In the plausible reporters, we observed that fibre from the groups of grains and flours, pasta and juices and nectars was higher in subjects without excess body weight and/or abdominal obesity than those with excess body weight and/or abdominal obesity, but these differences disappeared when an adjustment for age and PA was performed (Table S6). Taking into account sex and after adjusting for age and PA, fibre from fruits was significantly higher in individuals without excess body weight and/or abdominal obesity 20.2% (SE 1.042%) compared to subjects with excess body weight and/or abdominal obesity 16.9% (1.144%) ($p < 0.05$). Conversely, the fibre from ready-to-eat-meals was higher in those subjects with excess body weight and/or abdominal obesity 6.41 (SE 0.558%) than those without excess body weight and/or abdominal obesity 3.81% (SE 0.508%) ($p < 0.01$).

4. Discussion

The present study provides updated information on fibre intake and dietary sources and their association with the condition of excess body weight and abdominal obesity in a representative sample of the Spanish adult population. It is highlighted the ANIBES is the first national diet and nutrition survey in Spain that has taken into account the plausible reporters in the analysis of the data, based on well-harmonised procedures [33,34].

A great proportion of participants of the whole sample and of the plausible reporters had OW or OB, which is in concordance with other studies performed in the Spanish population [40,41]. Nonetheless, it is highlighted the prevalence of OW or OB was lower in the plausible reporters in comparison with the whole sample. When comparing our results with the FANPE study (carried out in 2009 on a representative sample of the Spanish population), we found that the combined prevalence of OW and OB of the study (47.80%) was lower than that observed in our study in the whole sample (55.70%) and higher than that observed in the plausible reporters (32.80%) [41], while the combined prevalence observed in the ENPE study, conducted in 2014–2015, also in Spain, was higher (60.9%) than that observed in the present study both in the whole sample and in the plausible reporters [40].

Some studies have indicated that the WHtR is a better predictor of metabolic syndrome or cardiovascular disease and mortality than the WC or BMI [21,23]. Possibly, the most important advantage of using the WHtR resides in the fact that this ratio takes into account the height of the subject, which avoids the overestimation or underestimation of individuals who have a high or low height [21,23,42]. In our study, the mean WHtR in the whole sample was 0.52 (SD 0.08) and 0.49 (SD 0.07) in the plausible reporters. These values are in line to those indicated by the FANPE and ENPE studies [40,43]. Using this parameter, 58.4% of the whole sample and 39.30%

of the plausible reporters had abdominal obesity, lower than those indicated in the DARIOS Study (conducted in 2013 in Spanish population), in which 89% of men and 77% of women had abdominal obesity [44]. Moreover, when the presence of excess body weight and/or the presence of abdominal obesity were examined, it was found that 63.93% of the whole sample and 42.70% of the plausible reporters had one or both of these problems.

Furthermore, we found that a high proportion of the studied population was sedentary, which has been already discussed in detail in a previous paper [45].

The mean dietary fibre intakes (raw, adjusted by energy intake and expressed in grams per 1000 kcal per day) both in the whole sample and in the plausible reporters were very similar and were lower in comparison with the observed in other studies performed in population with similar ages and characteristics [14,15,46,47]. When comparing the results of our study with those observed by the ENIDE study (carried out in a representative sample of the Spanish population aged 18 to 64 years in 2011), the fibre intake of the participants of our study was lower than the results of such study (men: 20.94 (SD 11.38) g/day and women: 18.85 (SD 10.06) g/day) [14]. Likewise, the mean fibre intakes shown in other study also performed in Spain 20.2 (SD 7.8) g/day and in a study carried out in Irish population 25.7 (SD 8.1) g/day were higher than that observed in our study [15,46]. However, our results were more similar to those observed in the National Health and Nutrition Examination Survey (NHANES 2009–2010) performed in United States adults aged 19 years and older where the fibre intake was 17.0 g/day [47].

The mean intake of fibre (raw) both in men and women was below the adequate intake established by the EFSA and IOM [29,30] in the whole sample and in the plausible reporters. This situation was close to the results shown in various studies performing in similar population [14,46,48,49].

We observed only in the whole sample that the fibre intake after adjusting for energy intake and the fibre per 1000 kcal per day were significantly higher in women than in men. This may be explained because women are usually more concerned about following healthy eating habits and tend to include more healthy foods in their diet compared to men [50]. The analysis of the source of daily fibre intake depending on the different meals throughout the day, revealed that nearly half came from lunch (47.46% and 42.98%) and almost a third from dinner (28.39% and 27.61%) in the whole sample and plausible reporters, respectively. It is noteworthy that the fibre from breakfast was too low in the whole sample (13.04%) and in the plausible reporters (14.27%). The number of frequency of meals per day, including snacks, has been positively related to the intake of various nutrients including the fibre intake [51]. In our study, the mid-morning and afternoon snacks provided the 11.08% and the 15.13% of the daily fibre in the whole sample and in the plausible reporters, respectively. In contrast to our results, the 2001–2010 NHANES study observed that most of the daily fibre came from dinner (37% for adults 19–50 years) [52]. Furthermore, the pattern of fibre intake from the different meals of the day differs according to sex. The proportion of fibre from breakfast and afternoon snacks was higher in women and from dinner in men only in the whole sample. These differences in the pattern of fibre intake are probably due to the differences in the food choices made by the subjects at each meal of the day [52]. A better contribution of fibre from breakfast or afternoon snack, with respect to other meals, could help to reduce appetite and food intake at subsequent meals [6,9]. This could be related to the better situation observed in women compared to men in connection with the presence of excess body weight and abdominal obesity described in a previous paper in more detail for the ANIBES Spanish adult population [53].

Regarding dietary sources of fibre, the main sources in the studied sample were grains, followed by vegetables, fruits, and pulses and were very similar in both studied samples. Similar food groups were identified as the major contributors in the Belgian population [49]. Unlike our study, the main sources of fibre in the ENIDE study were fruits (30%), followed by legumes and nuts (26%), cereals (22%), and vegetables (14%) [14]. Differences were also observed when compared to the results of the 2001–2010 NHANES study, where it was observed that the main sources were the vegetables, followed by cereals and fruits [52].

Some studies performed on populations from the United States [5], the Netherlands [4], and Spain [54] have observed an inverse association between fibre intake and BMI. In accordance with this, in our study, taking into account sex, and after adjusting for the age and physical activity of the participants, fibre intake (raw, adjusted by energy intake and expressed as grams per 1000 kcal per day) was different according to the BMI only in the whole sample. Participants with NW had a significantly higher intake of fibre (raw and expressed as grams per 1000 kcal per day) than those subjects with OW or OB. However, the differences on fibre intake adjusted by the energy intake only were observed in the male sex, where men with NW had a greater intake than those who had OW or OB, which is consistent with what is stated in the study conducted in the Dutch population, where they have found an inverse association between fibre intake and BMI only in men [4]. Moreover, the pattern of fibre intake in the different meals during the day varied depending on the body weight situation only in the whole sample. Specifically, we found that the percentage of fibre that comes from the afternoon snack was higher in individuals with NW than those with OW or OB, while the fibre from dinner was higher in individuals who had OB than those who had OW. The difference found regarding the contribution of fibre from the afternoon snack according to BMI, as previously mentioned, could be related, on the one hand, to the fact that a higher fibre content may favour a reduced appetite which, in turn, can help to take in less food at subsequent meals, in this case during dinner, thus balancing the daily energy intake [6,9]. On the other hand, this also could be explained due to an afternoon snack that contains a higher amount of fibre, which could also include healthier foods with a lower content of energy or fat.

An inverse relation between dietary fibre from cereals and fruits and body weight gain has been described in a study performed in male adults (40–75 years old) from the United States [55]. Although the fibre from grains was the most important fibre food source in the present study, there were no significant differences according to BMI in the whole sample. Conversely, we found that the intake of fibre coming from fruits was higher in men with NW compared to those who had OW or OB in the whole sample. These differences may be explained due to fruits that are rich in soluble fibre, which may help control appetite, or because people who consume fruits and vegetables regularly also tend to have a healthier lifestyle [9,49].

We only observed in the men of the group of plausible reporters that fibre from pasta was higher in those with UW than in those with NW or OW. This may be due to subjects who have an excessive body weight try to control their weight by the reduction of carbohydrates of the diet reducing the intake of this type of food.

When the data were analysed according to the presence or absence of abdominal obesity using the WHtR, we found that the intake of fibre (raw, adjusted by energy intake and express per 1000 kcal per day) only in the whole sample was higher in those subjects without abdominal obesity. In this manner, it becomes clear that the fibre intake may help to avoid the appearance of abdominal obesity, which has also been described in a study performed in Chinese adults that observed subjects with a lower WHtR had a higher fibre intake [56].

On the other hand, the pattern of fibre intake in the different meals during the day varied depending on the presence or absence of abdominal obesity only in the whole sample. The proportion of fibre from lunch was higher in the participants with abdominal obesity compared to their normal counterparts, which could be due to the style of eating in Spain, since in general, lunch is characterized by the presence of an abundant amount of foods like cereals, pulses and vegetables that provide a great amount of fibre, respect to other meals of the day. This type of lunch is largely respected by the general population regardless of individual food habits. However, in relation to the snack and dinner, in Spain is observed that there is a much more marked difference in the composition depending on the food habits of each person. On the other hand, the proportion of fibre from afternoon snacks was higher in individuals without abdominal obesity than in those who had this problem. This finding suggests that a higher intake of fibre in the afternoon could have a beneficial effect in relation to the abdominal accumulation of body fat and not only with respect to the body weight situation described previously. Nevertheless, further studies are needed to clarify this aspect.

Some studies have indicated that the consumption of whole grain foods seems to have benefits regarding weight control and abdominal adiposity, emphasizing that the consumption of whole grain products seems to have not promote weight gain, while refined-grain products are directly associated with the excess of weight and abdominal fat [7,57]. In our study, the contribution to the intake of fibre from bread and pasta was higher only in subjects with abdominal obesity of the whole sample. However, the information about the type of bread or pasta consumed by the population was not available in our study. Moreover, various studies have found an inverse association between dietary fibre from fruits and the WC, insulin resistance, and metabolic syndrome [58–60]. In line with this, in our study, the fibre from fruits was higher only in men of the whole sample without abdominal obesity than in those with this problem. This difference, as previously noted, could be explained because of the beneficial effect of soluble fibre on the reduction of the appetite or due to a healthier lifestyle [9,49]. A similar trend was also observed in relation to the group of sugars and sweets and, in particular, with the subgroup of chocolates. However, because the food groups disaggregated by food items have not been analysed, it was not possible to give an explanation. However, it is assumed that this difference may be due to participants without abdominal obesity selecting and consuming some type of chocolate or similar healthier product with a higher content of fibre, unlike the group who has abdominal obesity.

We only observed in the group of plausible reporters that fibre from ready-to-eat-meals was higher in individuals with abdominal obesity compared to subjects without abdominal obesity, which is according with following an unhealthy diet rich in ready-to-eat-meals, which is common in individuals with obesity.

Likewise, when analysing the excess body weight and abdominal obesity individually, it was confirmed that there was a greater fibre intake in subjects without excess body weight and abdominal obesity compared with those who had one or two of these problems only in the whole sample.

It is noted that the fibre from the afternoon snack seems to play a major role in the body weight situation and abdominal obesity. Even when considering the presence or absence of both problems in the same individual, we also found that those subjects in the whole sample with excess body weight or abdominal obesity had a lower proportion of fibre from the afternoon snack and higher from lunch than their counterparts. This suggests that, probably, the meal of the day in which the fibre is consumed is of relevance to obtaining the benefits of the fibre in relation to excess body weight or abdominal obesity.

In relation to the dietary fibre sources according to the excess body weight and/or abdominal obesity, we found a consistent tendency when the sources were analysed according to the excess body weight and abdominal obesity separately. A higher proportion of fibre from bread and pasta (in men and woman), and less from fruit (only in men), is associated with excess body weight and/or abdominal obesity in comparison with subjects with NW and without abdominal obesity.

As in the whole sample, in the plausible reporters we also observed that fibre from fruits was significantly higher in individuals without excess body weight and/or abdominal obesity compared to subjects with excess body weight and/or abdominal obesity. However, only in the plausible reporters, the fibre from ready-to-eat-meals was higher in those subjects with excess body weight and/or abdominal obesity than those without excess body weight and/or abdominal obesity, which is consistent with the results when the fibre dietary sources were analysed according to the presence or absence of abdominal obesity individually.

A limitation of our study was the inability to analyse the types of fibre (soluble and insoluble) and the food groups disaggregated by food items, since such information was not available. Nonetheless, this did not represent an impediment to achieve the aim of our work that was to study the intake and dietary food sources of fibre and analyse the differences in the fibre intake between people with different body weight situations, and with or without abdominal obesity. In contrast, the main strengths of our study include the methodological design used in the ANIBES study, such as the fact that all anthropometric data were measured and they were not self-reported by the participants, which improves the validity of the study, and the possibility of extrapolating our results to the Spanish population because it was conducted in a representative sample. It is important to highlight that this is the first Spanish study at national level that analyses the data for the whole population and the plausible reporters.

The findings regarding the association between diet and the health outcomes analysed in the present study should be interpreted with caution given the discrepancy observed between both samples. Further studies considering different methods to address misreporting are needed to confirm the association between the fibre intake and the excess body weight and/or abdominal obesity. At the same time, the information derived from our study can be useful in designing nutrition intervention strategies to increase the intake of fibre in our country that it was low both in the whole sample and in the plausible reporters, which in turn could prevent and control some health problems such as excess body weight and abdominal obesity.

5. Conclusions

The present study demonstrates an insufficient fibre intake among the Spanish adult population, both in the whole sample and in the plausible reporters. The main dietary sources were grains, followed by vegetables, fruits, and pulses for both samples. This study observed an association between the fibre intake and excess body weight and abdominal obesity in the whole sample but not in the plausible reporters. Further studies are needed to confirm the association between the fibre intake and the excess body weight and/or abdominal obesity. Nonetheless, it is advisable to increase the intake of foods rich in fibre in order to prevent diseases related with a low intake.

Supplementary Materials:
Table S1: Dietary food sources of total fibre (%) in the whole sample of the ANIBES study of the Spanish adult population (18–64 years) by body mass index., Table S2: Dietary food sources of total fibre (%) in the plausible reporters of the ANIBES study of the Spanish adult population (18–64 years) by body mass index, Table S3: Dietary food sources of total fibre (%) in the whole sample of the ANIBES Study Spanish adult population (18–64 years) by the presence or absence of abdominal obesity using the waist to height ratio, Table S4: Dietary food sources of total fibre (%) in the plausible reporters of the ANIBES Study Spanish adult population (18–64 years) by the presence or absence of abdominal obesity using the waist to height ratio, Table S5: Dietary food sources of total fibre (%) in the whole sample of the ANIBES study of the Spanish adult population (18–64 years) by the presence or absence of excess body weight and/or abdominal obesity using the body mass index and the waist to height ratio, Table S6: Dietary food sources of total fibre (%) in the plausible reporters of the ANIBES study of the Spanish adult population (18–64 years) by the presence or absence of excess body weight and/or abdominal obesity using the body mass index and the waist to height ratio.

Acknowledgments: The authors would like to thank Coca-Cola Iberia and IPSOS for its support and technical advice, particularly Rafael Urrialde and Javier Ruiz.

Author Contributions: L.G.G.-R., J.M.P.S and R.M.O. analysed the data. L.G.G.-R. also drafted and wrote the manuscript. J.M.P.S and R.M.O. contributed to the analysis and wrote the manuscript. J.A.-B., A.G., R.M.O., M.G.-G., and L.S.-M. are members of the Scientific Advisory Board of the ANIBES study and were responsible for careful review of the protocol, design, and methodology. These authors provided continuous scientific advice for the study and for the interpretation of results. These authors also critically reviewed the manuscript. G.V.-M., Principal Investigator of the ANIBES study, was responsible for the design, protocol, methodology, and follow-up checks of the study. All authors approved the final version of the manuscript.

Abbreviations

ANIBES	Anthropometric data, macronutrients and micronutrients intake, practice of physical activity, socioeconomic data and lifestyles
BMI	Body Mass Index
EFSA	European Food Safety Authority
GLP-1	Glucagon-like peptide-1
IOM	Institute of Medicine of the United States

IPAQ	International Physical Activity Questionnaire
NHANES	National Health and Nutrition Examination Survey
NW	Normal weight
OB	Obesity
OW	Overweight
PA	Physical activity
UW	Underweight
WC	Waist circumference
WHtR	Waist to height ratio

1. Tucker, L.A.; Thomas, K.S. Increasing Total Fiber Intake Reduces Risk of Weight and Fat Gains in Women. *J. Nutr.* **2009**, *139*, 576–581. [CrossRef] [PubMed]
2. Buil-Cosiales, P.; Toledo, E.; Salas-Salvado, J.; Zazpe, I.; Farras, M.; Basterra-Gortari, F.J.; Diez-Espino, J.; Estruch, R.; Corella, D.; Ros, E.; et al. Association between Dietary Fibre Intake and Fruit, Vegetable Or Whole-Grain Consumption and the Risk of CVD: Results from the PREvencion Con DIeta MEDiterranea (PREDIMED) Trial. *Br. J. Nutr.* **2016**, *116*, 534–546. [CrossRef] [PubMed]
3. Lin, Y.; Huybrechts, I.; Vereecken, C.; Mouratidou, T.; Valtuena, J.; Kersting, M.; Gonzalez-Gross, M.; Bolca, S.; Warnberg, J.; Cuenca-Garcia, M.; et al. Dietary Fiber Intake and its Association with Indicators of Adiposity and Serum Biomarkers in European Adolescents: The HELENA Study. *Eur. J. Nutr.* **2015**, *54*, 771–782. [CrossRef] [PubMed]
4. Van de Vijver, L.P.; van den Bosch, L.M.; van den Brandt, P.A.; Goldbohm, R.A. Whole-Grain Consumption, Dietary Fibre Intake and Body Mass Index in the Netherlands Cohort Study. *Eur. J. Clin. Nutr.* **2009**, *63*, 31–38. [CrossRef] [PubMed]
5. King, D.E.; Mainous, A.G., 3rd; Lambourne, C.A. Trends in Dietary Fiber Intake in the United States, 1999–2008. *J. Acad. Nutr. Diet.* **2012**, *112*, 642–648. [CrossRef] [PubMed]
6. Hamedani, A.; Akhavan, T.; Samra, R.A.; Anderson, G.H. Reduced Energy Intake at Breakfast is Not Compensated for at Lunch if a High-Insoluble-Fiber Cereal Replaces a Low-Fiber Cereal. *Am. J. Clin. Nutr.* **2009**, *89*, 1343–1349. [CrossRef] [PubMed]
7. Serra-Majem, L.; Bautista-Castano, I. Relationship between Bread and Obesity. *Br. J. Nutr.* **2015**, *113*, S29–S35. [CrossRef] [PubMed]
8. Slavin, J.L. Dietary Fiber and Body Weight. *Nutrition* **2005**, *21*, 411–418. [CrossRef] [PubMed]
9. Guess, N.D.; Dornhorst, A.; Oliver, N.; Bell, J.D.; Thomas, E.L.; Frost, G.S. A Randomized Controlled Trial: The Effect of Inulin on Weight Management and Ectopic Fat in Subjects with Prediabetes. *Nutr. Metab. (Lond.)* **2015**, *12*, 36. [CrossRef] [PubMed]
10. Lupton, J.R. Sugar and Fiber Intake and Type of Adiposity: Are they Related? *Am. J. Clin. Nutr.* **2009**, *90*, 1119–1120. [CrossRef] [PubMed]
11. Barczynska, R.; Bandurska, K.; Slizewska, K.; Litwin, M.; Szalecki, M.; Libudzisz, Z.; Kapusniak, J. Intestinal Microbiota, Obesity and Prebiotics. *Pol. J. Microbiol.* **2015**, *64*, 93–100. [PubMed]
12. Sleeth, M.L.; Thompson, E.L.; Ford, H.E.; Zac-Varghese, S.E.; Frost, G. Free Fatty Acid Receptor 2 and Nutrient Sensing: A Proposed Role for Fibre, Fermentable Carbohydrates and Short-Chain Fatty Acids in Appetite Regulation. *Nutr. Res. Rev.* **2010**, *23*, 135–145. [CrossRef] [PubMed]
13. St-Pierre, D.H.; Rabasa-Lhoret, R.; Lavoie, M.E.; Karelis, A.D.; Strychar, I.; Doucet, E.; Coderre, L. Fiber Intake Predicts Ghrelin Levels in Overweight and Obese Postmenopausal Women. *Eur. J. Endocrinol.* **2009**, *161*, 65–72. [CrossRef] [PubMed]
14. Agencia Española de Seguridad Alimentaria y Nutrición (AESAN). Evaluación Nutricional De La Dieta Española. I Energía Y Macronutrientes. Sobre Datos De La Encuesta Nacional De Ingesta Dietética (ENIDE), 2011. Available online: http://www.Aesan.Msc.Es/AESAN/Docs/Docs/Notas_prensa/Presentacion_ENIDE.Pdf (accessed on 15 February 2016).
15. Moreno Franco, B.; Leon Latre, M.; Andres Esteban, E.M.; Ordovas, J.M.; Casasnovas, J.A.; Penalvo, J.L. Soluble and Insoluble Dietary Fibre Intake and Risk Factors for Metabolic Syndrome and Cardiovascular Disease in Middle-Aged Adults: The AWHS Cohort. *Nutr. Hosp.* **2014**, *30*, 1279–1288. [PubMed]
16. Ruiz, E.; Avila, J.M.; Castillo, A.; Valero, T.; del Pozo, S.; Rodriguez, P.; Bartrina, J.A.; Gil, A.; Gonzalez-Gross, M.; Ortega, R.M.; et al. The ANIBES Study on Energy Balance in Spain: Design, Protocol and Methodology. *Nutrients* **2015**, *7*, 970–998. [CrossRef] [PubMed]

17. Moreiras, G.V.; Avila, J.M.; Ruiz, E. Energy Balance, a New Paradigm and Methodological Issues: The ANIBES Study in Spain. *Nutr. Hosp.* **2015**, *31*, 101–112.
18. Marfell-Jones, M.; Olds, T.; Stewart, A.; Carter, L. *International Standards for Anthropometric Assessment*; International Society for the Advancement of Kinanthropometry: Potchefstroom, South Africa, 2006; pp. 1–137.
19. WHO. Obesity: Preventing and Managing the Global Epidemic. Report of a WHO Consultation. *World Health. Organ. Tech. Rep. Ser.* **2000**, *894*, 1–253.
20. Srinivasan, S.R.; Wang, R.; Chen, W.; Wei, C.Y.; Xu, J.; Berenson, G.S. Utility of Waist-to-Height Ratio in Detecting Central Obesity and Related Adverse Cardiovascular Risk Profile among Normal Weight Younger Adults (from the Bogalusa Heart Study). *Am. J. Cardiol.* **2009**, *104*, 721–724. [CrossRef] [PubMed]
21. Browning, L.M.; Hsieh, S.D.; Ashwell, M. A Systematic Review of Waist-to-Height Ratio as a Screening Tool for the Prediction of Cardiovascular Disease and Diabetes: 0.5 could be a Suitable Global Boundary Value. *Nutr. Res. Rev.* **2010**, *23*, 247–269. [CrossRef] [PubMed]
22. Ashwell, M.; Hsieh, S.D. Six Reasons Why the Waist-to-Height Ratio is a Rapid and Effective Global Indicator for Health Risks of Obesity and how its use could Simplify the International Public Health Message on Obesity. *Int. J. Food Sci. Nutr.* **2005**, *56*, 303–307. [CrossRef] [PubMed]
23. Schneider, H.J.; Friedrich, N.; Klotsche, J.; Pieper, L.; Nauck, M.; John, U.; Dorr, M.; Felix, S.; Lehnert, H.; Pittrow, D.; et al. The Predictive Value of Different Measures of Obesity for Incident Cardiovascular Events and Mortality. *J. Clin. Endocrinol. Metable* **2010**, *95*, 1777–1785. [CrossRef] [PubMed]
24. Craig, C.L.; Marshall, A.L.; Sjostrom, M.; Bauman, A.E.; Booth, M.L.; Ainsworth, B.E.; Pratt, M.; Ekelund, U.; Yngve, A.; Sallis, J.F.; et al. International Physical Activity Questionnaire: 12-Country Reliability and Validity. *Med. Sci. Sports Exerc.* **2003**, *35*, 1381–1395. [CrossRef] [PubMed]
25. Moreiras, O.; Carbajal, A.; Cabrera, L.; Cuadrado, C. *Tablas De Composición De Alimentos/Guía De Prácticas*, 16th ed.; Ediciones Pirámide: Madrid, Spain, 2013.
26. Hercberg, S.; Deheeger, M.; Preziosi, P. *Portions Alimentaires. Manuel Photos Pour L'estimation Des Quantités. SUVIMAX*; Polytechnica: Paris, France, 1994.
27. Willett, W.; Stampfer, M.J. Total Energy Intake: Implications for Epidemiologic Analyses. *Am. J. Epidemiol.* **1986**, *124*, 17–27. [CrossRef] [PubMed]
28. Willett, W.C.; Sampson, L.; Stampfer, M.J.; Rosner, B.; Bain, C.; Witschi, J.; Hennekens, C.H.; Speizer, F.E. Reproducibility and Validity of a Semiquantitative Food Frequency Questionnaire. *Am. J. Epidemiol.* **1985**, *122*, 51–65. [CrossRef] [PubMed]
29. EFSA Panel on Dietetic Products, Nutrition, and Allergies (NDA). Scientific Opinion on Dietary Reference Values for Carbohydrates and Dietary Fibre. *EFSA J.* **2010**, *8*, 1462.
30. Institute of Medicine. *Reference Intakes for Energy, Carbohydrate, Fiber, Fat, Fatty Acids, Cholesterol, Protein and Aminoacids*; The National Academies Press: Washington, DC, USA, 2005.
31. Krebs-Smith, S.M.; Kott, P.S.; Guenther, P.M. Mean Proportion and Population Proportion: Two Answers to the Same Question? *J. Am. Diet. Assoc.* **1989**, *89*, 671–676. [PubMed]
32. Rhee, J.J.; Sampson, L.; Cho, E.; Hughes, M.D.; Hu, F.B.; Willett, W.C. Comparison of Methods to Account for Implausible Reporting of Energy Intake in Epidemiologic Studies. *Am. J. Epidemiol.* **2015**, *181*, 225–233. [CrossRef] [PubMed]
33. Ambrus, Á.; Horváth, Z.; Farkas, Z.; Dorogházi, E.; Cseh, J.; Petrova, S.; Dimitrov, P.; Duleva, V.; Rangelova, L.; Chikova-Iscener, E. Pilot Study in the View of a Pan-European Dietary survey—Adolescents, Adults and Elderly. *EFSA Support. Publ.* **2013**, *EN-485*, 1–85.
34. European Food Safety Authority (EFSA). Example of a Protocol for Identification of Misreporting (Under- and Over-Reporting of Energy Intake) Based on the PILOT-PANEU Project. *EFSA J.* **2013**, *11*, 1–17. Available online: http://www.efsa.europa.eu/sites/default/files/efsa_rep/blobserver_assets/3944A-8-2-1.pdf (Accessed on 1 March 2017).
35. Goldberg, G.R.; Black, A.E.; Jebb, S.A.; Cole, T.J.; Murgatroyd, P.R.; Coward, W.A.; Prentice, A.M. Critical Evaluation of Energy Intake Data using Fundamental Principles of Energy Physiology: 1. Derivation of Cut-Off Limits to Identify Under-Recording. *Eur. J. Clin. Nutr.* **1991**, *45*, 569–581. [PubMed]
36. Black, A.E. Critical Evaluation of Energy Intake using the Goldberg Cut-Off for Energy Intake:Basal Metabolic Rate. A Practical Guide to its Calculation, use and Limitations. *Int. J. Obes. Relat. Metab. Disord.* **2000**, *24*, 1119–1130. [CrossRef] [PubMed]

37. Black, A.E. The Sensitivity and Specificity of the Goldberg Cut-Off for EI:BMR for Identifying Diet Reports of Poor Validity. *Eur. J. Clin. Nutr.* **2000**, *54*, 395–404. [CrossRef] [PubMed]
38. Schofield, W.N. Predicting Basal Metabolic Rate, New Standards and Review of Previous Work. *Hum. Nutr. Clin. Nutr.* **1985**, *39*, 5–41. [PubMed]
39. Olza, J.; Aranceta-Bartrina, J.; Gonzalez-Gross, M.; Ortega, R.M.; Serra-Majem, L.; Varela-Moreiras, G.; Gil, A. Reported Dietary Intake, Disparity between the Reported Consumption and the Level Needed for Adequacy and Food Sources of Calcium, Phosphorus, Magnesium and Vitamin D in the Spanish Population: Findings from the ANIBES Study Dagger. *Nutrients* **2017**. [CrossRef] [PubMed]
40. Aranceta-Bartrina, J.; Perez-Rodrigo, C.; Alberdi-Aresti, G.; Ramos-Carrera, N.; Lazaro-Masedo, S. Prevalence of General Obesity and Abdominal Obesity in the Spanish Adult Population (Aged 25–64 Years) 2014–2015: The ENPE Study. *Rev. Esp. Cardiol. (Engl. Ed.)* **2016**, *69*, 579–587. [CrossRef] [PubMed]
41. Ortega Anta, R.M.; Lopez-Solaber, A.M.; Perez-Farinos, N. Associated Factors of Obesity in Spanish Representative Samples. *Nutr. Hosp.* **2013**, *28*, 56–62. [PubMed]
42. Ashwell, M.; Gunn, P.; Gibson, S. Waist-to-Height Ratio is a Better Screening Tool than Waist Circumference and BMI for Adult Cardiometabolic Risk Factors: Systematic Review and Meta-Analysis. *Obes. Rev.* **2012**, *13*, 275–286. [CrossRef] [PubMed]
43. Navia, B.; Aparicio, A.; Perea, J.M.; Perez-Farinos, N.; Villar-Villalba, C.; Labrado, E.; Ortega, R.M. Sodium Intake may Promote Weight Gain; Results of the FANPE Study in a Representative Sample of the Adult Spanish Population. *Nutr. Hosp.* **2014**, *29*, 1283–1289. [PubMed]
44. Felix-Redondo, F.J.; Grau, M.; Baena-Diez, J.M.; Degano, I.R.; de Leon, A.C.; Guembe, M.J.; Alzamora, M.T.; Vega-Alonso, T.; Robles, N.R.; Ortiz, H.; et al. Prevalence of Obesity and Associated Cardiovascular Risk: The DARIOS Study. *BMC Public Health* **2013**, *13*, 542. [CrossRef] [PubMed]
45. Mielgo-Ayuso, J.; Aparicio-Ugarriza, R.; Castillo, A.; Ruiz, E.; Avila, J.M.; Aranceta-Batrina, J.; Gil, A.; Ortega, R.M.; Serra-Majem, L.; Varela-Moreiras, G.; et al. Physical Activity Patterns of the Spanish Population are mostly Determined by Sex and Age: Findings in the ANIBES Study. *PLoS ONE* **2016**, *11*, e0149969. [CrossRef] [PubMed]
46. Galvin, M.A.; Kiely, M.; Harrington, K.E.; Robson, P.J.; Moore, R.; Flynn, A. The North/South Ireland Food Consumption Survey: The Dietary Fibre Intake of Irish Adults. *Public Health Nutr.* **2001**, *4*, 1061–1068. [CrossRef] [PubMed]
47. Reicks, M.; Jonnalagadda, S.; Albertson, A.M.; Joshi, N. Total Dietary Fiber Intakes in the US Population are Related to Whole Grain Consumption: Results from the National Health and Nutrition Examination Survey 2009 to 2010. *Nutr. Res.* **2014**, *34*, 226–234. [CrossRef] [PubMed]
48. McGill, C.R.; Birkett, A.; Fulgonii Iii, V.L. Healthy Eating Index-2010 and Food Groups Consumed by US Adults Who Meet Or Exceed Fiber Intake Recommendations NHANES 2001–2010. *Food Nutr. Res.* **2016**, *60*, 29977. [CrossRef] [PubMed]
49. Lin, Y.; Huybrechts, I.; Vandevijvere, S.; Bolca, S.; De Keyzer, W.; De Vriese, S.; Polet, A.; De Neve, M.; Van Oyen, H.; Van Camp, J.; et al. Fibre Intake among the Belgian Population by Sex-Age and Sex-Education Groups and its Association with BMI and Waist Circumference. *Br. J. Nutr.* **2011**, *105*, 1692–1703. [CrossRef] [PubMed]
50. Grunert, K.G.; Wills, J.M.; Fernandez-Celemin, L. Nutrition Knowledge, and use and Understanding of Nutrition Information on Food Labels among Consumers in the UK. *Appetite* **2010**, *55*, 177–189. [CrossRef] [PubMed]
51. Kerver, J.M.; Yang, E.J.; Obayashi, S.; Bianchi, L.; Song, W.O. Meal and Snack Patterns are Associated with Dietary Intake of Energy and Nutrients in US Adults. *J. Am. Diet. Assoc.* **2006**, *106*, 46–53. [CrossRef] [PubMed]
52. McGill, C.R.; Fulgoni, V.L., 3rd; Devareddy, L. Ten-Year Trends in Fiber and Whole Grain Intakes and Food Sources for the United States Population: National Health and Nutrition Examination Survey 2001–2010. *Nutrients* **2015**, *7*, 1119–1130. [CrossRef] [PubMed]
53. Lopez-Sobaler, A.M.; Aparicio, A.; Aranceta-Bartrina, J.; Gil, A.; Gonzalez-Gross, M.; Serra-Majem, L.; Varela-Moreiras, G.; Ortega, R.M. Overweight and General and Abdominal Obesity in a Representative Sample of Spanish Adults: Findings from the ANIBES Study. *Biomed. Res. Int.* **2016**, *2016*, 8341487. [CrossRef] [PubMed]

54. Bes-Rastrollo, M.; Martinez-Gonzalez, M.A.; Sanchez-Villegas, A.; de la Fuente Arrillaga, C.; Martinez, J.A. Association of Fiber Intake and Fruit/Vegetable Consumption with Weight Gain in a Mediterranean Population. *Nutrition* **2006**, *22*, 504–511. [CrossRef] [PubMed]
55. Koh-Banerjee, P.; Franz, M.; Sampson, L.; Liu, S.; Jacobs, D.R., Jr.; Spiegelman, D.; Willett, W.; Rimm, E. Changes in Whole-Grain, Bran, and Cereal Fiber Consumption in Relation to 8-Y Weight Gain among Men. *Am. J. Clin. Nutr.* **2004**, *80*, 1237–1245. [PubMed]
56. Thompson, A.L.; Adair, L.; Gordon-Larsen, P.; Zhang, B.; Popkin, B. Environmental, Dietary, and Behavioral Factors Distinguish Chinese Adults with High Waist-to-Height Ratio with and without Inflammation. *J. Nutr.* **2015**, *145*, 1335–1344. [CrossRef] [PubMed]
57. Liu, S.; Willett, W.C.; Manson, J.E.; Hu, F.B.; Rosner, B.; Colditz, G. Relation between Changes in Intakes of Dietary Fiber and Grain Products and Changes in Weight and Development of Obesity among Middle-Aged Women. *Am. J. Clin. Nutr.* **2003**, *78*, 920–927. [PubMed]
58. Du, H.; van der, A.D.L.; Boshuizen, H.C.; Forouhi, N.G.; Wareham, N.J.; Halkjaer, J.; Tjonneland, A.; Overvad, K.; Jakobsen, M.U.; Boeing, H.; et al. Dietary Fiber and Subsequent Changes in Body Weight and Waist Circumference in European Men and Women. *Am. J. Clin. Nutr.* **2010**, *91*, 329–336. [CrossRef] [PubMed]
59. Hosseinpour-Niazi, S.; Mirmiran, P.; Mirzaei, S.; Azizi, F. Cereal, Fruit and Vegetable Fibre Intake and the Risk of the Metabolic Syndrome: A Prospective Study in the Tehran Lipid and Glucose Study. *J. Hum. Nutr. Diet.* **2015**, *28*, 236–245. [CrossRef] [PubMed]
60. McKeown, N.M.; Meigs, J.B.; Liu, S.; Saltzman, E.; Wilson, P.W.; Jacques, P.F. Carbohydrate Nutrition, Insulin Resistance, and the Prevalence of the Metabolic Syndrome in the Framingham Offspring Cohort. *Diabetes Care* **2004**, *27*, 538–546. [CrossRef] [PubMed]

16

Dietary Fiber and the Human Gut Microbiota: Application of Evidence Mapping Methodology

Caleigh M. Sawicki [1,2], Kara A. Livingston [1], Martin Obin [3], Susan B. Roberts [4], Mei Chung [5] and Nicola M. McKeown [1,2,*]

1 Nutritional Epidemiology, Jean Mayer USDA Human Nutrition Research Center on Aging at Tufts University, Boston, MA 02111, USA; caleigh.sawicki@tufts.edu (C.M.S.); kara.livingston@tufts.edu (K.A.L.)
2 Friedman School of Nutrition Science and Policy, Tufts University, Boston, MA 02111, USA
3 Nutrition & Genomics Laboratory, Jean Mayer USDA Human Nutrition Research Center on Aging at Tufts University, Boston, MA 02111, USA; martin.obin@tufts.edu
4 Energy Metabolism Laboratory, Jean Mayer USDA Human Nutrition Research Center on Aging at Tufts University, Boston, MA 02111, USA; susan.roberts@tufts.edu
5 Nutrition/Infection Unit, Department of Public Health and Community Medicine, Tufts University School of Medicine, Boston, MA 02111, USA; Mei_Chun.Chung@tufts.edu
* Correspondence: nicola.mckeown@tufts.edu;

Abstract: Interest is rapidly growing around the role of the human gut microbiota in facilitating beneficial health effects associated with consumption of dietary fiber. An evidence map of current research activity in this area was created using a newly developed database of dietary fiber intervention studies in humans to identify studies with the following broad outcomes: (1) modulation of colonic microflora; and/or (2) colonic fermentation/short-chain fatty acid concentration. Study design characteristics, fiber exposures, and outcome categories were summarized. A sub-analysis described oligosaccharides and bacterial composition in greater detail. One hundred eighty-eight relevant studies were identified. The fiber categories represented by the most studies were oligosaccharides (20%), resistant starch (16%), and chemically synthesized fibers (15%). Short-chain fatty acid concentration (47%) and bacterial composition (88%) were the most frequently studied outcomes. Whole-diet interventions, measures of bacterial activity, and studies in metabolically at-risk subjects were identified as potential gaps in the evidence. This evidence map efficiently captured the variability in characteristics of expanding research on dietary fiber, gut microbiota, and physiological health benefits, and identified areas that may benefit from further research. We hope that this evidence map will provide a resource for researchers to direct new intervention studies and meta-analyses.

Keywords: dietary fiber; gut microbiota; evidence map; colonic fermentation; oligosaccharides; resistant starch; cereal fiber; *Bifidobacteria*; *Lactobacilli*

---

1. Introduction

According to the 2009 Codex Alimentarius definition of dietary fiber, which aims to unify the definition among all countries, dietary fiber includes all carbohydrate polymers of three or more monomeric units that resist digestion in the small intestine [1,2]. A further stipulation of this definition is that isolated or chemically synthesized fibers need to show a physiological health benefit. Epidemiological evidence consistently shows that higher intake of dietary fiber is associated with a reduced risk of chronic diseases, such as cardiovascular disease (CVD), type 2 diabetes, and cancer [3]. However, new research is interested in the role of the gut microbiota with respect to observed beneficial effects [4,5].

Research on the human gut microbiota, sometimes referred to as the "forgotten organ" [6], has exponentially increased over the past decade with recent advances in technology. There has been growing evidence that the microbiota not only produces metabolites that can influence host physiology, but these metabolites also play an integral role in the host immune system and metabolism through a complex array of chemical interactions and signaling pathways [7–9]. These interactions can greatly impact host health and risk of disease [7,10], and the microbiota have been linked to numerous diseases such as irritable bowel syndrome (IBS), asthma, allergy, metabolic syndrome, diabetes, obesity, cardiovascular disease, and colorectal cancer [11].

A number of factors can cause the composition of the microbiota to shift, including changes in diet [10]. Consumption of dietary fiber has been shown to influence the gut microbiota by altering bacterial fermentation, colony size, and species composition [12]. Non-digestible carbohydrates are the primary energy source for most gut microbes and, therefore, can directly impact those species that heavily depend on that substrate [13]. There can also be indirect impacts through cross-feeding, where some types of microbes depend on the by-products, or metabolites, of other types of microbes [14,15]. In addition to substrate availability, the magnitude and diversity of the microbiota are also greatly influenced by other aspects of the gut environment, including pH, host secretions, and transit time [11,12,16–19]. While certain dietary components play an important role in the gut environment, products of microbial fermentation can also have an influence [10,20]. For example, consumption of fermentable dietary fiber will provide substrates for microbial activity but will also increase the concentrations of fermentation products, such as short-chain fatty acids (SCFAs). A buildup of SCFAs subsequently lowers the colonic pH, which can then have dramatic effects on the composition of the microbiota [16,20,21]. Therefore, the relationship between diet, the gut microbiota, microbial activity, and gut physiology is complex.

The distribution of different strains or species of bacteria within the gut will determine the metabolic profile of the microbiota, which could have potential physiologic effects on health [10]. SCFAs, such as butyrate, acetate, and propionate produced by the fermentation of dietary fibers, may play a role in energy homeostasis, immune function, and host-microbe signaling [7,22,23], and prevention of diseases, such as bowel disease, colon cancer, and metabolic syndrome [20,24–26]. Therefore, fiber-induced modulation of the gut microbiota has gained interest for its potential impact on health and disease [27]. However, it is not well understood how and to what extent these changes may happen in a predictable way [28]. The first step toward answering these questions is to gather and summarize the current literature on dietary fiber and the gut microbiota, which can be done effectively using evidence mapping.

Evidence mapping is a new technique being applied in nutritional epidemiology to review and characterize the published research on a broad topic of interest, allowing for the identification of gaps and prioritizing new research questions [29–31]. Evidence maps may be considered as the first few steps in a systematic review but are generally more comprehensive in the scope of the research question [31,32]. Instead of a specific, targeted question, an evidence map aims to determine the research "landscape" of the topic area. Evidence mapping can provide a context for systematic reviews and meta-analyses by presenting a wide range of study designs and methods being utilized in the area of interest [29]. While systematic reviews are the method of choice for synthesizing study results, evidence mapping is a more efficient methodology for visualizing the evidence and is a particularly useful technique in fast-paced or rapidly growing areas of research, such as the human gut microbiota.

Our objective was to describe existing research on dietary fiber intake and the gut microbiota. Through the creation of an evidence map, we identify potential gaps in the research and highlight areas where new hypotheses may be addressed in future studies. Furthermore, we extended our evidence mapping to summarize broad study findings in a focused area regarding the effects of the oligosaccharide interventions on the gut microbial composition. In doing so, we demonstrate how this evidence map can be used as a platform to build on the existing evidence by answering the following two questions: (1) Can we identify specific gut microbial species that are modulated by dietary fiber? (2) Is there evidence that modulation of the gut microbiota is correlated with fermentation or physiological effects on host health?

2. Materials and Methods

Evidence mapping involves three major steps: (1) clearly defining a topic area and setting criteria around the questions of interest; (2) systematically searching for and selecting relevant studies based on pre-defined criteria, such as study design and outcomes of interest and, thereby, creating a "map" of available evidence; and (3) reporting on study characteristics and the extent of existing research [30–32].

To develop the dietary fiber and human gut microbiota evidence map, we utilized a newly developed Dietary Fiber Database (Version 3.0), containing data on published dietary fiber interventions [33]. The database, housed in the Systematic Review Data Repository (SRDR) [34], contains descriptive data extracted from dietary fiber intervention studies that were identified by a systematic literature search. It includes all human studies published from 1946 to May 2016 that examined the effect of dietary fiber on at least one of nine pre-defined physiological health outcomes. For the complete list of the inclusion/exclusion criteria, including the nine health outcomes, refer to Supplementary Materials Table S1.

The database includes two specific outcomes related to the gut microbiota: (1) modulation of colonic microflora; and (2) colonic fermentation/short-chain fatty acid concentration. Keywords used to identify these specific outcomes in the development of the database are provided in the Supplementary Methods. Our evidence map is comprised of all publications in the database reporting on at least one of these two outcomes.

Descriptive analyses were performed to examine the range of study designs, fiber interventions, and types of outcomes examined. Because evidence mapping is meant to capture the wider landscape of evidence and is, therefore, more inclusive and less homogenous than is usually required for a meta-analysis, results are specifically not represented. Due to the large variety of fiber interventions identified, fiber intervention exposures were grouped into categories according to structure or source, depending on how they were described in the original publication. If the same fiber intervention was given at different doses within the same study, that fiber type was only counted once for that study.

Microbiota outcomes identified by the database were examined in more detail and were re-classified into three categories: (1) fermentation, which included measures of SCFAs, breath markers (such as H_2 and CH_4), bacterial enzyme activity and metabolites, bile acid metabolism, and fiber digestibility (measured by fecal recovery); (2) bacterial composition, which included relative or absolute bacterial counts; and (3) colonic and fecal pH.

Weighted scatter plots were used to visualize the available evidence on different fiber types by outcome groups and sample size. Each bubble in the plot represents a single publication with the size of the bubble corresponding to the study sample size. Publications may be represented more than once throughout the plot if multiple fiber interventions or outcomes were reported but are not repeated within any single cross-sectional area.

To further explore the information captured in this evidence map, we isolated publications on the top most reported fiber type, oligosaccharides. We examined oligosaccharides in relation to bacterial composition and extracted more detailed information on the study characteristics, bacterial strains and/or species identified in the publication and the direction of change in strain/species frequency (increased, decreased, or remained the same) in response to the fiber intervention.

3. Results

A total of 188 distinct studies with at least one outcome related to the gut microbiota were identified in the Dietary Fiber Database (Version 3.0). The study design and population characteristics of these studies are summarized in Table 1.

Table 1. Study Design Characteristics.

Characteristic, *n* (% of Studies)	Total	Top Three Fiber Types		
		Oligosaccharides	Resistant Starch	Chemically Synthesized
n	188	38	30	28
Design				
Randomized, parallel	54 (29%)	14 (37%)	3 (10%)	10 (36%)
Randomized, crossover	127 (67%)	24 (63%)	27 (3%)	16 (57%)
Randomized, combined parallel and crossover	2 (1%)	0 (0%)	0 (0%)	1 (4%)
Non-Randomized	2 (1%)	0 (0%)	0 (0%)	0 (0%)
Unspecified Randomization	3 (2%)	0 (0%)	0 (0%)	1 (4%)
Sample size				
Less than 10	19 (10%)	1 (3%)	6 (20%)	2 (7%)
10 to 49	145 (77%)	29 (76%)	23 (77%)	23 (82%)
50 to 100	20 (11%)	6 (16%)	0 (0%)	2 (7%)
More than 100	4 (2%)	2 (5%)	1 (3%)	1 (4%)
Duration				
Acute (<1 week)	36 (19%)	4 (11%)	9 (30%)	6 (21%)
1–4 weeks	126 (67%)	26 (68%)	21 (70%)	20 (71%)
1–6 months	25 (13%)	8 (21%)	0 (0%)	2 (7%)
More than 6 months	1 (1%)	0 (0%)	0 (0%)	0 (0%)
Diet type				
Acute	36 (19%)	4 (11%)	9 (30%)	6 (21%)
Isocaloric/Maintenance	115 (61%)	26 (68%)	17 (57%)	12 (43%)
Weight Loss	2 (1%)	0 (0%)	0 (0%)	0 (0%)
Other/Unspecified	35 (19%)	8 (21%)	4 (13%)	10 (36%)
Age				
Adults (≥17 years *)	185 (98%)	37 (97%)	30 (100%)	27 (96%)
Adolescents (12–17 years)	1 (1%)	0 (0%)	0 (0%)	1 (4%)
Children (3–11 years)	2 (1%)	1 (3%)	0 (0%)	0 (0%)
Baseline Health				
Healthy	153 (81%)	34 (89%)	26 (87%)	27 (96%)
Overweight or Obese	7 (4%)	1 (3%)	0 (0%)	1 (4%)
Diabetic	1 (1%)	0 (0%)	0 (0%)	0 (0%)
Metabolically at Risk	8 (4%)	1 (3%)	2 (7%)	0 (0%)
Hyperlipidemia	6 (3%)	1 (3%)	1 (3%)	0 (0%)
GI/Digestive Issues	6 (3%)	0 (0%)	0 (0%)	0 (0%)
Other	7 (4%)	1 (1%)	1 (3%)	0 (0%)
Region				
Asia	6 (3%)	2 (5%)	1 (3%)	3 (11%)
Australia/New Zealand	16 (8%)	1 (3%)	7 (23%)	1 (4%)
Europe	114 (61%)	31 (81%)	17 (57%)	12 (43%)
North America	51 (27%)	4 (11%)	5 (17%)	12 (43%)
South America	1 (1%)	0 (0%)	0 (0%)	0 (0%)

* Only one study had an age range of 17–61 years, all other studies in adults included subjects ≥18 years.

The majority (96%) were randomized, controlled studies, with only two studies not randomized, and three studies with unknown randomization. The majority of studies used a crossover design compared to a parallel design (67% randomized, crossover; 29% randomized, parallel; and 1% combination of crossover and parallel designs). The size of the study samples ranged from 4 to 435 subjects, but the majority of studies (87%) had fewer than 50 subjects. Few studies (14%) had an intervention duration exceeding four weeks. Most (67%) lasted 1–4 weeks, and 19% were acute feeding interventions, which usually consisted of a single test meal. The subjects were described as healthy in the majority of studies (81%). Fewer studies involved subjects that were overweight or obese (4%), diabetic (1%), hyperlipidemic (3%), had metabolic syndrome or "at-risk" for metabolic syndrome (4%), digestive issues (3%), or risk factors for developing colon cancer (2%).

Within the 188 studies, 47 different fiber types were captured. These fiber interventions fell into 11 different categories, as detailed in Table 2.

Table 2. Fiber types (total studies = 188), 324 unique exposures.

Group	Studies (%)	Fiber Types	*n*
Oligosaccharide	38 (20%)	Fructooligosaccharide	22
		Galactooligosaccharide	11
		Arabinoxylan-oligosaccharides	6
		Xylo-oligosaccharide	2
		Soybean oligosaccharides	1
Resistant Starch	30 (16%)	Resistant starch type 1	1
		Resistant starch type 2 [a]	20
		Resistant starch type 3	11
		Resistant Starch, mixed or unspecified	4
Chemically synthesized	28 (15%)	Polydextrose	12
		Dextrin [g]	9
		Soluble corn fiber	7
		PolyGlycopleX (PGX)	2
		Resistant starch type 4	2
		Microcrystalline cellulose	1
		Solubilized potato polysaccharide	1
		Pullulan	1
		Butyrylated high amylose maize starch	1
Inulin	25 (13%)	Inulin	18
		Oligofructose-enriched inulin (OF-IN)	7
Bran	24 (13%)	Wheat Bran	12
		Oat Bran	9
		Corn bran	2
		Barley bran	1
		Rye Bran	1
		Bran	2
Cereal fiber	21 (11%)	Cereal fiber, wheat [b]	9
		Cereal fiber, barley [c]	8
		Cereal fiber, oat [d]	4
		Cereal fiber, rye [e]	4
		Cereal fiber [f]	3
Fruit/Vegetable/Plant fibers	15 (8%)	Vegetable fiber	6
		Lupin Kernel Fiber	3
		Sugar cane fiber	2
		Sugar Beet fiber	1
		Bean fiber	1
		Citrus fiber	2
		Fruit fiber	1
Combination	13 (7%)	Combination/Mixture	13
Gums and Mucilages	10 (5%)	Gums [h]	7
		Psyllium [i]	6
Other non-starch polysaccharides	9 (5%)	Pectin	4
		Cellulose	3
		Hemicellulose [j]	3
		Beta-glucan, barley	1
		Polysaccharide, non starch	1
High fiber diet	4 (2%)	Dietary fiber	4

More specific fiber types described include [a] high-amylose maize starch; [b] whole-grain wheat; [c] barley flour, barley kernels; [d] oat kernels; [e] whole-grain rye, rye kernels; [f] whole-grain, mixture, or unspecified cereal fiber; [g] wheat dextrin, resistant dextrin, resistant maltodextrin, soluble fiber dextrin; [h] guar gum, gum arabic; [i] ispaghula, Metamucil; [j] arabinogalactan, xylans, glucomannan.

The fibers most frequently studied were oligosaccharides (20% of studies), resistant starch (16%), and chemically synthesized fibers (15%), followed closely by inulin (13%), bran (13%) and cereal fiber (11%). The study design characteristics for studies examining the top three fibers are also presented in Table 1. Notably, resistant starch had a higher proportion of studies with a sample size of fewer than 10 subjects, while oligosaccharides were more often examined in studies of much larger sample sizes and longer duration.

Table 3 reports the frequency and percentage of three major microbiota outcomes: bacterial composition (47% of studies), colonic/fecal pH (32%), and fermentation (76%). Fermentation is further broken down by the specific measurement used to determine the degree of fermentation. SCFA concentration (52%) and breath gas excretion (27%) were the most commonly measured markers of fermentation, but others included bacterial enzyme activity, bile acid metabolism, and fecal starch recovery.

Table 3. Microbiota outcomes (total studies = 188).

Outcome Group	Studies (%)
Fermentation	142 (76%)
SCFA concentration	98 (52%)
Breath gas excretion	50 (27%)
Bacterial enzyme activity	18 (10%)
Bile acids	15 (8%)
Fecal fiber/starch recovery	13 (7%)
Bacterial composition	88 (47%)
Colonic/fecal pH	60 (32%)

Figure 1 is a weighted scatter plot of the microbiota outcomes by fiber group. It provides a visual representation summarizing the research activity in this field. For example, while SCFA concentration and bacterial composition are studied often, fewer and less sizeable studies measure breath gas excretion and other markers of fermentation. Specific gaps in the research are readily identified. Notably, we can see that there are currently no published studies examining the effect of a high fiber whole-diet intervention on bacterial composition of the microbiota. This plot also shows active areas of interest. We can see, for example, that a large number of relatively larger studies have been published on bacterial composition and oligosaccharide interventions.

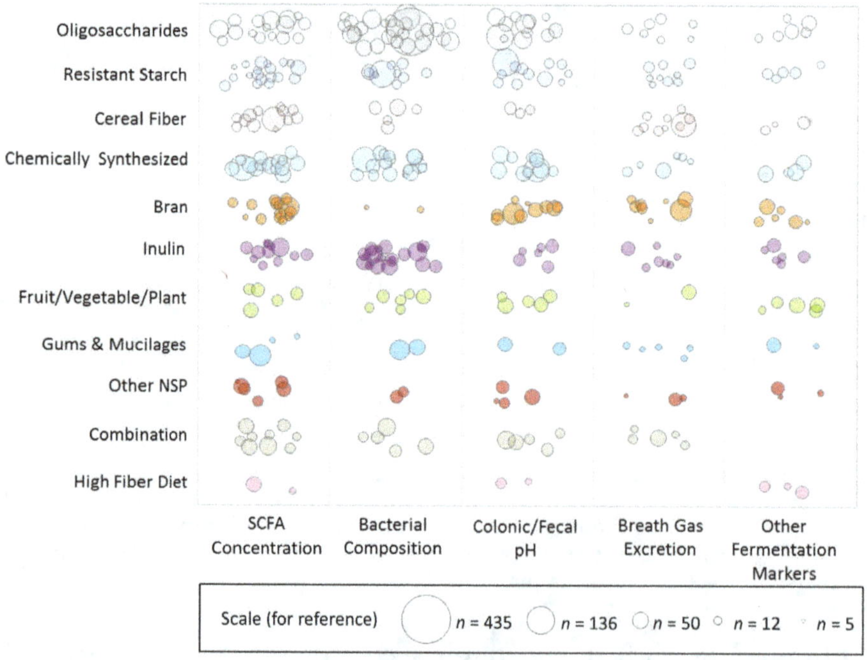

Figure 1. Weighted scatter plot of microbiota outcomes by fiber group. Each bubble in the plot represents a single publication with the size of the bubble corresponding to the study sample size. Studies may be represented more than once throughout the plot if multiple fiber interventions or outcomes were reported but are not repeated within any single cross-sectional area. Note that the outcome effect is not represented in this graphic, i.e., this does not reflect the effect of the fiber on the outcome.

Figure 2 is a weighted scatter plot displaying the other physiological health outcomes captured in this evidence map. Not surprisingly, gastrointestinal (GI) health, which includes measures of fecal bulking, laxation, and transit time, is very frequently studied along with the gut microbiota, but there is less evidence on satiety, adiposity, and blood pressure. There is also just one study published so far examining bone health in the context of dietary fiber and the gut microbiota, a very new emerging area of interest. Supplementary Materials Figures S1 and S2 present weighted scatter plots similar to those in Figure 2, restricted by study duration. The acute studies (Figure S1) exclusively examine the short-term fermentation response by measuring SCFA concentration and/or breath gas excretion, most frequently in cereal fibers, whereas studies of greater duration (Figure S2) examine more outcomes in a larger array of fiber types. Notably, however, there are no longer duration (>4 weeks) studies on resistant starch.

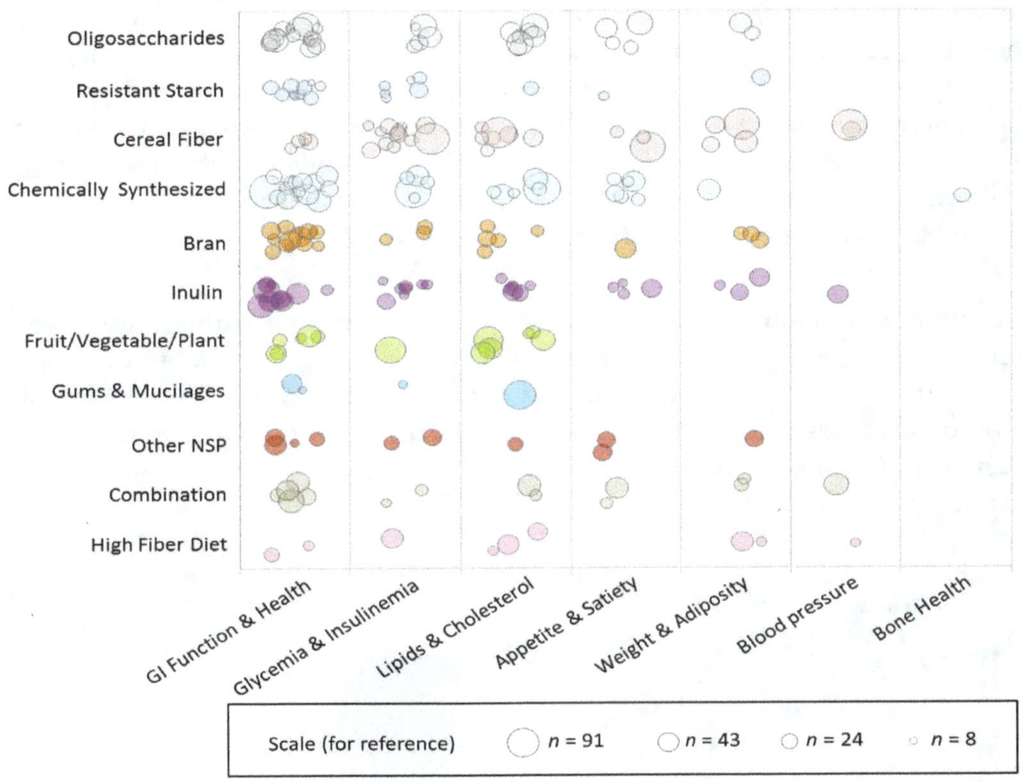

Figure 2. Weighted scatter plot of other physiological health outcomes by fiber group. Each bubble in the plot represents a single publication with the size of the bubble corresponding to the study sample size. Studies may be represented more than once throughout the plot if multiple fiber interventions or outcomes were reported but are not repeated within any single cross-sectional area. Note that the outcome effect is not represented in this graphic, i.e., this does not reflect the effect of the fiber on the outcome.

We extended our evidence mapping of the fiber–microbiota research landscape by examining one of the most active areas in more detail: oligosaccharide interventions and bacterial composition. There were 26 studies (from 25 publications) on this topic. Three of the studies utilized a dose of antibiotics to specifically examine the use of oligosaccharides to assist recolonization of the gut, and, for comparison purposes, we excluded these from this sub-analysis. Details of the remaining 23 studies are shown in Table 4. Studies were published between 1996 and 2015, and all were randomized controlled trials (9 parallel, 14 crossovers). Intervention durations ranged from 1 to 12 weeks, and sample size ranged from 15 to 136 (mean of 46) subjects. Notably, only one study recruited subjects that were overweight with metabolic syndrome, and one study recruited subjects that were overweight, while all the other studies reported on healthy subjects. Most studies had a similar age range, but there was one study in children and one specifically in older adults.

Among these 23 studies, there are 26 fiber interventions: eight fructooligosaccharides (FOS), nine galactooligosaccharides (GOS), six arabinoxylan-oligosaccharides (AX-OS), two xylo-oligosaccharide (XOS), and one soybean oligosaccharide. All but one study found a bifidogenic effect of oligosaccharides, with doses as small as 1.4 g/day (XOS) and a range of treatment forms, including tablets, beverages, and whole foods. Many studies also examined oligosaccharide impacts on *Lactobacilli* or *Lactobacillus–Enterococcus* frequency, with 19 studies reporting no effect, three reporting a positive effect, and one reporting a negative effect. Few publications reported decreases in bacterial strains/species, but among those that did, it was most often *Bacteroides*, with four studies finding a significant decrease in response to a GOS intervention. However, two intervention studies found no effect of GOS on *Bacteroides*, five interventions using other oligosaccharides also found no effect, and one XOS intervention found a significant increase in *Baceroides fragilis*. There were a number of other strains/species reported; however, it is important to note that some studies used targeted culturing techniques, whereas others used DNA sequencing to attempt to identify all species present.

Table 5 summarizes the other physiological outcomes examined within these studies. Ten out of the 26 interventions also significantly increased markers of fermentation, but only one intervention had a significant effect on fecal bulking, and only two had significant effects on transit time. Of the other physiologic outcomes examined in these studies, most were related to GI health. Only a few studies measured lipids, glucose, or insulin, and of those that did, only one study found a significant effect on total cholesterol and insulin.

Table 4. Characteristics of oligosaccharide interventions and direction of evidence on bacteria composition.

Reference	*n*	Design	Duration	Age, Mean (Range)	% Male	BL Health	BMI, Mean (Range)	Fiber Type (g/Day)	Form	Control	Method	Bacterial Composition Reported Measures
[35]	20	RCT, P, DB	12 days	(22–39)	50	Healthy	NR	FOS (12.5)	NR (3 oral doses)	Saccharose placebo	Stool (whole), Wilkins-Chalgren agar, Beerens' medium	↑ *Bifidobacteria* NS Total anaerobes
[36]	40	RCT, P	7 days	29.6 (18–47)	45	Healthy	NR	FOS (2.5, 5, 10, 20)	Powder	Saccharose powder	Stool (whole), Wilkins-Chalgren, Beeren's medium	↑ *Bifidobacteria* (at doses 5–20 g) NS Total anaerobes
[37]	15	RCT, C, DB	3 weeks	NR	~47	Healthy	NR	FOS (2.5)	Biscuits	Matched biscuits without FOS	Stool (partial), PCR-DGGE (denaturing gradient gel electrophoresis), fluorescent in situ hybridization (FISH)	NS *Bifidobacteria* NS Lactobaccilli NS Lactose-fermenting enterobacteria NS Total enterobacteria NS Enterococci
								GOS (2.5)	Biscuits			NS *Bifidobacteria* NS *Lactobaccilli* NS Lactose-fermenting enterobacteria NS Total enterobacteria NS *Enterococci*
[38]	136	RCT, P, DB	7 days	~30 (~18–54)	~41	Healthy	NR	FOS (2.5, 5.0, 7.5, 10)	NR (2 oral doses)	Sucrose and fully digestible maltodextrin placebo	Stool (partial), Wilkins-Chalgren agar. Beerens's medium, Bacteroides Bile Esculin agar, Lactobacillus agar, MRS agar, and McConkey agar	↑ *Bifidobacteria* NS Total anaerobes NS *Lactobacillus* NS *Baceroides* NS *Enterobacteria*
								GOS (2.5, 5.0, 7.5, 10)	NR (2 oral doses)			↑ *Bifidobacteria* NS Total anaerobes NS *Lactobacillus* NS *Baceroides* NS *Enterobacteria*
								SB-OS (2.5, 5.0, 7.5, 10)	NR (2 oral doses)			↑ *Bifidobacteria* NS Total anaerobes NS *Lactobacillus* NS *Baceroides* NS *Enterobacteria*
[39]	39	RCT, P, DB	30 days	60.4	0	Healthy	NR	FOS (7)	Cereal bars and gelified milk	Matched cereal bars and gelified milk without FOS	Stool (partial), temperature-gradient gel electrophoresis (TTGE), FISH	↑ *Bifidobacterium* spp. ↑ Bifidobacterium Animalis and related species NS Bacteroides and relatives NS Clostridium coccoides-Eubacterium rectale cluster NS Faecalibacterium prausnitzi subgroup NS Lactobacillus-Enterocococcus group NS Atopobium group

Table 4. *Cont.*

Reference	*n*	Design	Duration	Age, Mean (Range)	% Male	BL Health	BMI, Mean (Range)	Fiber Type (g/Day)	Form	Control	Method	Bacterial Composition Reported Measures
[40]	34	RCT, C, DB	2 weeks	27.7	100	Healthy	23.2	FOS (20)	Beverage (lemonade)	Matched lemonade with sucrose placebo	Stool (whole), RT-qPCR	↑ *Bifidobacteria* ↑ *Lactobacilli* NS *E. coli*
[41]	40	RCT, P	7 days	29	~45	Healthy	NR	FOS (2.5, 5.0, 7.5, 10)	Tablet	Sucrose and fully digestible maltodextrin placebo	Stool (partial), Wilkins-Chalgren agar, Beerens' medium, MRS agar, BBE agar, McConkey agar	↑ *Bifidobacteria* (all doses) ↑ Total Anaerobes (10 g only) NS *Lactobacilli* NS *Bacteroides* NS *Enterobacteria*
[42]	30	RCT, C, DB	7 days	36.3 (21–59)	~40	Healthy	NR	GOS (3.6, 7)	Powder, mixed with water	Matched sucrose placebo powder	Stool (whole), FISH	↑ *Bifidobacterium* ↑ Clostridium perfringens-histolyticum subgroup (3.6 g only) NS *Lactobacillus-Enterococcus* spp. NS Bacteroides-prevotella
	29			32.5 (19–55)	~45	Healthy	NR	GOS (7)	Powder, mixed with water	Matched powder without GOS		↑ *Bifidobacterium* ↓ Bacteroides-prevotella NS *Lactobacillus-Enterococcus* spp. NS Clostridium perfringens-histolyticum subgroup
[43]	44	RCT, C, DB	10 weeks	69.3 (64–79)	~36	Healthy	(22–31)	GOS (5.5)	Powder, mixed with water	Matched maltodextrin placebo	Stool (partial), FISH	↑ Bifidobacterium spp. ↑ *Lactobacillus-Enterococcus* spp. ↑ Clostridium coccoides-Eubacterium rectale group ↓ *Bacteroides* spp. ↓ Clostridium histolyticum group ↓ *Escherchia coli* ↓ *Desulfovibrio* spp.
[44]	64	RCT, P, DB	30 days	33 (22–51)	~41	Healthy	NR	FOS (5)	Powder, used to prepare a jelly	Commercial dessert (jelly, lemon flavored)	Stool (partial), Beerens' agar, Chromocult Coliform agar, Slanetz and Bartley medium, Rogosa agar, Wilkins-Chalgren anaerobe agar with 5% (v/v) defibrinated horse blood and G-N anaerobe selective supplement (OXOID), Perfringens agar with D-cycloserine.	↑ *Bifidobacterium* spp. ↓ Total coliforms ↓ *Escherichia coli* NS Total aerobes NS *Enterococcus* spp. NS Total anaerobes NS *Bacteroides* spp. NS *Lactobacillus* spp. NS *Clostridium perfringens*

Table 4. *Cont.*

Reference	*n*	Design	Duration	Age, Mean (Range)	% Male	BL Health	BMI, Mean (Range)	Fiber Type (g/Day)	Form	Control	Method	Bacterial Composition Reported Measures
[45]	20	RCT, C	3 weeks	24	30	Healthy	20.9	AX-OS (10)	Beverage (orange juice drink)	Matched maltodextrin placebo beverage	Stool (partial), real-time PCR, real-time PCR TaqMan, real-time PCR SYBR Green technology	↑ *Bifidobacteria* ↑ *Bifidobacterium adolescentis* ↓ *Lactobacilli* NS Total bacteria NS Roseburia-Eubacterium rectale NS *Enterobacteria*
[46]	39	RCT, C, DB	3 weeks	58.9 (50–81)	~46	Healthy	26.1 (19.7–38.4)	GOS (~8)	Beverage (orange juice drink)	Matched placebo beverage	Stool (partial), quantitative PCR, FISH	↑ *Bifidobacterium* ↓ *Bacteroides* NS *Total bacteria* NS *Lactobacillus* NS *Escherichia coli* NS Eubacterium rectales group NS Clostridium histolyticum group
[47]	60	RCT, P, DB	4 weeks	~20 (18–24)	~43	Healthy	~21.3	X-OS (5)	Beverage (orange juice drink)	Matched wheat maltodextrin placebo beverage	Stool (partial), quantitative PCR	↑ *Bifidobacterium* NS *Lactobacillus* NS *Peptostreptococcus* NS *Clostridium* NS *Firmicutes* NS *Bacteroidetes* NS Faecalibacterium prausnitzii NS *Roseburia* spp.
[48]	27	RCT, C, DB	3 weeks	25	~37	Healthy	20.9	AX-OS (2.14)	Wheat/rye bread	Matched wheat/rye or refined wheat bread, no AX-OS	Stool (partial), FISH	↑ *Bifidobacterium* NS Total bacteria NS Lactobacillus NS Lactobacillus rods NS Enterobacteriaceae NS *Clostridium* histolyticym/lituburiense
[49]	63	RCT, C, DB	3 weeks	42	~52	Healthy	23.3	AX-OS (2.4, 8)	Beverage (non-carbonated soft drink)	Placebo beverage with 0.25 g tricalcium phosphate, no AX-OS	Stool (partial), FISH, 4′-6-diamidino-2-phenylindole (DAPI)	↑ Bifidobacterium (8 g only) NS Total bacteria NS Lactobacilli NS Faecalibacterium prausnitzii NS Clostridium histolyticum-lituseburense NS Roseburia-Eubacterium rectale
[50]	40	RCT, C, DB	21 days	31.4 (18–55)	50	Healthy	23.3 (18.5–30.0)	AX-OS (2.2)	Wheat/rye bread	Matched wheat/rye bread without AX-OS	Stool (whole), FISH	↑ *Bifidobacterium* spp. ↑ *Escherichia coli* ↑ *Lactobacillus-Enterococcus* ↑ Total bacteria ↑ Bacteroides NS Clostridium histolyticum group NS Atopobium-Coriobacterium group NS Eubacterium rectale group NS Roseburia-Eubacteria NS Faecalibacterium prausnitzii cluster

Table 4. *Cont.*

Reference	n	Design	Duration	Age, Mean (Range)	% Male	BL Health	BMI, Mean (Range)	Fiber Type (g/Day)	Form	Control	Method	Bacterial Composition Reported Measures
[51]	65	RCT, C, DB	21 days	53.1 (18–75)	46	Healthy	27.8 (18.5–35.0)	AX-OS (2.2, 4.8)	Wheat-based ready-to-eat cereal	Wheat-based ready-to-eat cereal without AXOS	Stool (partial), FISH	↑ Bifidobacterium (4.8 g only, significant dose trend) NS Total bacteria NS *Lactobacillus* spp. NS Bacertoides NS Clostridium coccoides NS Roseburia intestinalis-Eubacterium rectale group NS Faecalibacterium prausnitzii NS Clostridium clusters I and II
[52]	48	RCT, C, DB	12 weeks	~44.6	36	OW, metabolic syndrome	~31.4	GOS (5.5)	Powder, mixed with water	Maltodextrin placebo	Stool (partial), FISH	↑ *Bifidobacteria* ↓ *Bacteroides* spp. ↓ *Clostridium histolyticum* group ↓ *Desulfovibrio* spp. NS Total bacteria NS *Lactobacillus-Enterococcus* spp. NS Clostridium coccoides-Eubacterium rectale group NS Atopobium cluster NS Eubacterium cylindroides NS Eubacterium hallii NS Beta-proteobacteria NS Clostridium cluster IX NS Faecalibacterium prausnizii cluster
[53]	28	RCT, C, DB	3 weeks	9.8 (8–12)	64	Healthy	NR	AX-OS (5.0)	Beverage	Placebo beverage with 0.25 g tricalcium phosphate, no AX-OS	Stool (partial), FISH	↑ Bifidobacteria NS Clostridium histolyticum/lituseburense NS Faecalibacterium prausnitzii NS Lactobacillus/Enterococcus NS Roseburia/Eubacterium rectale NS Total bacteria
[54]	32	RCT, P, DB	8 weeks	~32.4 (21–49)	~34.4	Healthy	~24.6	XOS (1.4, 2.8)	Tablet	Maltodextrin placebo	Stool (partial), 16 rRNA gene sequencing, pyrosequencing	↑ Bifidobacterium ↑ Total anaerobic flora ↑ Bacteroides fragilis (2.8 g only) ↑ Faecalibacterium (2.8 g only) ↑ Akkermansia (2.8 g only) ↓ Enterobacteriaceae (placebo only) NS Lactobacillus NS Clostridium NS Clustering
[55]	44	RCT, P, DB	14 d	~37 (18–60)	50	OW	~26.5 (25–28)	GOS (12.0)	Beverage (oolong tea)	Matched beverage with glucose	Stool, real-time quantitative PCR	↑ Bifidobacteria NS Total bacteria

Table 4. *Cont.*

Reference	*n*	Design	Duration	Age, Mean (Range)	% Male	BL Health	BMI, Mean (Range)	Fiber Type (g/Day)	Form	Control	Method	Bacterial Composition Reported Measures
[56]	40	RCT, C, DB	10 weeks	70 (65–80)	38	Healthy	NR	GOS (5.5)	Powder, mixed with water	Maltodextrin placebo	Stool (partial), FISH	↑ *Bifidobacterium* spp. ↑ *Bacteroides* spp. NS Atopobium cluster NS Clostridium coccoides/*E. rectale* NS Clostridium histolyticum group NS *Desulfovibrio* spp. NS *Escherichia coli* NS *Lactobacillus/Enterococcus* spp. NS Faecalibacterium prausnitzii NS Roseburia/Eubacterium rectale NS Total bacteria

Abbreviations: AX-OS, arabinoxylan-oligosaccharides; BL, baseline; C, crossover; DB, double-blind; FOS, fructooligosaccharides; GOS, galactooligosaccharides; MS, metabolic syndrome; NR, not reported; NS, no significant change; OW, overweight; P, parallel; RCT, randomized controlled trial; SB-OS, soybean oligosaccharides; X-OS, xylo-oligosaccharides; ~denotes a value that was calculated or estimated from the data available in the publication; ↑ significantly increased; ↓ significantly decreased.

Table 5. Other outcomes reported in oligosaccharide interventions reporting on bacterial composition.

Reference	Fiber Type	Evidence of Fermentation	Evidence of Fecal Bulking	Evidence of Changes in Transit Time	Evidence of Other Changes in Host Physiology
[35]	FOS	S	NS	–	S: GI symptoms (mild bloating) NS: Fecal pH
[36]	FOS	NS	–	–	S: GI symptoms (excess flatus) NS: Fecal pH
[37]	FOS	S	–	–	NS: GI symptoms
	GOS	S	–	–	NS: GI symptoms
[38]	FOS	–	–	NS	NS: GI symptoms, fecal pH
	GOS	–	–	NS	NS: GI symptoms, fecal pH
	SB-OS	–	–	NS	NS: GI symptoms, fecal pH
[39]	FOS	–	–	–	–
[40]	FOS	S	S	–	S: GI symptoms (flatulence and intestinal bloating) NS: fecal water pH
[41]	FOS	–	–	–	S: GI symptoms NS: fecal pH
[42]	GOS	–	–	–	–
	GOS	–	–	–	–
[43]	GOS	–	–	–	NS: Total and HDL cholesterol #
[44]	FOS	–	–	–	S: GI symptoms
[45]	AX-OS	–	NS	–	NS: Total, LDL, and HDL cholesterol #
[46]	GOS	–	–	–	NS: GI symptoms, stool consistency #
[47]	X-OS	S	–	–	NS: Stool consistency #
[48]	AX-OS	S	–	S	NS: Stool consistency #
[49]	AX-OS	S	–	NS	NS: Total energy intake, total and LDL cholesterol #, stool consistency
[50]	AX-OS	S	–	–	–
[51]	AX-OS	S	NS	NS	NS: LDL cholesterol #, fasting insulin and glucose, stool consistency
[52]	GOS	–	–	–	S: Total cholesterol and insulin NS: LDL, and HDL cholesterol, triglycerides, or fasting glucose
[53]	AX-OS	S	–	NS	NS: GI symptoms
[54]	X-OS	NS	–	NS	NS: Fecal pH, GI symptoms
[55]	GOS	–	NS	S	S: Satiety, total energy intake NS: Weight/Adiposity
[56]	GOS	S	NS	NS	–

Abbreviations: AX-OS, arabinoxylan-oligosaccharides; FOS, fructooligosaccharides; GOS, galactooligosaccharides; NS, no statistically significant health benefit was observed; S, a significant effect was observed; SB-OS, soybean oligosaccharides; X-OS, xylo-oligosaccharides; # No significant effect of intervention, but the effect was in a direction opposite to providing a health benefit.

4. Discussion

Observational/epidemiologic evidence shows that diets higher in fiber are associated with reduced risk of certain chronic diseases, such as heart disease, diabetes, and obesity [3,57], and these may be related to the effect of dietary fiber on the gut microbiota [4,5]. However, the present evidence map reveals that there is insufficient data from well-controlled dietary fiber interventions that study the gut microbiota in relation to intermediate risk factors of cardiometabolic disease or in relation to chronic conditions such as obesity. In fact, we found little evidence on the intersection of dietary fiber, the microbiota, and adiposity. Much of the current literature has shown positive effects of dietary fiber on gut function or beneficial bacterial species, or positive effects of dietary fiber on specific health outcomes, but few seem to be directly measuring these outcomes together, to provide evidence of a dietary fiber-modulated gut microbiota and health outcome [58,59].

Over the last 25 years, there has been a rapid increase in interest on dietary fiber and the microbiota, particularly with respect to prebiotics, such as oligosaccharides and inulin, as well as chemically synthesized fibers such as Polydextrose (PDX), soluble corn fiber, and PolyGlycopleX (PGX). From this map, we can see that the most actively researched fibers are oligosaccharides, resistant starch, and chemically synthesized fibers, followed closely by inulin, bran, and cereal fiber (Table 2), and the most common measures of the gut microbiota are SCFA concentration and bacterial composition (Table 3). The fiber and outcome most frequently studied together were oligosaccharides and bacterial composition, and we, therefore, examined these studies in more detail in summarizing our evidence map.

Oligosaccharides are short-chain saccharide polymers, generally made up of 3–10 carbohydrate monomers [60,61], and are known for their prebiotic activity. Prebiotics are defined as non-digestible foods that, when metabolized, alter the composition and/or activity of the microbiota in a such a way that promotes the health of the host [4,62,63]. Randomized controlled trials have consistently shown that oligosaccharides, and FOS in particular, increase *Bifidobacterium* (Table 4), a genus of oligosaccharide fermenting gut bacteria that may be beneficial to human health [64–66]. Despite the considerable number of studies showing this bifidogenic effect, few have actually examined direct relationships of this modulation of the gut microbiota to other physiological health outcomes. In our sub-analysis on oligosaccharides, we found that only five [43,45,51–53] of the 26 oligosaccharide interventions measuring bacterial composition also measured changes in lipids, and only two [51,52] measured glucose and insulin response. Additionally, only one study [52] found a small statistically significant beneficial effect on total cholesterol and insulin, while the rest found no beneficial effect. These findings are consistent with reviews by McRorie et al. [67–70], which conclude that clinical evidence does not support a link between soluble, non-viscous, readily fermentable fibers (such as oligosaccharides) and physiological health benefits on cholesterol, glycemic control, or laxation. Rather, these benefits are attributed to the physical properties of soluble, viscous/gel-forming fibers that are not readily fermented (such as beta glucan and raw guar gum).

However, readily-fermented fiber types, such as oligosaccharides and resistant starch, may have other important physiologic effects via the metabolites produced from microbial fermentation. The most studied products of fermentation are SCFAs, mainly butyrate, propionate, and acetate [25]. Up to 95% of SCFAs are absorbed by the colonocytes of the large intestine [20], and recent evidence has shown that they may play a role in health and prevention of disease, such as bowel disease, colon cancer, and metabolic syndrome [20,24–26]. SCFAs have been shown to affect gut health, immune function, energy metabolism, stimulation of the sympathetic nervous system, and serotonin release [4,7,20].

This evidence map also highlights areas where evidence is lacking. For instance, high-fiber diet interventions, where total dietary fiber was increased from a variety of sources, have the least number of publications. As more emphasis is put on the importance of dietary patterns rather than individual foods or food components [71], more whole-diet intervention studies need to be conducted to understand how these relationships among diet, the gut microbiota, and health work in the context of a whole diet. With respect to microbiota outcomes, fewer studies have measured bacterial enzyme activity, which may be more important than simply measuring changes in the bacterial composition because some strains or species may alter their function, and, therefore, their metabolites, in response to changes in the gut environment rather than their absolute number. Well-controlled human intervention trials incorporating "next generation" metagenomics, meta-transcriptomics and metabolomics will be vital to further understanding these changes in microbial activity. In addition, the microbiota composition or activity may be altered in people with chronic diseases such as obesity [58], and future research should consider whether diet may have differential effects depending on underlying health status. Based on this evidence map, the majority of fiber research on the gut microbiota was conducted in healthy adults (81%).

The definition of fiber has been a moving target, and fibers, being one of the most heterogeneous groups of associated molecules, have been categorized in many different contexts, including by source, structure, or physical properties (solubility, fermentability, etc.). Further, fibers may be delivered/consumed as isolated supplements, but they are more often consumed intact in whole foods (such as in raw fruits and vegetables), or in processed foods (including processes such as cooking, milling, and baking). The food matrix is important to consider because other components of the food, such as phytochemicals, may provide synergistic effects [72,73], and the degree of processing can alter the structure and physical attributes of the fiber [70]. All of these factors contribute to the type and extent of microbial utilization [28]. Therefore, it is important for future studies to describe the dietary fiber intervention in as much detail as possible, and, where applicable, define the characteristics of the fibers being studied.

Creating an updatable evidence map of microbiota-related outcomes allows researchers to obtain a more global view of the research landscape, including its history, current trajectory, and specific areas or research questions lacking data or consensus. Since the Dietary Fiber Database used for this evidence map captures literature going back to 1946, it is important to note that the literature in the database often represents evolving knowledge about particular fiber types. This is both a strength and limitation of the database and the evidence mapping process overall, and it highlights the importance of reviewing the totality of available evidence. For instance, bran is well represented in the evidence map, and although the effect of bran on the microbiota was of interest in earlier publications, it is now well-established that insoluble bran is not very readily fermented and may have less of an effect on the microbiota. Instead, interest has shifted toward more fermentable fibers such as the prebiotics and chemically synthesized fibers.

Unlike systematic reviews, which generally address a narrower, focused question with extensive quality analysis and risk of bias assessment, the primary goal of evidence mapping is to identify patterns and provide a broader context within which systematic reviews may occur. As such, in Tables 4 and 5, we did not provide information on effect size of the significance, as this information was not reported in the published fiber database [33]. Furthermore, because of the complex nature of dietary fiber and the size of the literature on dietary fiber, the database which this evidence map is based on has some inherent limitations, which are detailed in a separate publication [33]. Notably, the database was limited to publications in PubMed, and studies were only included if there was a well-defined dietary fiber intervention with a concurrent control. Further, because this database was designed to specifically capture certain health outcomes, other publications of interest to microbiota research may not be represented.

A major strength of this evidence map is that it is a cost effective way of summarizing the data on dietary fiber and the gut microbiota. For instance, the data presented in Tables 4 and 5 may be used to guide future work, such as a meta-analysis, which would provide more specific information to quantify statistical significance. We were able to use a previously created database in order to efficiently identify potentially relevant literature. Although we closely reviewed the subset of relevant literature identified via the database, we saved significant resources in conducting initial, broad searches which would inevitably yield a large amount of irrelevant literature to screen through. The result is a'useful platform to visualize the current evidence, which can be used to summarize the volume of existing research, generate new hypotheses, direct systematic reviews and meta-analyses, and can be continually updated.

5. Conclusions

In conclusion, this evidence map summarizes the existing literature on dietary fiber interventions and the human gut microbiota. This is a rapidly growing area of interest, but well-controlled human interventions are needed to support the associations being seen in animal and observational studies. We hope that this evidence map will provide a resource for researchers to direct new intervention studies and meta-analyses.

Supplementary Materials:
Table S1: Inclusion/Exclusion Criteria. Supplementary Methods. Figure S1: Acute studies: weighted scatter plot of other microbiota outcomes by fiber group presents weighted scatter. The acute studies exclusively examine the short-term fermentation response by measuring SCFA concentration and/or breath gas excretion, most frequently in cereal fibers. Figure S2: Longer duration studies: weighted scatter plot of other microbiota outcomes by fiber group. Studies of greater duration examine more outcomes in a larger array of fiber types. Notably, however, there are no longer duration (>4 weeks) studies on resistant starch.

Acknowledgments: Funding support provided by a research grant from the International Life Science Institute, North America Branch, Technical Committee on Carbohydrates and from the USDA Agricultural Research Service (agreement 58-1950-0-014). We acknowledge Katherine Rancaño for her assistance with the tables.

Author Contributions: N.M.M. and M.C. designed research; C.M.S. and K.A.L. conducted research; M.C., S.B.R. and M.O. provided expertise on the following areas: evidence mapping methodology, dietary fibers, and gut microbiota; C.M.S. and K.A.L. analyzed data; C.M.S. and N.M.M. wrote paper; and N.M.M. had primary responsibility for final content. All authors have read and approved the final manuscript.

References

1. Codex Alimentarius Commission. *Codex Alimentarius Commission Report of the 30th Session of the Codex Committee on Nutrition and Foods for Special Dietary Uses*; Codex Alimentarius Commission: Cape Town, South Africa, 2008.
2. Jones, J.M. CODEX-aligned dietary fiber definitions help to bridge the "fiber gap". *Nutr. J.* **2014**, *13*, 34. [CrossRef] [PubMed]
3. Dahl, W.J.; Stewart, M.L. Position of the Academy of Nutrition and Dietetics: Health implications of dietary fiber. *J. Acad. Nutr. Diet.* **2015**, *115*, 1861–1870. [CrossRef] [PubMed]
4. Slavin, J. Fiber and prebiotics: Mechanisms and health benefits. *Nutrients* **2013**, *5*, 1417–1435. [CrossRef] [PubMed]
5. Conlon, M.A.; Bird, A.R. The impact of diet and lifestyle on gut microbiota and human health. *Nutrients* **2014**, *7*, 17–44. [CrossRef] [PubMed]
6. O'Hara, A.M.; Shanahan, F. The gut flora as a forgotten organ. *EMBO Rep.* **2006**, *7*, 688–693. [CrossRef] [PubMed]
7. Nicholson, J.K.; Holmes, E.; Kinross, J.; Burcelin, R.; Gibson, G.; Jia, W.; Pettersson, S. Host-gut microbiota metabolic interactions. *Science* **2012**, *336*, 1262–1267. [CrossRef] [PubMed]
8. Hooper, L.V.; Littman, D.R.; Macpherson, A.J. Interactions between the microbiota and the immune system. *Science* **2012**, *336*, 1268–1273. [CrossRef] [PubMed]
9. Clemente, J.C.; Ursell, L.K.; Parfrey, L.W.; Knight, R. The impact of the gut microbiota on human health: An integrative view. *Cell* **2012**, *148*, 1258–1270. [CrossRef] [PubMed]
10. Flint, H.J.; Duncan, S.H.; Scott, K.P.; Louis, P. Links between diet, gut microbiota composition and gut metabolism. *Proc. Nutr. Soc.* **2015**, *74*, 13–22. [CrossRef] [PubMed]
11. Blumberg, R.; Powrie, F. Microbiota, disease, and back to health: A metastable journey. *Sci. Transl. Med.* **2012**, *4*, 137rv7. [CrossRef] [PubMed]
12. Flint, H.J. The impact of nutrition on the human microbiome. *Nutr. Rev.* **2012**, *70* (Suppl. 1), S10–S13. [CrossRef] [PubMed]

13. David, L.A.; Maurice, C.F.; Carmody, R.N.; Gootenberg, D.B.; Button, J.E.; Wolfe, B.E.; Ling, A.V.; Devlin, A.S.; Varma, Y.; Fischbach, M.A.; et al. Diet rapidly and reproducibly alters the human gut microbiome. *Nature* **2014**, *505*, 559–563. [CrossRef] [PubMed]
14. Belenguer, A.; Duncan, S.H.; Calder, A.G.; Holtrop, G.; Louis, P.; Lobley, G.E.; Flint, H.J. Two routes of metabolic cross-feeding between *Bifidobacterium adolescentis* and butyrate-producing anaerobes from the human gut. *Appl. Environ. Microbiol.* **2006**, *72*, 3593–3599. [CrossRef] [PubMed]
15. Falony, G.; Vlachou, A.; Verbrugghe, K.; De Vuyst, L. Cross-feeding between *Bifidobacterium longum* BB536 and acetate-converting, butyrate-producing colon bacteria during growth on oligofructose. *Appl. Environ. Microbiol.* **2006**, *72*, 7835–7841. [CrossRef] [PubMed]
16. El Oufir, L.; Flourié, B.; Bruley des Varannes, S.; Barry, J.L.; Cloarec, D.; Bornet, F.; Galmiche, J.P. Relations between transit time, fermentation products, and hydrogen consuming flora in healthy humans. *Gut* **1996**, *38*, 870–877. [CrossRef] [PubMed]
17. Stephen, A.M.; Wiggins, H.S.; Cummings, J.H. Effect of changing transit time on colonic microbial metabolism in man. *Gut* **1987**, *28*, 601–609. [CrossRef] [PubMed]
18. Lewis, S.J.; Heaton, K.W. Increasing butyrate concentration in the distal colon by accelerating intestinal transit. *Gut* **1997**, *41*, 245–251. [CrossRef] [PubMed]
19. Graf, D.; Di Cagno, R.; Fåk, F.; Flint, H.J.; Nyman, M.; Saarela, M.; Watzl, B. Contribution of diet to the composition of the human gut microbiota. *Microb. Ecol. Health Dis.* **2015**, *26*, 26164. [CrossRef] [PubMed]
20. Den Besten, G.; van Eunen, K.; Groen, A.K.; Venema, K.; Reijngoud, D.-J.; Bakker, B.M. The role of short-chain fatty acids in the interplay between diet, gut microbiota, and host energy metabolism. *J. Lipid Res.* **2013**, *54*, 2325–2340. [CrossRef] [PubMed]
21. Duncan, S.H.; Louis, P.; Thomson, J.M.; Flint, H.J. The role of pH in determining the species composition of the human colonic microbiota. *Environ. Microbiol.* **2009**, *11*, 2112–2122. [CrossRef] [PubMed]
22. Samuel, B.S.; Shaito, A.; Motoike, T.; Rey, F.E.; Backhed, F.; Manchester, J.K.; Hammer, R.E.; Williams, S.C.; Crowley, J.; Yanagisawa, M.; et al. Effects of the gut microbiota on host adiposity are modulated by the short-chain fatty-acid binding G protein-coupled receptor, Gpr41. *Proc. Natl. Acad. Sci. USA* **2008**, *105*, 16767–16772. [CrossRef] [PubMed]
23. Wong, J.M.W.; de Souza, R.; Kendall, C.W.C.; Emam, A.; Jenkins, D.J.A. Colonic health: Fermentation and short chain fatty acids. *J. Clin. Gastroenterol.* **2006**, *40*, 235–243. [CrossRef] [PubMed]
24. Tan, J.; McKenzie, C.; Potamitis, M.; Thorburn, A.N.; Mackay, C.R.; Macia, L. The role of short-chain fatty acids in health and disease. *Adv. Immunol.* **2014**, *121*, 91–119. [PubMed]
25. Birt, D.F.; Boylston, T.; Hendrich, S.; Jane, J.-L.; Hollis, J.; Li, L.; McClelland, J.; Moore, S.; Phillips, G.J.; Rowling, M.; et al. Resistant starch: Promise for improving human health. *Adv. Nutr. Int. Rev. J.* **2013**, *4*, 587–601. [CrossRef] [PubMed]
26. Hamer, H.M.; Jonkers, D.; Venema, K.; Vanhoutvin, S.; Troost, F.J.; Brummer, R.-J. Review article: The role of butyrate on colonic function. *Aliment. Pharmacol. Ther.* **2008**, *27*, 104–119. [CrossRef] [PubMed]
27. Flint, H.J.; Scott, K.P.; Louis, P.; Duncan, S.H. The role of the gut microbiota in nutrition and health. *Nat. Rev. Gastroenterol. Hepatol.* **2012**, *9*, 577–589. [CrossRef] [PubMed]
28. Hamaker, B.R.; Tuncil, Y.E. A perspective on the complexity of dietary fiber structures and their potential effect on the gut microbiota. *J. Mol. Biol.* **2014**, *426*, 3838–3850. [CrossRef] [PubMed]
29. Althuis, M.D.; Weed, D.L. Evidence mapping: Methodologic foundations and application to intervention and observational research on sugar-sweetened beverages and health outcomes. *Am. J. Clin. Nutr.* **2013**, *98*, 755–768. [CrossRef] [PubMed]
30. Bragge, P.; Clavisi, O.; Turner, T.; Tavender, E.; Collie, A.; Gruen, R.L. The global evidence mapping initiative: Scoping research in broad topic areas. *BMC Med. Res. Methodol.* **2011**, *11*, 92. [CrossRef] [PubMed]
31. Hetrick, S.E.; Parker, A.G.; Callahan, P.; Purcell, R. Evidence mapping: Illustrating an emerging methodology to improve evidence-based practice in youth mental health. *J. Eval. Clin. Pract.* **2010**, *16*, 1025–1030. [CrossRef] [PubMed]
32. Wang, D.D.; Shams-White, M.; Bright, O.J.M.; Parrott, J.S.; Chung, M. Creating a literature database of low-calorie sweeteners and health studies: Evidence mapping. *BMC Med. Res. Methodol.* **2016**, *16*, 1. [CrossRef] [PubMed]

33. Livingston, K.A.; Chung, M.; Sawicki, C.M.; Lyle, B.J.; Wang, D.D.; Roberts, S.B.; McKeown, N.M. Development of a publicly available, comprehensive database of fiber and health outcomes: Rationale and methods. *PLoS ONE* **2016**, *11*, e0156961. [CrossRef] [PubMed]
34. McKeown, N.M.; Chung, M.; Livingston, K.A.; Sawicki, C.M.; Wang, D.D.; Blakeley, C.; Jia, Y.; Baruch, N.; Karlsen, M.; Brown, C. Project: Diet-Related Fibers and Human Health Outcomes, Version 1 (Retired Version). Available online: http://srdr.ahrq.gov/projects/564 (accessed on 7 September 2015).
35. Bouhnik, Y.; Flourié, B.; Riottot, M.; Bisetti, N.; Gailing, M.F.; Guibert, A.; Bornet, F.; Rambaud, J.C. Effects of fructo-oligosaccharides ingestion on fecal bifidobacteria and selected metabolic indexes of colon carcinogenesis in healthy humans. *Nutr. Cancer* **1996**, *26*, 21–29. [CrossRef] [PubMed]
36. Bouhnik, Y.; Vahedi, K.; Achour, L.; Attar, A.; Salfati, J.; Pochart, P.; Marteau, P.; Flourié, B.; Bornet, F.; Rambaud, J.C. Short-chain fructo-oligosaccharide administration dose-dependently increases fecal bifidobacteria in healthy humans. *J. Nutr.* **1999**, *129*, 113–116. [PubMed]
37. Tannock, G.W.; Munro, K.; Bibiloni, R.; Simon, M.A.; Hargreaves, P.; Gopal, P.; Harmsen, H.; Welling, G. Impact of consumption of oligosaccharide-containing biscuits on the fecal microbiota of humans. *Appl. Environ. Microbiol.* **2004**, *70*, 2129–2136. [CrossRef] [PubMed]
38. Bouhnik, Y.; Raskine, L.; Simoneau, G.; Vicaut, E.; Neut, C.; Flourié, B.; Brouns, F.; Bornet, F.R. The capacity of nondigestible carbohydrates to stimulate fecal bifidobacteria in healthy humans: A double-blind, randomized, placebo-controlled, parallel-group, dose-response relation study. *Am. J. Clin. Nutr.* **2004**, *80*, 1658–1664. [PubMed]
39. Clavel, T.; Fallani, M.; Lepage, P.; Levenez, F.; Mathey, J.; Rochet, V.; Sérézat, M.; Sutren, M.; Henderson, G.; Bennetau-Pelissero, C.; et al. Isoflavones and functional foods alter the dominant intestinal microbiota in postmenopausal women. *J. Nutr.* **2005**, *135*, 2786–2792. [PubMed]
40. Ten Bruggencate, S.J.M.; Bovee-Oudenhoven, I.M.J.; Lettink-Wissink, M.L.G.; Katan, M.B.; van der Meer, R. Dietary fructooligosaccharides affect intestinal barrier function in healthy men. *J. Nutr.* **2006**, *136*, 70–74. [PubMed]
41. Bouhnik, Y.; Raskine, L.; Simoneau, G.; Paineau, D.; Bornet, F. The capacity of short-chain fructo-oligosaccharides to stimulate faecal bifidobacteria: A dose-response relationship study in healthy humans. *Nutr. J.* **2006**, *5*, 8. [CrossRef] [PubMed]
42. Depeint, F.; Tzortzis, G.; Vulevic, J.; I'anson, K.; Gibson, G.R. Prebiotic evaluation of a novel galactooligosaccharide mixture produced by the enzymatic activity of *Bifidobacterium bifidum* NCIMB 41171, in healthy humans: A randomized, double-blind, crossover, placebo-controlled intervention study. *Am. J. Clin. Nutr.* **2008**, *87*, 785–791. [PubMed]
43. Vulevic, J.; Drakoularakou, A.; Yaqoob, P.; Tzortzis, G.; Gibson, G.R. Modulation of the fecal microflora profile and immune function by a novel trans-galactooligosaccharide mixture (B-GOS) in healthy elderly volunteers. *Am. J. Clin. Nutr.* **2008**, *88*, 1438–1446. [PubMed]
44. Mitsou, E.K.; Turunen, K.; Anapliotis, P.; Zisi, D.; Spiliotis, V.; Kyriacou, A. Impact of a jelly containing short-chain fructo-oligosaccharides and *Sideritis euboea* extract on human faecal microbiota. *Int. J. Food Microbiol.* **2009**, *135*, 112–117. [CrossRef] [PubMed]
45. Cloetens, L.; Broekaert, W.F.; Delaedt, Y.; Ollevier, F.; Courtin, C.M.; Delcour, J.A.; Rutgeerts, P.; Verbeke, K. Tolerance of arabinoxylan-oligosaccharides and their prebiotic activity in healthy subjects: A randomised, placebo-controlled cross-over study. *Br. J. Nutr.* **2010**, *103*, 703–713. [CrossRef] [PubMed]
46. Walton, G.E.; van den Heuvel, E.G.H.M.; Kosters, M.H.W.; Rastall, R.A.; Tuohy, K.M.; Gibson, G.R. A randomised crossover study investigating the effects of galacto-oligosaccharides on the faecal microbiota in men and women over 50 years of age. *Br. J. Nutr.* **2012**, *107*, 1466–1475. [CrossRef] [PubMed]
47. Lecerf, J.-M.; Dépeint, F.; Clerc, E.; Dugenet, Y.; Niamba, C.N.; Rhazi, L.; Cayzeele, A.; Abdelnour, G.; Jaruga, A.; Younes, H.; et al. Xylo-oligosaccharide (XOS) in combination with inulin modulates both the intestinal environment and immune status in healthy subjects, while XOS alone only shows prebiotic properties. *Br. J. Nutr.* **2012**, *108*, 1847–1858. [CrossRef] [PubMed]
48. Damen, B.; Cloetens, L.; Broekaert, W.F.; François, I.; Lescroart, O.; Trogh, I.; Arnaut, F.; Welling, G.W.; Wijffels, J.; Delcour, J.A.; et al. Consumption of breads containing in situ-produced arabinoxylan oligosaccharides alters gastrointestinal effects in healthy volunteers. *J. Nutr.* **2012**, *142*, 470–477. [CrossRef] [PubMed]

49. François, I.E.J.A.; Lescroart, O.; Veraverbeke, W.S.; Marzorati, M.; Possemiers, S.; Evenepoel, P.; Hamer, H.; Houben, E.; Windey, K.; Welling, G.W.; et al. Effects of a wheat bran extract containing arabinoxylan oligosaccharides on gastrointestinal health parameters in healthy adult human volunteers: A double-blind, randomised, placebo-controlled, cross-over trial. *Br. J. Nutr.* **2012**, *108*, 2229–2242. [CrossRef] [PubMed]
50. Walton, G.E.; Lu, C.; Trogh, I.; Arnaut, F.; Gibson, G.R. A randomised, double-blind, placebo controlled cross-over study to determine the gastrointestinal effects of consumption of arabinoxylan-oligosaccharides enriched bread in healthy volunteers. *Nutr. J.* **2012**, *11*, 36. [CrossRef] [PubMed]
51. Maki, K.C.; Gibson, G.R.; Dickmann, R.S.; Kendall, C.W.C.; Chen, C.-Y.O.; Costabile, A.; Comelli, E.M.; McKay, D.L.; Almeida, N.G.; Jenkins, D.; et al. Digestive and physiologic effects of a wheat bran extract, arabino-xylan-oligosaccharide, in breakfast cereal. *Nutrition* **2012**, *28*, 1115–1121. [CrossRef] [PubMed]
52. Vulevic, J.; Juric, A.; Tzortzis, G.; Gibson, G.R. A mixture of trans-galactooligosaccharides reduces markers of metabolic syndrome and modulates the fecal microbiota and immune function of overweight adults. *J. Nutr.* **2013**, *143*, 324–331. [CrossRef] [PubMed]
53. François, I.E.J.A.; Lescroart, O.; Veraverbeke, W.S.; Marzorati, M.; Possemiers, S.; Hamer, H.; Windey, K.; Welling, G.W.; Delcour, J.A.; Courtin, C.M.; et al. Effects of wheat bran extract containing arabinoxylan oligosaccharides on gastrointestinal parameters in healthy preadolescent children. *J. Pediatr. Gastroenterol. Nutr.* **2014**, *58*, 647–653. [CrossRef] [PubMed]
54. Finegold, S.M.; Li, Z.; Summanen, P.H.; Downes, J.; Thames, G.; Corbett, K.; Dowd, S.; Krak, M.; Heber, D. Xylooligosaccharide increases bifidobacteria but not lactobacilli in human gut microbiota. *Food Funct.* **2014**, *5*, 436–445. [CrossRef] [PubMed]
55. Morel, F.B.; Dai, Q.; Ni, J.; Thomas, D.; Parnet, P.; Fança-Berthon, P. α-Galacto-oligosaccharides dose-dependently reduce appetite and decrease inflammation in overweight adults. *J. Nutr.* **2015**, *145*, 2052–2059. [CrossRef] [PubMed]
56. Vulevic, J.; Juric, A.; Walton, G.E.; Claus, S.P.; Tzortzis, G.; Toward, R.E.; Gibson, G.R. Influence of galacto-oligosaccharide mixture (B-GOS) on gut microbiota, immune parameters and metabonomics in elderly persons. *Br. J. Nutr.* **2015**, *114*, 586–595. [CrossRef] [PubMed]
57. Hur, I.Y.; Reicks, M. Relationship between whole-grain intake, chronic disease risk indicators, and weight status among adolescents in the National Health and Nutrition Examination Survey, 1999–2004. *J. Acad. Nutr. Diet.* **2012**, *112*, 46–55. [CrossRef] [PubMed]
58. Ley, R.E.; Bäckhed, F.; Turnbaugh, P.; Lozupone, C.A.; Knight, R.D.; Gordon, J.I. Obesity alters gut microbial ecology. *Proc. Natl. Acad. Sci. USA* **2005**, *102*, 11070–11075. [CrossRef] [PubMed]
59. Kalliomäki, M.; Collado, M.C.; Salminen, S.; Isolauri, E. Early differences in fecal microbiota composition in children may predict overweight. *Am. J. Clin. Nutr.* **2008**, *87*, 534–538. [PubMed]
60. Carbohydrates in Human Nutrition. *Report of a Joint FAO/WHO Expert Consultation*; Food and Agriculture Organization, World Health Organization (FAO/WHO): Rome, Italy, 1997; pp. 1–140.
61. American Association of Cereal Chemists (AACC). The Definition of Dietary Fiber. Report of the Dietary Fiber Definition Committee to the Board of Directors of the American Association of Cereal Chemists. *Cereal Foods World* **2001**, *46*, 112–126.
62. Valcheva, R.; Dieleman, L.A. Prebiotics: Definition and protective mechanisms. *Best Pract. Res. Clin. Gastroenterol.* **2016**, *30*, 27–37. [CrossRef] [PubMed]
63. Bindels, L.B.; Delzenne, N.M.; Cani, P.D.; Walter, J. Towards a more comprehensive concept for prebiotics. *Nat. Rev. Gastroenterol. Hepatol.* **2015**, *12*, 303–310. [CrossRef] [PubMed]
64. Cummings, J.H.; Antoine, J.-M.; Azpiroz, F.; Bourdet-Sicard, R.; Brandtzaeg, P.; Calder, P.C.; Gibson, G.R.; Guarner, F.; Isolauri, E.; Pannemans, D.; et al. PASSCLAIM—Gut health and immunity. *Eur. J. Nutr.* **2004**, *43* (Suppl. 2), II118–II173. [CrossRef] [PubMed]
65. Meyer, D. Inunlin, gut microbes, and health. In *Dietary Fiber and Health*; Cho, S.S., Almeida, N., Eds.; CRC Press Taylor & Francis Group: Boca Raton, FL, USA, 2012; pp. 169–183.
66. Tojo, R.; Suárez, A.; Clemente, M.G.; de los Reyes-Gavilán, C.G.; Margolles, A.; Gueimonde, M.; Ruas-Madiedo, P. Intestinal microbiota in health and disease: Role of bifidobacteria in gut homeostasis. *World J. Gastroenterol.* **2014**, *20*, 15163–15176. [CrossRef] [PubMed]
67. McRorie, J.W. Evidence-based approach to fiber supplements and clinically meaningful health benefits, part 1: What to look for and how to recommend an effective fiber therapy. *Nutr. Today* **2015**, *50*, 82–89. [CrossRef] [PubMed]

68. McRorie, J.W. Evidence-based approach to fiber supplements and clinically meaningful health benefits, part 2: What to look for and how to recommend an effective fiber therapy. *Nutr. Today* **2015**, *50*, 90–97. [CrossRef] [PubMed]
69. Mcrorie, J.W.; Fahey, G.C. A review of gastrointestinal physiology and the mechanisms underlying the health benefits of dietary fiber: Matching an effective fiber with specific patient needs. *Clin. Nurs. Stud.* **2013**, *1*, 82–92. [CrossRef]
70. McRorie, J.W.; McKeown, N.M. Understanding the physics of functional fibers in the gastrointestinal tract: An evidence-based approach to resolving enduring misconceptions about insoluble and soluble fiber. *J. Acad. Nutr. Diet.* **2017**, *17*, 251–264. [CrossRef] [PubMed]
71. 2015–2020 Dietary Guidelines—Health.gov. Available online: https://health.gov/dietaryguidelines/2015/guidelines/ (accessed on 15 December 2016).
72. Okarter, N.; Liu, R.H. Health benefits of whole grain phytochemicals. *Crit. Rev. Food Sci. Nutr.* **2010**, *50*, 193–208. [CrossRef] [PubMed]
73. Vitaglione, P.; Mennella, I.; Ferracane, R.; Rivellese, A.A.; Giacco, R.; Ercolini, D.; Gibbons, S.M.; La Storia, A.; Gilbert, J.A.; Jonnalagadda, S.; et al. Whole-grain wheat consumption reduces inflammation in a randomized controlled trial on overweight and obese subjects with unhealthy dietary and lifestyle behaviors: Role of polyphenols bound to cereal dietary fiber. *Am. J. Clin. Nutr.* **2015**, *101*, 251–261. [CrossRef] [PubMed]

17

Cell-Surface and Nuclear Receptors in the Colon as Targets for Bacterial Metabolites and its Relevance to Colon Health

Sathish Sivaprakasam, Yangzom D. Bhutia, Sabarish Ramachandran and Vadivel Ganapathy *

Department of Cell Biology and Biochemistry, Texas Tech University Health Sciences Center, Lubbock, TX 79430, USA; sathish.sivaprakasam@ttuhsc.edu (S.S.); yangzom.d.bhutia@ttuhsc.edu (Y.D.B.); s.ramachandran@ttuhsc.edu (S.R.)

* Correspondence: vadivel.ganapathy@ttuhsc.edu;

Abstract: The symbiotic co-habitation of bacteria in the host colon is mutually beneficial to both partners. While the host provides the place and food for the bacteria to colonize and live, the bacteria in turn help the host in energy and nutritional homeostasis, development and maturation of the mucosal immune system, and protection against inflammation and carcinogenesis. In this review, we highlight the molecular mediators of the effective communication between the bacteria and the host, focusing on selective metabolites from the bacteria that serve as messengers to the host by acting through selective receptors in the host colon. These bacterial metabolites include the short-chain fatty acids acetate, propionate, and butyrate, the tryptophan degradation products indole-3-aldehyde, indole-3-acetic, acid and indole-3-propionic acid, and derivatives of endogenous bile acids. The targets for these bacterial products in the host include the cell-surface G-protein-coupled receptors GPR41, GPR43, and GPR109A and the nuclear receptors aryl hydrocarbon receptor (AhR), pregnane X receptor (PXR), and farnesoid X receptor (FXR). The chemical communication between these bacterial metabolite messengers and the host targets collectively has the ability to impact metabolism, gene expression, and epigenetics in colonic epithelial cells as well as in mucosal immune cells. The end result, for the most part, is the maintenance of optimal colonic health.

Keywords: colonic bacteria; symbiotic relationship; bacterial metabolites; molecular targets; cell-surface receptors; nuclear receptors; immune tolerance; colitis; colon cancer

---

1. Introduction

Over millions of years, humans have co-evolved with microorganisms through co-habitation. Adult human harbors microflora that is equal or even greater than their human cells in number [1,2]. These microorganisms colonize different parts of the body that are exposed to external environment, which include skin, oral cavity, airway lumen, intestinal tract, and vagina. Among these, the colon is the site where the microorganisms are most abundant, with bacteria as the principal component. There are 800–1000 different species of colonic bacteria under normal physiological conditions, but the presence or absence of specific strains and the relative abundance of any given strain might vary from individual to individual, primarily influenced by the environmental factors such as the diet, air and water quality, medications, and mode of delivery (vaginal or Cesarean section) [3]. Because of the impact of multiple variables, the colonic bacteria might not remain the same even in a given individual over a long period of time. Despite these interpersonal variations, colonic bacteria are in general dominated by two phyla: Bacteroidetes and Firmicutes [4,5]. Normal microflora in the colon elicit significant influence on the host, in the colon and in other organs. Recent studies have implicated colonic bacteria in brain function (gut-brain axis), liver function (gut-liver axis), mucosal and systemic immune function, diabetes (type 1 and type 2) (gut-pancreas axis), nutrition and obesity, and cardiovascular diseases [6–10]. This broad spectrum of biological impact of colonic bacteria on the host is possible because of active communication between the two co-habitants. The impact of colonic bacteria on the host is not limited locally to the colon because of the changes the bacteria bring in terms of gene expression and biological function in colonic epithelial cells as well as mucosal immune cells. The colon releases a wide variety of biologically active molecules into circulation in response to changes in the density and phylogenic makeup of the bacterial population; these active molecules include hormones and cytokines that impact on the functions of distant organs including the liver, pancreas, and brain. Similarly, mucosal immune cells are also influenced in their behavior and function in response to colonic bacteria, which then travel to distant sites to modulate immune function and disease processes [11,12]. Furthermore, colonic bacteria themselves elaborate different classes of metabolites, which enter the portal and systemic circulations to regulate the biology of cells and tissues at distant sites through specific molecular targets that include enzymes and receptors [10,13,14].

Because of its close proximity to the bacteria, the colon is the most influenced organ as the result of this co-habitation. The presence of bacteria in the colon is absolutely necessary for optimal colonic health; normal bacteria in the colon offer protection against inflammation and cancer. As such, the beneficial effects of colonic bacteria are undeniable. Any imbalance in the normal density and phylogenetic composition in colonic bacteria, generally referred to as dysbiosis, is detrimental to colonic health [15–18]. Inflammatory bowel diseases (IBD) are chronic inflammatory disorders of the intestinal tract that develop as a result of deregulation of the immune response toward the intestinal/colonic bacteria. In particular, there is a marked decrease in the colonization of Firmicutes and Bacteroidetes in the gut microbiota in association with IBD. Crohn's disease and ulcerative colitis are the two major types of IBD, which are distinct diseases with different histological features and etiology that involve different immune cell types. Animal studies have shown that neither of these diseases develops under germ-free conditions, indicating that the presence of bacteria is obligatory for the disease process [19,20]. The findings that normal bacteria are essential for colonic health and that IBD does not develop in the absence of bacteria are not necessarily contradictory. The epithelial cells of the intestine/colon form an effective barrier between the bacteria and the host, and the communication between the two co-habitants occurs solely via chemical messengers to make sure that the mucosal immune system is not overly active in response to the bacterial antigens. However, if the barrier function is compromised for any reason, the ability of the mucosal immune system to tolerate the bacteria is at risk [21–23]. What causes the breakdown of the barrier in IBD is not completely understood, but changes in the normal bacterial phylogenetic composition are believed to be major determinants in the process. When the phylogenetic composition (i.e., dysbiosis) is altered in the colon, the chemical communication between the bacteria and the host also undergoes changes, thus initiating the inflammatory disease process. This phenomenon is also relevant to carcinogenesis in the colon because chronic inflammation as occurs in ulcerative colitis increases the risk of colorectal cancer [24].

2. Relationship between Microbiota and the Host: Parasitism, Commensalism, or Mutualism?

The relationship between the host and the microbiota could fall into three categories—parasitism, commensalism, and mutualism—depending on the specifics of the interaction. In parasitism, one of the co-habitants gets the benefits, while the other is harmed. In commensalism, one of the co-habitants reaps the benefits, while the co-habitation is neither beneficial nor harmful to the other partner. In mutualism, both partners get the benefits from the co-existence. The relationship between the host and the colonic bacteria falls under the third category, mutualism. The benefits to the bacteria as a result of this co-habitation include the availability of the colonic lumen for colonization and proliferation and provision of the nutrients by the host necessary for survival and growth. The host also benefits from the relationship [25–27]. Colonic bacteria synthesize a variety of vitamins (folic acid, biotin, vitamin K, etc.) that are made available to the host. The principal fermentation products of bacterial metabolism, called short-chain fatty acids, that are present in normal colonic lumen at concentrations as high as 100 mM serve as preferential metabolic fuel to colonic epithelial cells [28]. These short-chain fatty acids also function as signaling molecules eliciting a broad range of biological effects in colonic epithelium by targeting enzymes such histone deacetylases (HDACs), cell-surface receptors such as GPR109A and GPR43, and nuclear receptors such as AhR, PXR, FXR, and peroxisome proliferator-activated receptors (PPARs) [29]. The end result of this mutually beneficial co-habitation is a symbiotic relationship between the two partners. Notwithstanding this overwhelming evidence for mutualism between the host and colonic bacteria, too many investigators and published reports still continue to describe the relationship between the host and the bacteria as commensalism and the bacteria as commensals [30–32]. Surprisingly, the terms "commensalism" and "commensals" appear even in publications that provide data in support of the mutually beneficial relationship between the host and the colonic bacteria [25,30–32].

3. Bacterial Dysbiosis as a Cause of Colonic Diseases

Dysbiosis in the colon is a critical determinant in the pathogenesis of IBD. Research on colitis induction in germ-free mice with introduction of specific strains of bacteria has shown that microbial dysbiosis, rather than genetic factors, is the major factor for IBD pathogenesis. Many genetically-engineered mouse models that develop spontaneous colitis in the presence of bacteria in the colon are resistant to colitis when raised under germ-free conditions [33,34]. This suggests that the presence of bacteria in the intestinal tract is a critical requirement for IBD development. Most animal models of colitis show altered bacterial composition in the colon, providing evidence of dysbiosis [16,35]. However, the link between dysbiosis and IBD is only associative, and the cause-effect relationship has not yet been established beyond doubt. Nonetheless, administration of probiotics to patients with colonic inflammation has beneficial effects in terms of slowing or preventing progression of the disease process [36–38]. As these probiotics tend to favor colonization of normal bacterial flora and suppress the growth of pathogenic bacteria in the colon, the preventive effects of probiotics suggest effective reversal of the disease-associated dysbiosis and may actually point to a mechanistic model in which the dysbiosis is most likely the cause, rather than the result, of colonic inflammation [37,39,40].

4. Bacterial Metabolites with Impact on the Host: Relevance to Colitis and Colon Cancer

The communication between colonic bacteria and the host could be contact-dependent as well as contact-independent. The phylogenetic composition of the microflora in colonic lumen is not exactly the same as that of the microflora on the surface of the colonic epithelium. Which bacterial strains adhere to the colonic epithelial cells depends on multiple factors such as the presence or absence of cell-surface receptors for a given strain, ability of bacterial strains to traverse the thick mucin present on the luminal surface of the epithelial cell layer, as well as susceptibility of the bacterial strains to the bactericidal and bacteriostatic actions of the various molecules secreted by the epithelial cells and mucosal immune cells. The physical contact followed by insertion of specific bacterial proteins into the epithelial cell membrane could elicit signaling changes in the epithelium as a means of communication. Another mode of communication, probably more prevalent than the former, is through metabolites released into the lumen from live bacteria or from dead bacterial cells. The colon provides a favorable environment for anaerobic microbial growth, resulting in fermentation by resident bacteria of dietary constituents that reach the colon. The microbiota population in the colon is highly variable depending on the intestinal physiology, substrate availability, oxygen tension, and pH [28]. As a result, the microorganisms present in the colon are not the same all through the length of the large intestine. The phylogenetic composition of the bacteria is significantly different between the proximal colon and the distal colon [41]. As the metabolites elaborated by these bacteria depend on the repertoire of metabolic pathways in a given strain of the bacteria, different regions of the colon are exposed to different bacterial metabolites and hence respond differently. Furthermore, the phylogenetic composition of the colonic bacteria varies from individual to individual and also in the same individual in health and disease; this again impacts the biological response of the host colon to the presence of bacteria that could be significantly different on an individual basis and also depend on the health status of the individual.

Among these bacterial metabolites responsible for communication between the bacteria and the host, short-chain fatty acids (SCFAs) have received the most attention [42–45]. SCFAs are organic acids consisting of 2–4 carbon atoms. The principal components of SCFAs are acetate (C2), propionate (C3), and butyrate (C4). These fatty acids arise in the colon by bacterial fermentation of carbohydrates that reach the colon either in the form of dietary fiber or due to ineffective digestion and absorption in the small intestine. The relative ratio of acetate, propionate, and butyrate in colon is 6:3:1, and the total concentration of these three SCFAs in colonic lumen is in the range of 50–100 mM. SCFAs serve as an important energy source for colonocytes. These fatty acids enter the colonic epithelium across the lumen–facing apical membrane by diffusion, anion-exchange, $H^+/SCFA^-$ symport, and $Na^+/SCFA^-$ symport [46–49]. The relative contributions of each of these entry mechanisms might vary depending on the luminal concentrations of SCFAs because of the marked differences in the substrate affinities for the transport processes. Under physiological conditions with luminal concentrations of SCFAs in the range of 50–100 mM, diffusion is probably the major entry mechanism. When the concentrations decrease due to changes in the dietary intake of fibers or due to dysbiosis under disease conditions, the carrier-mediated entry mechanisms probably play the major role. Irrespective of the entry mechanism, most of the SCFAs generated by the bacteria are absorbed in the colon, with only a minimal amount excreted in feces. The biological effects of SCFAs in the colon are not restricted to their role as energy substrates for the epithelial cells. These bacterial metabolites promote water and electrolyte absorption in the colon, thus providing protection against potential diarrheagenic diseases [48]. They also modulate the mucosal immune system by helping the development of a tolerant environment to facilitate the co-habitation of the bacteria and the host [50–52]. They aid in the maintenance of the mucosal barrier, thus preventing the direct exposure of systemic organs to colonic bacteria. SCFAs also suppress colonic inflammation and carcinogenesis [43,46,53–56].

As the cell-surface receptors for SCFAs are located on the lumen-facing apical membrane of colonic epithelial cells (see below), the luminal concentrations of these agonists are physiologically relevant. SCFAs are low-affinity agonists for these receptors, and the normal luminal concentrations of these bacterial metabolites are in the millimolar levels, sufficient to activate these receptors from the luminal side. However, some of the molecular targets for these metabolites are either inside the cells (e.g., HDACs) or on the surface of the immune cells located in the lamina propria. Therefore, concentrations of these metabolites inside the colonic epithelial cells and in the lamina propria are relevant to impact these molecular targets. The intracellular target HDAC is inhibited by butyrate and propionate at low micromolar concentrations. There are effective transport systems for SCFAs in the apical membrane of colonic epithelial cells (e.g., proton-coupled and sodium-coupled monocarboxylate transporters) [47], thus making it very likely for these SCFAs to reach intracellular levels sufficient to inhibit HDACs. Even though the luminal concentrations of SCFAs are in the millimolar range, it is unlikely that they reach lamina propria at significant levels to activate the cell-surface receptors present on the mucosal immune cells. These metabolites are present only at micromolar levels in the portal blood [57], indicating that they undergo robust metabolism inside the colonic epithelial cells. This raises the question as to the physiological relevance of these bacterial metabolites to the activation of the cell-surface SCFA receptors in immune cells located in the lamina propria. With regard to this issue, it is important to note that colonic epithelial cells are highly ketogenic; they use acetate and butyrate to generate the ketone body β-hydroxybutyrate [58]. This ketone body is released from the cells into portal blood. As β-hydroxybutyrate is 3–4 times more potent than butyrate in activating its receptor GPR109A, it can be speculated that the colon-derived ketone body is most likely involved in the activation of the SCFA receptor in mucosal immune cells.

Lactate is another bacterial metabolite that is important to colonic health but has received much less attention than the SCFAs. Lactobacilli that generate lactate as a fermentation product form a significant constituent of normal bacterial flora in the colon. As such, in addition to the dietary sources of lactate from yogurt and other dairy products, bacterial metabolism constitutes an important source of lactate in the colonic lumen [36,59].

Bacterial metabolites arising from protein catabolism are receiving increasing attention in recent years, particularly the metabolites resulting from tryptophan degradation [60,61]. This includes indole, indole-3-aldehyde, indole-3-acetic acid, and indole-3-propionic acid. These metabolites also elicit beneficial effects on the host colon; they suppress inflammation and carcinogenesis [14,62]. Another important class of bacterial metabolites that impact on colonic health is the secondary bile acids [63]. Liver synthesizes two different bile acids, namely cholic acid and chenodeoxycholic acid, which are called primary bile acids. These bile acids are secreted into the bile and reach the small intestine to facilitate the digestion and absorption of dietary fat. Almost 95% of these bile acids are reabsorbed in the ileum to undergo entero-hepatic circulation. The remaining bile acids reach the colon where the resident bacteria metabolize them into secondary bile acids (deoxycholic acid and lithocholic acid). The bacteria-generated secondary bile acids get absorbed in the colon and enter the entero-hepatic circulation similar to the primary bile acids produced by the liver. Colonic bacteria also act on dietary lipids, generating metabolites such as conjugated linoleic and linolenic acids and trimethylamine [64–66]. All these molecules have marked biological effects on the host colon. In addition to these metabolites, the bacterial cell-wall components such as lipopolysaccharide, peptidoglycans, and polysaccharide A also serve signaling molecules in the colon.

5. Molecular Targets for Bacterial Metabolites in the Host

Even though the beneficial effects of colonic bacteria and their metabolites on the host have been recognized for a long time, it was not until recently that we began to understand the molecular mechanisms that underlie this important biological phenomenon. This was true even in the case of SCFAs for which there is a long history of investigations focusing on the role of these bacterial metabolites as the molecular link between colonic bacteria and the host. Inhibition of histone deacetylases (HDACs) by the SCFA butyrate is an exception; HDAC is probably the first molecular target discovered for bacterial metabolites in the colon to provide a mechanistic insight into the communication between colonic bacteria and the host [67]. HDACs are enzymes that modulate the epigenetics of the target cells, including the colonic epithelium. Butyrate is an inhibitor of HDAC1 and HDAC3, which belong to class I HDACs [68,69]. Propionate also possesses this inhibitory effect [68,69]. There is overwhelming evidence in the literature for overexpression of HDACs in cancer and for the therapeutic rationale and efficacy of HDAC inhibitors in cancer treatment [70,71]. As such, the biologic phenomenon of protection against colon carcinogenesis by SCFAs can be explained, at least in part, by the functions of butyrate and propionate as inhibitors of HDACs. This also provided a mechanistic explanation for the tumor-suppressive function of the Na^+-coupled SCFA transporter SMCT1 (SLC5A8) in the colon [46]. HDACs being intracellular enzymes, entry of SCFAs from the lumen into colonic epithelial cells is a prerequisite for these bacterial metabolites to reach their molecular targets inside the cells. As inhibition of HDACs causes tumor suppression, it is understandable why the transporter that facilitates this process functions as a tumor suppressor.

In the past decade, we have witnessed a burgeoning of literature describing identification of new and novel molecular targets in the colon for bacterial metabolites [29,50,51,60,61]. These new discoveries have expanded our current understanding and knowledge of the molecular mechanisms as the basis of effective communication between the colonic bacteria and the host. The newly identified molecular targets include the cell-surface G-protein-coupled receptors GPR109A, GPR43, GPR41, GPR 81, and GPR91, and the nuclear receptors AhR (aryl hydrocarbon receptor), PXR (pregnane X receptor), and FXR (farnesoid X receptor). Table 1 lists the bacterial metabolites and the corresponding endogenous metabolites that function as agonists for each of these molecular targets. There are additional molecular targets for bacterial metabolites such as the receptors for bacterial cell-wall components (TLR4 for lipopolysaccharide, NOD1/NOD2 for peptidoglycans, and TLR2 for polysaccharide A) and the receptors for lipid metabolites from bacteria (TAAR5 for trimethylamine and PPARs for conjugated linoleic and linolenic acids) [29]. The present review however will focus on the cell-surface G-protein-coupled receptors GPR109A, GPR43, GPR41, GPR81, and GPR91, and the nuclear receptors AhR, PXR, and FXR.

Table 1. Receptors involved in host-bacteria communication in the colon.

Receptor	Agonist	
	Bacterial Metabolite	**Endogenous Metabolite**
Cell-surface receptors		
GPR109A	Butyrate [72,73]	β-Hydroxybutyrate [74]
GPR43	Acetate, Propionate, Butyrate [75–77]	Acetate, Propionate [75–77]
GPR41	Acetate, Propionate, Butyrate [75]	Acetate, Propionate [75]
GPR81	Lactate [78]	Lactate [78]
GPR91	Succinate [79]	Succinate [79]
Nuclear receptors		
AhR	Tryptamine, Indole, Indole-3-aldehyde, Indole-3-acetic acid, Indole-3-propionic acid [60,61], Indole-3-acrylic acid [80]	Kynurenine [81]
PXR	Lithocholic acid, Indole-3-propionic acid [82]	Steroids [82]
FXR	Deoxycholic acid, Lithocholic acid [83–86]	Cholic acid, Chenodeoxycholic acid [83–86]

6. G-Protein-Coupled Receptors for Bacterial Metabolites

G-protein-coupled receptors are seven transmembrane domain–containing proteins involved in cellular signaling; most of them are expressed on the cell surface to interact with extracellular signals and transmit the signals into the cells via second messengers. The human genome encodes ~700 G-protein-coupled receptors. Even though physiological agonists have been identified for many of these receptors, a significant number of them still remain as orphan receptors with no information on the identity of their agonists. In the last decade, however, a distinct class of these "orphan" receptors has been found to be activated by normal physiological metabolites, which were never considered as signaling molecules; these include long-chain fatty acids, the ketone body β-hydroxybutyrate, the ubiquitous metabolite lactate, and the citric-acid-cycle intermediate succinate. Many of these metabolites are also found in the bacterial kingdom and hence are present in colonic lumen; consequently, if these receptors are expressed on the lumen-facing apical membrane of colonic epithelial cells, bacterial metabolites serve as the agonists for these receptors rather than the metabolites arising from the host metabolism. Examples of this category include GPR81, GPR91, GPR43, and GPR41 (Table 1). In some cases, the endogenous agonists for the receptors in non-colonic tissues are different from the bacterial metabolites, which activate the same receptors in the colon; in these cases, metabolites from bacteria that are structurally similar to endogenous agonists "hijack" the receptors for bacteria-host communication. Examples of this category include GPR109A, AhR, PXR, and FXR (Table 1).

7. GPR109A: Expression and Function in the Colon and the Mucosal Immune System

GPR109A was originally identified as a high-affinity receptor for the B-complex vitamin niacin (nicotinic acid) [87–89]. This provided a molecular mechanism for the niacin-induced correction of dyslipidemia because activation of the receptor in adipocytes inactivates the hormone-sensitive lipase and inhibits lipolysis. However, niacin is only a pharmacological agonist as the affinity of the receptor for niacin (~1 μM) is such that plasma concentrations of niacin under normal physiological conditions (~0.1 μM) are not sufficient to activate the receptor. Subsequently, β-hydroxybutyrate, the major ketone body in blood, was identified as the physiological agonist for the receptor [74]. GPR109A is expressed in a wide variety of tissues/cells including adipose tissue, skin, hepatocytes, retinal cells, and bones; it is also highly expressed in immune cells such as macrophages and dendritic cells [90,91]. Butyrate is the only known SCFA agonist for GPR109A, but it activates the receptor only with low affinity (EC_{50} value in low millimolar range) [72,73]. Acetate and propionate do not interact with the receptor. The receptor is expressed in the intestinal tract, most robustly in the colon where butyrate is present at concentrations high enough to activate the receptor [72,73]. The expression is restricted to the lumen-facing apical membrane of intestinal and colonic epithelial cells, thus having direct access to butyrate in the lumen. As such, the bacterial metabolite butyrate appears to be the principal agonist for GPR109A in the intestinal tract. Colonic bacteria regulate the expression of the receptor in the colon; the expression is markedly reduced in germ-free mice, but the expression comes back to normal when the colon gets re-colonized [73].

Upon ligand binding, GPR109A couples through the Gi pathway in most tissues, resulting in decreased levels of cAMP inside the cells [87,88]. The receptor functions as a suppressor of inflammation and carcinogenesis in the colon [72,92,93]. Deletion of the receptor in mice accelerates the progression of colonic inflammation and colon cancer in multiple experimental model systems [92,93]. The receptor is also expressed on mucosal immune cells, particularly in dendritic cells. Activation of the receptor in dendritic cells promotes the ability of these cells to convert naïve T cells into immunosuppressive Tregs and potentiates the production of the anti-inflammatory cytokine IL-10; Gpr109a-null mice have reduced number of Tregs in the colon, reduced levels of IL-10, and increased levels of the pro-inflammatory cytokine IL-17 [92,93]. Studies with NLRP6 knockout mice have shown that increased Prevotellaceae and decreased IL-18 levels are associated with colitis [94]. Gpr109a-null mice also show decreased IL-18 production and increased population of Prevotellaceae, both alterations leading to potentiation of experimentally induced colitis [92]. Recent studies show that NLRP3-mediated inflammasome plays an important role in IL-18 secretion and regulation of microbiota through GPR109A [93].

8. GPR43: Expression and Function in the Colon and the Mucosal Immune System

GPR43 was discovered in a cluster of four novel GPRs located in close proximity to CD22 on human chromosome 19 [95] and then cloned from mouse leukemia cells [96]. It has a widespread expression pattern, with most prominent expression in the adipose tissue, gastrointestinal tract, leukocytes and neutrophils [75]. The receptor is coupled to both Gq and Gi/o, leading to a decrease in cAMP levels and the activation of phospholipase-C [50,75]. Studies with reporter mice have shown that Gpr43 is highly expressed not only in colonic epithelial cells but also in immune cells present in the colon lamina propria [76]. The receptor is activated by all three major SCFAs, acetate, propionate, and butyrate [77], which is in contrast to GPR109A that is activated solely by butyrate.

The exact biological role of GPR43 under normal physiological conditions remains controversial with regard to whether the receptor suppresses or promotes inflammation and carcinogenesis in the colon. Several studies have demonstrated that the receptor plays a role in promoting inflammation and cancer [77,97–99]. GPR43 is expressed at higher levels in colorectal and gastric cancers and overexpression of the receptor in cancer cells potentiates their growth when xenografted in nude mice [97]. The receptor has also been shown to induce neutrophil chemotaxis and promote inflammation [77,98,99]. However, there are other reports that show the opposite; the receptor functions as a suppressor of colonic inflammation and carcinogenesis [55,100,101]. Tang et al. [100] have reported that GPR43 is silenced in colon cancer, both at the primary site and in metastatic spreads. Most colon cancer cells do not express the receptor, and when engineered to express the receptor ectopically, the cells undergo apoptosis upon exposure to the receptor agonists propionate or butyrate. These studies strongly demonstrate a tumor-suppressive function for the receptor. Maslowski et al. [55] and Masui et al. [101] have shown that Gpr43- null mice are more susceptible to experimental colitis, indicating an anti-inflammatory role for the receptor. Our own studies [102] also corroborated the function of the receptor as a suppressor of inflammation and carcinogenesis. The anti-inflammatory role is further supported by the findings that Gpr43 blocks inflammasomes [93] and deletion of the receptor in mice leads to dysbiosis in colonic microflora and increased susceptibility to colon cancer [102].

In contrast to GPR109A, which is expressed only in colonic epithelial cells, GPR43 is expressed in epithelial cells and in enteroendocrine cells, particularly L-cells [103–105]. This has significant biological implications. L-cells secrete two important gut hormones: glucagon-like peptide 1 and Peptide YY. Activation of GPR43 by SCFAs increases the secretion of both these gut hormones. As these hormones impact on the function of pancreas (insulin secretion) and brain (appetite control), SCFAs influence the biology of distant organs via GPR43 expressed in the intestinal tract.

9. GPR41: Expression and Function in the Colon

GPR41 is also a receptor for SCFAs: all three SCFAs activate the receptor [50]. However, similar to GPR43, GPR41 is expressed in enteroendocrine cells, but unlike GPR43, GPR41 is not expressed in colonic epithelial cells [104–106]. Furthermore, unlike GPR109A and GPR43, GPR41 is also in enteric neurons [107]. However, the intracellular signaling mechanism seems to be similar for all three SCFA receptors, which involve a decrease intracellular levels of cAMP in response to receptor activation. Activation of GPR41 by SCFAs present in the colonic lumen is capable of altering secretion of gut hormones to impact biology at distant organs. Studies have shown that activation of Gpr41 by SCFAs induces secretion of glucagon-like peptide 1 and Peptide YY to alter insulin secretion and appetite control [104,105].

10. GPR81 and GPR91: Expression and Function in the Colon

GPR81 is a cell-surface, G-protein-coupled receptor for the ubiquitous metabolite lactate [78] whereas GPR91, also present on cell-surface, is a G-protein-coupled receptor for the citric-acid cycle intermediate succinate [79]. Relatively less is known about the role of these receptors in the colon. Both these receptors are expressed in colonic epithelial cells and are likely to play a role in colonic biology because lactate is a major metabolite generated by normal colonic bacteria, particularly by Lactobacilli, and succinate is released by dead bacterial cells. The presence of these receptors in the colon and their ligands in the colonic lumen strongly suggest a potential connection between these receptors and colonic health. Further investigations are needed to understand the biological significance of these two receptors and their role in the communication between colonic bacteria and the host.

11. Nuclear Receptors AhR, PXR, and FXR and Their Modulation by Bacterial Metabolites

There are bacterial metabolites other than the SCFAs that are also important for the communication between the host and colonic bacteria and hence for optimal colonic health. These include tryptophan metabolites and bile acids (Table 1). While the SCFAs elicit their biological effects on the colon by serving as agonists for the cell-surface G-protein-coupled receptors GPR109A, GPR43, and GPR41, tryptophan metabolites and bile acids impact colonic health by serving as the ligands for the nuclear receptors AhR (aryl hydrocarbon receptor), PXR (pregnane X receptor), and FXR (farnesoid X receptor). Unlike the G-protein-coupled receptors, which regulate cellular function via changes in intracellular levels of the second messengers such as cAMP and calcium, the nuclear receptors modulate cellular function by altering gene transcription as they all function as transcription factors. However, the ability of these nuclear receptors to bind to their target genes is ligand-dependent; the receptors reside in the cytoplasm when not bound to their ligands, but in the presence of the ligands, the receptor-ligand complex translocates into the nucleus to act on the target genes.

AhR is expressed in colonic epithelial cells and functions as a suppressor of inflammation and carcinogenesis [62,108,109]. The bacterial metabolites that activate this receptor originate from tryptophan catabolism; these include tryptamine, indole, indole-3-aldehyde, indole-3-acetic acid, and indole-3-propionic acid (Table 1). Activation of AhR by these metabolites occurs at doses that are relevant to their concentrations found in the colonic lumen under normal physiological conditions [60,61]. AhR has received considerable attention for its activation by xenobiotics as a process related to xenobiotic biotransformation and their subsequent elimination from the body. However, recent studies have identified the endogenous tryptophan metabolite kynurenine as the physiological agonist for the receptor [81]. Kynurenine is a catabolic product of tryptophan in mammalian cells, generated by the intracellular enzyme indoleamine-2,3-dioxygenase-1 (IDO1); this enzyme is expressed at high levels in colonic epithelial cells. IDO1 is an immunosuppressive enzyme [110] and its robust expression in the colon contributes to the tolerance of the colonic bacteria by the host. Activation of AhR by kynurenine in the colon is obviously essential for the host-bacteria symbiotic relationship. The tryptophan metabolites produced by the colonic bacteria also contribute to this process via their ability to activate the same receptor. A more recent study has identified another tryptophan metabolite, indole-3-acrylic acid, in colonic lumen that is generated by a specific bacterial species, Peptostreptococcus [80]. This metabolite is an agonist for AhR and is also a potent activator of antioxidant machinery in cells [80]. Through these mechanisms, indole-3-acrylic acid promotes intestinal barrier function and attenuates inflammation.

PXR and FXR are also nuclear receptors and they are also activated by various xenobiotics. However, the endogenous agonists for these receptors are steroids and bile acids, respectively (Table 1). The bacterial metabolites that activate these receptors include the secondary bile acids deoxycholic acid and lithocholic acid and the tryptophan metabolite indole-3-propionic acid. The activation of both these receptors elicits protective effects in the colon against inflammation and cancer [82–86].

12. Relevance of Dietary Fiber to the Production of Tryptophan Metabolites in Colon

Colonic bacteria generate tryptophan metabolites via protein metabolism. In contrast, the short-chain fatty acids are generated via fermentation of carbohydrates that reach the colon mostly in the form of dietary fiber. However, the quantity and quality of dietary fiber can potentially impact the generation of tryptophan metabolites because fiber as the source of carbon and energy is a major determinant of the composition of bacterial species in the colon. It has been documented that restriction of sugar in the diet promotes expansion of Lactobacilli species that possess enzymatic machinery to generate selective tryptophan metabolites to activate AhR and stimulate IL22 production [14]. This cytokine alters mucosal immune response in such a manner that it facilitates colonization of selective bacterial species and at the same time prevents colonization of the fungus Candida albicans [14]. As such, alterations in dietary fiber intake have a major impact on the generation of tryptophan metabolites and possibly other metabolites as well.

13. Conclusions

The symbiotic relationship between colonic bacteria and the host is undeniable, and this mutually beneficial coexistence is made possible through effective communication between the two partners in this co-habitation. The primary mode of this communication is chemical, mediated by specific bacterial metabolites that elicit their biological effects on the host by activating selective molecular targets in the host colon. Some of these molecular targets (GPR41, GPR43, GPR109A, GPR81, and GPR91) are located on the lumen-facing apical membrane of colonic epithelial cells where they have direct access to bacterial metabolites generated in the lumen. Some are located intracellularly (e.g., HDACs, AhR, FXR, PXR, and PPARs), and there is evidence that the bacterial metabolites generated in the lumen enter the colonic epithelial cells, many of them via selective transporters expressed in the apical membrane of these cells. Mucosal immune cells present in the lamina propria also express the same molecular targets as in colonic epithelial cells for these bacterial metabolites, but it is questionable if all of these metabolites reach lamina propria at concentrations sufficient to act on these targets in immune cells. This question seems particularly appropriate for SCFAs because these metabolites are actively metabolized in colonic epithelial cells. This might not be an issue for tryptophan metabolites. Taken collectively, there is an overwhelming evidence for active dialogue between colonic bacteria and the host with selective bacterial metabolites functioning as messengers. The end result of this chemical communication is the tolerance of colonic bacteria by the host immune system, which is obligatory for the symbiosis. A beneficial byproduct of this co-habitation and symbiosis is the maintenance of optimal colonic health with a decreased risk of colonic inflammation and carcinogenesis.

Acknowledgments: This work was supported by the National Institutes of Health grant CA190710 and by the Welch Endowed Chair in Biochemistry, Grant No. BI-0028, at the Texas Tech University Health Sciences Center.

Author Contributions: Sathish Sivaprakasam prepared the first draft of the review; Yangzom D. Bhutia and Sabarish Ramachandran helped in the literature search and also worked on the first draft; Vadivel Ganapathy corrected, edited, and revised the first draft and prepared the final version.

References

1. Sender, R.; Fuchs, S.; Milo, R. Revised estimates for the number of human and bacterial cells in the body. *PLoS Biol.* **2016**, *14*, e1002533. [CrossRef] [PubMed]
2. Sender, R.; Fuchs, S.; Milo, R. Are we really vastly outnumbered? Revisiting the ratio of bacterial to host cells in humans. *Cell* **2016**, *164*, 337–340. [CrossRef] [PubMed]
3. Lozupone, C.A.; Stombaugh, J.I.; Gordon, J.I.; Jansson, J.K.; Knight, R. Diversity and resilience of the human gut microbiota. *Nature* **2012**, *489*, 220–230. [CrossRef] [PubMed]
4. Qin, J.; Li, R.; Raes, J.; Arumugam, M.; Burgdorf, K.S.; Manichanh, C.; Nielsen, T.; Pons, N.; Levenez, F.; Yamada, T.; et al. A human gut microbial gene catalogue established by metagenomic sequencing. *Nature* **2010**, *464*, 59–65. [CrossRef] [PubMed]
5. Arumugam, M.; Raes, J.; Pelletier, E.; Le Paslier, D.; Yamada, T.; Mende, D.R.; Fernandes, G.R.; Tap, J.; Bruls, T.; Batto, J.M.; et al. Enterotypes of the human gut microbiome. *Nature* **2011**, *473*, 174–180. [CrossRef] [PubMed]
6. Mu, C.; Yang, Y.; Zhu, W. Gut microbiota: The brain peacekeeper. *Front. Microbiol.* **2016**, *7*, 345. [CrossRef] [PubMed]
7. Haque, T.R.; Barritt, A.S. Intestinal microbiota in liver disease. *Best Pract. Res. Clin. Gastroenterol.* **2016**, *30*, 133–142. [CrossRef] [PubMed]
8. Leal-Lopes, C.; Velloso, F.J.; Campopiano, J.C.; Sogayar, M.C.; Correa, R.G. Roles of commensal microbiota in pancreas homeostasis and pancreatic pathologies. *J. Diabetes Res.* **2015**, *2015*, 284680. [CrossRef] [PubMed]
9. Khan, M.J.; Gerasimidis, K.; Edwards, C.A.; Shaikh, M.G. Role of gut microbiota in the aetiology of obesity: Proposed mechanisms and review of the literature. *J. Obes.* **2016**, *2016*, 7353642. [CrossRef] [PubMed]
10. Jonsson, A.L.; Backhed, F. Role of gut microbiota in atherosclerosis. *Nat. Rev. Cardiol.* **2017**, *14*, 79–87. [CrossRef] [PubMed]
11. Haghikia, A.; Jorg, S.; Duscha, A.; Berg, J.; Manzel, A.; Waschbisch, A.; Hammer, A.; Lee, D.H.; May, C.; Wilck, N.; et al. Dietary fatty acids directly impact central nervous system autoimmunity via the small intestine. *Immunity* **2015**, *43*, 817–829. [CrossRef] [PubMed]
12. Bhutia, Y.D.; Ganapathy, V. Short, but smart: SCFAs train T cells in the gut to fight autoimmunity in the brain. *Immunity* **2015**, *43*, 629–631. [CrossRef] [PubMed]
13. Rothhammer, V.; Mascanfroni, I.D.; Bunse, L.; Takenaka, M.C.; Kenison, J.E.; Mayo, L.; Chao, C.C.; Patel, B.; Yan, R.; Blain, M.; et al. Type I interferons and microbial metabolites of tryptophan modulate astrocyte activity and central nervous system inflammation via the aryl hydrocarbon receptor. *Nat. Med.* **2016**, *22*, 586–597. [CrossRef] [PubMed]
14. Zelante, T.; Iannitti, R.G.; Cunha, C.; De Luca, A.; Giovannini, G.; Pieraccini, G.; Zecchi, R.; D'Angelo, C.; Massi-Benedetti, C.; Fallarino, F.; et al. Tryptophan catabolites from microbiota engage aryl hydrocarbon receptor and balance mucosal reactivity via interleukin-22. *Immunity* **2013**, *39*, 372–385. [CrossRef] [PubMed]
15. Ohland, C.L.; Jobin, C. Microbial activities and intestinal homeostasis: A delicate balance between health and disease. *Cell. Mol. Gastroenterol. Hepatol.* **2015**, *1*, 28–40. [CrossRef] [PubMed]
16. Buttó, L.F.; Haller, D. Dysbiosis in intestinal inflammation: Cause or consequence. *Int. J. Med. Microbiol.* **2016**, *306*, 302–309. [CrossRef] [PubMed]
17. Gao, Z.; Guo, B.; Gao, R.; Zhu, Q.; Qin, H. Microbiota disbiosis is associated with colorectal cancer. *Front. Microbiol.* **2015**, *6*, 20. [CrossRef] [PubMed]

18. Arthur, J.C.; Jobin, C. The struggle within: Microbial influences on colorectal cancer. *Inflamm. Bowel Dis.* **2011**, *17*, 396–409. [CrossRef] [PubMed]
19. Sadlack, B.; Merz, H.; Schorle, H.; Schimpl, A.; Feller, A.C.; Horak, I. Ulcerative colitis-like disease with a disrupted interleukin-2 gene. *Cell* **1993**, *75*, 253–261. [CrossRef]
20. Madsen, K.L. Inflammatory bowel disease: Lessons from the IL-10 gene-deficient mouse. *Clin. Investig. Med.* **2001**, *24*, 250–257.
21. Cani, P.D.; Everard, A. Talking microbes: When gut bacteria interact with diet and host organs. *Mol. Nutr. Food Res.* **2016**, *60*, 58–66. [CrossRef] [PubMed]
22. Velcich, A.; Yang, W.; Heyer, J.; Fragale, A.; Nicholas, C.; Viani, S.; Kucherlapati, R.; Lipkin, M.; Yang, K.; Augenlicht, L. Colorectal cancer in mice genetically deficient in the mucin Muc2. *Science* **2002**, *295*, 1726–1729. [CrossRef] [PubMed]
23. Salim, S.Y.; Söderholm, J.D. Importance of disrupted intestinal barrier in inflammatory bowel diseases. *Inflamm. Bowel Dis.* **2011**, *17*, 362–381. [CrossRef] [PubMed]
24. Yashiro, M. Ulcerative colitis-associated colorectal cancer. *World J. Gastroenterol.* **2014**, *20*, 16389–16397. [CrossRef] [PubMed]
25. Mueller, C.; Macpherson, A.J. Layers of mutualism with commensal bacteria protect us from intestinal inflammation. *Gut* **2006**, *55*, 276–284. [CrossRef] [PubMed]
26. Shapira, M. Gut microbiotas and host evolution: Scaling up symbiosis. *Trends Ecol. Evol.* **2016**, *31*, 539–549. [CrossRef] [PubMed]
27. Cogen, A.L.; Nizet, V.; Gallo, R.L. Skin microbiota: A source of disease or defence? *Br. J. Dermatol.* **2008**, *158*, 442–455. [CrossRef] [PubMed]
28. Macfarlane, S.; Macfarlane, G.T. Regulation of short-chain fatty acid production. *Proc. Nutr. Soc.* **2003**, *62*, 67–72. [CrossRef] [PubMed]
29. Bhutia, Y.D.; Ogura, J.; Sivaprakasam, S.; Ganapathy, V. Gut microbiome and colon cancer: Role of bacterial metabolites and their molecular targets in the host. *Curr. Colorectal Cancer Rep.* **2017**, *13*, 111–118. [CrossRef]
30. Cario, E. Microbiota and innate immunity in intestinal inflammation and neoplasia. *Curr. Opin. Gastroenterol.* **2013**, *29*, 85–91. [CrossRef] [PubMed]
31. Shanahan, F. The colonic microbiota in health and disease. *Curr. Opin. Gastroenterol.* **2013**, *29*, 49–54. [CrossRef] [PubMed]
32. Wang, X.; Huycke, M.M. Colorectal cancer: Role of commensal bacteria and bystander effects. *Gut Microbes* **2015**, *6*, 370–376. [CrossRef] [PubMed]
33. Peloquin, J.M.; Nguyen, D.D. The microbiota and inflammatory bowel disease: Insights from animal models. *Anaerobe* **2013**, *24*, 102–106. [CrossRef] [PubMed]
34. Seksik, P.; Sokol, H.; Lepage, P.; Vasquez, N.; Manichanh, C.; Mangin, I.; Pochart, P.; Dore, J.; Marteau, P. Review article: The role of bacteria in onset and perpetuation of inflammatory bowel disease. *Aliment. Pharmacol. Ther.* **2006**, *24* (Suppl. 3), 11–18. [CrossRef] [PubMed]
35. Butto, L.F.; Schaubeck, M.; Haller, D. Mechanisms of microbe-host interaction in Crohn's disease: Dysbiosis vs. pathobiont selection. *Front. Immunol.* **2015**, *6*, 555. [CrossRef] [PubMed]
36. De Moreno de LeBlanc, A.; Del Carmen, S.; Chatel, J.M.; Miyoshi, A.; Azevedo, V.; Langella, P.; Bermudez-Humaran, L.G.; LeBlanc, J.G. Current review of genetically modified lactic acid bacteria for the prevention and treatment of colitis using murine models. *Gasteroenterol. Res. Pract.* **2015**, *2015*, 146972. [CrossRef] [PubMed]
37. Wasilewski, A.; Zielinska, M.; Storr, M.; Fichna, J. Beneficial effects of probiotics, prebiotics, synbiotics, and psychobiotics in inflammatory bowel disease. *Inflamm. Bowel Dis.* **2015**, *21*, 1674–1682. [CrossRef] [PubMed]
38. Bellaguarda, E.; Chang, E.B. IBD and the gut microbiota—From bench to personalized medicine. *Curr. Gastroenterol. Rep.* **2015**, *17*, 15. [CrossRef] [PubMed]
39. Patel, R.; DuPont, H.L. New approaches for bacteriotherapy: Prebiotics, new-generation probiotics, and synbiotics. *Clin. Infect. Dis.* **2015**, *60* (Suppl. 2), S108–S121. [CrossRef] [PubMed]
40. Grimm, V.; Riedel, C.U. Manipulation of the microbiota using probiotics. *Adv. Exp. Med. Biol.* **2016**, *902*, 109–117. [PubMed]

41. Stearns, J.C.; Lynch, M.D.; Senadheera, D.B.; Tenenbaum, H.C.; Goldberg, M.B.; Cvitkovitch, D.G.; Croitoru, K.; Moreno-Hagelsieb, G.; Neufeld, J.D. Bacterial biogeography of the human digestive tract. *Sci. Rep.* **2011**, *1*, 170. [CrossRef] [PubMed]
42. Vinolo, M.A.; Rodrigues, H.G.; Nachbar, R.T.; Curi, R. Regulation of inflammation by short-chain fatty acids. *Nutrients* **2011**, *3*, 858–876. [CrossRef] [PubMed]
43. Leonel, A.J.; Alvarez-Leite, J.I. Butyrate: Implications for intestinal function. *Curr. Opin. Clin. Nutr. Metab. Care* **2012**, *15*, 474–479. [CrossRef] [PubMed]
44. O'Keefe, S.J. Diet, microorganisms and their metabolites, and colon cancer. *Nat. Rev. Gastroenterol. Hepatol.* **2016**, *13*, 691–706. [CrossRef] [PubMed]
45. Rios-Covian, D.; Ruas-Madeido, P.; Margolles, A.; Gueimonde, M.; de Los Reyes-Gavilan, C.G.; Salazar, N. Intestinal short chain fatty acids and their link with diet and human health. *Front. Microbiol.* **2016**, *7*, 185. [CrossRef] [PubMed]
46. Gupta, N.; Martin, P.M.; Prasad, P.D.; Ganapathy, V. SLC5A8 (SMCT1)-mediated transport of butyrate forms the basis for the tumor-suppressive function of the transporter. *Life Sci.* **2006**, *78*, 2419–2425. [CrossRef] [PubMed]
47. Ganapathy, V.; Thangaraju, M.; Gopal, E.; Martin, P.M.; Itagaki, S.; Miyauchi, S.; Prasad, P.D. Sodium-coupled monocarboxylate transporters in normal tissues and in cancer. *AAPS J.* **2008**, *10*, 193–199. [CrossRef] [PubMed]
48. Binder, H.J. Role of colonic short-chain fatty acid transport in diarrhea. *Annu. Rev. Physiol.* **2010**, *72*, 297–313. [CrossRef] [PubMed]
49. Goncalves, P.; Martel, F. Butyrate and colorectal cancer: The role of butyrate transport. *Curr. Drug Metab.* **2013**, *14*, 994–1008. [CrossRef] [PubMed]
50. Tazoe, H.; Otomo, Y.; Kaji, I.; Tanaka, R.; Karaki, S.I.; Kuwahara, A. Roles of short-chain fatty acids receptors, GPR41 and GPR43 on colonic functions. *J. Physiol. Pharmacol.* **2008**, *59* (Suppl. 2), 252–262.
51. Ganapathy, V.; Thangaraju, M.; Prasad, P.D.; Martin, P.M.; Singh, N. Transporters and receptors for short-chain fatty acids as the molecular link between colonic bacteria and the host. *Curr. Opin. Pharmacol.* **2013**, *13*, 869–874. [CrossRef] [PubMed]
52. Tan, J.; McKenzie, C.; Potamitis, M.; Thorburn, A.N.; Mackay, C.R.; Macia, L. The role of short-chain fatty acids in health and disease. *Adv. Immunol.* **2014**, *121*, 91–119. [PubMed]
53. Arpaia, N.; Campbell, C.; Fan, X.; Dikiy, S.; van der Veeken, J.; deRoos, P.; Liu, H.; Cross, J.R.; Pfeffer, K.; Coffer, P.J.; et al. Metabolites produced by commensal bacteria promote peripheral regulatory T-cell generation. *Nature* **2013**, *504*, 451–455. [CrossRef] [PubMed]
54. Smith, P.M.; Howitt, M.R.; Panikov, N.; Michaud, M.; Gallini, C.A.; Bohlooly-Y, M.; Glickman, J.N.; Garrett, W.S. The microbial metabolites, short-chain fatty acids, regulate colonic Treg cell homeostasis. *Science* **2013**, *341*, 569–573. [CrossRef] [PubMed]
55. Maslowski, K.M.; Vieira, A.T.; Ng, A.; Kranich, J.; Sierro, F.; Yu, D.; Schilter, H.C.; Rolph, M.S.; Mackay, F.; Artis, D.; et al. Regulation of inflammatory responses by gut microbiota and chemoattractant receptor GPR43. *Nature* **2009**, *461*, 1282–1286. [CrossRef] [PubMed]
56. Sengupta, S.; Muir, J.G.; Gibson, P.R. Does butyrate protect from colorectal cancer? *J. Gastroenterol. Hepatol.* **2006**, *21*, 209–218. [CrossRef] [PubMed]
57. Cummings, J.H.; Pomare, E.W.; Branch, W.J.; Naylor, C.P.; Macfarlane, G.T. Short chain fatty acids in human large intestine, portal, hepatic and venous blood. *Gut* **1987**, *28*, 1221–1227. [CrossRef] [PubMed]
58. Helenius, T.O.; Misiorek, J.O.; Nystrom, J.H.; Fortelius, L.E.; Habtezion, A.; Liao, J.; Asghar, M.N.; Zhang, H.; Azhar, S.; Omary, M.B.; et al. Keratin 8 absence down-regulates colonocyte HMGCS2 and modulates colonic ketogenesis and energy metabolism. *Mol. Biol. Cell* **2015**, *26*, 2298–2310. [CrossRef] [PubMed]
59. Pace, F.; Pace, M.; Quartarone, G. Probiotics in digestive diseases: Focus on Lactobacillus GG. *Minerva Gastroenterol. Dietol.* **2015**, *61*, 273–292. [PubMed]
60. Hubbard, T.D.; Murray, I.A.; Perdew, G.H. Indole and tryptophan metabolism: Endogenous and dietary routes to Ah receptor activation. *Drug Metab. Dispos.* **2015**, *43*, 1522–1535. [CrossRef] [PubMed]
61. Jin, U.H.; Lee, S.O.; Sridharan, G.; Lee, K.; Davidson, L.A.; Jayaraman, A.; Chapkin, R.S.; Alaniz, R.; Safe, S. Microbiome-derived tryptophan metabolites and their aryl hydrocarbon receptor-dependent agonist and antagonist activities. *Mol. Pharmacol.* **2014**, *85*, 777–788. [CrossRef] [PubMed]

62. Díaz-Díaz, C.J.; Ronnekleiv-Kelly, S.M.; Nukaya, M.; Geiger, P.G.; Balbo, S.; Dator, R.; Megna, B.W.; Carney, P.R.; Bradfield, C.A.; Kennedy, G.D. The aryl hydrocarbon receptor is a repressor of inflammation-associated colorectal tumorigenesis in mouse. *Ann. Surg.* **2016**, *264*, 429–436. [CrossRef] [PubMed]
63. Ridlon, J.M.; Harris, S.C.; Bhowmik, S.; Kang, D.J.; Hylemon, P.B. Consequences of bile salt biotransformations by intestinal bacteria. *Gut Microbes* **2016**, *7*, 22–39. [CrossRef] [PubMed]
64. Brown, J.M.; Hazen, S.L. The gut microbial endocrine organ: Bacterially derived signals driving cardiometabolic diseases. *Annu. Rev. Med.* **2015**, *66*, 343–359. [CrossRef] [PubMed]
65. Wilson, A.; McLean, C.; Kim, R.B. Trimethylamine-N-oxide: A link between the gut microbiome, bile acid metabolism, and atherosclerosis. *Curr. Opin. Lipidol.* **2016**, *27*, 148–154. [CrossRef] [PubMed]
66. Gorissen, L.; Leroy, F.; De Vuyst, L.; De Smet, S.; Raes, K. Bacterial production of conjugated linoleic and linolenic acid in foods: A technological challenge. *Crit. Rev. Food Sci. Nutr.* **2015**, *55*, 1561–1574. [CrossRef] [PubMed]
67. Davie, J.R. Inhibition of histone deacetylase activity by butyrate. *J. Nutr.* **2003**, *133* (Suppl. 7), S2485–S2493.
68. Thangaraju, M.; Gopal, E.; Martin, P.M.; Ananth, S.; Smith, S.B.; Prasad, P.D.; Sterneck, E.; Ganapathy, V. SLC5A8 triggers tumor cell apoptosis through pyruvate-dependent inhibition of histone deacetylases. *Cancer Res.* **2006**, *66*, 11560–11564. [CrossRef] [PubMed]
69. Singh, N.; Thangaraju, M.; Prasad, P.D.; Martin, P.M.; Lambert, N.A.; Boettger, T.; Offermanns, S.; Ganapathy, V. Blockade of dendritic cell development by bacterial fermentation products butyrate and propionate through a transporter (Slc5a8)-dependent inhibition of histone deacetylases. *J. Biol. Chem.* **2010**, *285*, 27601–27608. [CrossRef] [PubMed]
70. Montezuma, D.; Henrique, R.M.; Jeronimo, C. Altered expression of histone deacetylases in cancer. *Crit. Rev. Oncog.* **2015**, *20*, 19–34. [CrossRef] [PubMed]
71. West, A.C.; Johnstone, R.W. New and emerging HDAC inhibitors for cancer treatment. *J. Clin. Investig.* **2014**, *124*, 30–39. [CrossRef] [PubMed]
72. Thangaraju, M.; Cresci, G.A.; Liu, K.; Ananth, S.; Gnanaprakasam, J.P.; Browning, D.D.; Mellinger, J.D.; Smith, S.B.; Digby, G.J.; Lambert, N.A.; et al. GPR109A is a G-protein-coupled receptor for the bacterial fermentation product butyrate and functions as a tumor suppressor in colon. *Cancer Res.* **2009**, *69*, 2826–2832. [CrossRef] [PubMed]
73. Cresci, G.A.; Thangaraju, M.; Mellinger, J.D.; Liu, K.; Ganapathy, V. Colonic gene expression in conventional and germ-free mice with a focus on the butyrate receptor GPR109A and the butyrate transporter SLC5A8. *J. Gastrointest. Surg.* **2010**, *14*, 449–461. [CrossRef] [PubMed]
74. Taggart, A.K.; Kero, J.; Gan, X.; Cai, T.Q.; Cheng, K.; Ippolito, M.; Ren, N.; Kaplan, R.; Wu, K.; Wu, T.J.; et al. (D)-β-hydroxybutyrate inhibits adipocyte lipolysis via the nicotinic acid receptor PUMA-G. *J. Biol. Chem.* **2005**, *280*, 26649–26652. [CrossRef] [PubMed]
75. Brown, A.J.; Goldsworthy, S.M.; Barnes, A.A.; Eilert, M.M.; Tcheang, L.; Daniels, D.; Muir, A.I.; Wigglesworth, M.J.; Kinghorn, I.; Fraser, N.J.; et al. The Orphan G protein-coupled receptors GPR41 and GPR43 are activated by propionate and other short chain carboxylic acids. *J. Biol. Chem.* **2003**, *278*, 11312–11319. [CrossRef] [PubMed]
76. Nøhr, M.K.; Pedersen, M.H.; Gille, A.; Egerod, K.L.; Engelstoft, M.S.; Husted, A.S.; Sichlau, R.M.; Grunddal, K.V.; Poulsen, S.S.; Han, S.; et al. GPR41/FFAR3 and GPR43/FFAR2 as cosensors for short-chain fatty acids in enteroendocrine cells vs. FFAR3 in enteric neurons and FFAR2 in enteric leukocytes. *Endocrinology* **2013**, *154*, 3552–3564. [CrossRef] [PubMed]
77. Le Poul, E.; Loison, C.; Struyf, S.; Springael, J.Y.; Lannoy, V.; Decobecq, M.E.; Brezillon, S.; Dupriez, V.; Vassart, G.; Van Damme, J.; et al. Functional characterization of human receptors for short chain fatty acids and their role in polymorphonuclear cell activation. *J. Biol. Chem.* **2003**, *278*, 25481–25489. [CrossRef] [PubMed]
78. Liu, C.; Wu, J.; Zhu, J.; Kuei, C.; Yu, J.; Shelton, J.; Sutton, S.W.; Li, X.; Yun, S.J.; Mirzadegan, T.; et al. Lactate inhibits lipolysis in fat cells through activation of an orphan G-protein-coupled receptor. *J. Biol. Chem.* **2009**, *284*, 2811–2822. [CrossRef] [PubMed]
79. He, W.; Miao, F.J.; Lin, D.C.; Schwandner, R.T.; Wang, Z.; Gao, J.; Chen, J.L.; Tian, H.; Ling, L. Citric acid cycle intermediates as ligands for orphan G-protein-coupled receptors. *Nature* **2004**, *429*, 188–193. [CrossRef] [PubMed]

80. Wlodarska, M.; Luo, C.; Kolde, R.; d'Hennezel, E.; Annand, J.W.; Heim, C.E.; Krastel, P.; Schmitt, E.K.; Omar, A.S.; Creasey, E.A.; et al. Indoleacrylic acid produced by commensal Peptostrreptococcus species suppresses inflammation. *Cell Host Microbe* **2017**, *22*, 25–37. [CrossRef] [PubMed]
81. Opitz, C.A.; Litzenburger, U.M.; Sahm, F.; Ott, M.; Tritschler, I.; Trump, S.; Schumacher, T.; Jestaedt, L.; Schrenk, D.; Weller, M.; et al. An endogenous tumour-promoting ligand of the human aryl hydrocarbon receptor. *Nature* **2011**, *478*, 197–203. [CrossRef] [PubMed]
82. Cheng, J.; Shah, Y.M.; Gonzalez, F.J. Pregnane X receptor as a target for treatment of inflammatory bowel disorders. *Trends Pharmacol. Sci.* **2012**, *33*, 323–330. [CrossRef] [PubMed]
83. Cheng, J.; Fang, Z.Z.; Nagaoka, K.; Okamoto, M.; Qu, A.; Tanaka, N.; Kimura, S.; Gonzalez, F.J. Activation of intestinal human pregnane X receptor protects against azoxymethane/dextran sulfate sodium-induced colitis. *J. Pharmacol. Exp. Ther.* **2014**, *351*, 559–567. [CrossRef] [PubMed]
84. Modica, S.; Murzilli, S.; Salvatore, L.; Schmidt, D.R.; Moschetta, A. Nuclear bile acid receptor FXR protects against intestinal tumorigenesis. *Cancer Res.* **2008**, *68*, 9589–9594. [CrossRef] [PubMed]
85. Maran, R.R.; Thomas, A.; Roth, M.; Sheng, Z.; Esterly, N.; Pinson, D.; Gao, X.; Zhang, Y.; Ganapathy, V.; Gonzalez, F.J.; et al. Farnesoid X receptor deficiency in mice leads to increased intestinal epithelial cell proliferation and tumor development. *J. Pharmacol. Exp. Ther.* **2009**, *328*, 469–477. [CrossRef] [PubMed]
86. Stojancevic, M.; Stankov, K.; Mikov, M. The impact of farnesoid X receptor activation on intestinal permeability in inflammatory bowel disease. *Can. J. Gastroenterol.* **2012**, *26*, 631–637. [CrossRef] [PubMed]
87. Tunaru, S.; Kero, J.; Schaub, A.; Wufka, C.; Blaukat, A.; Pfeffer, K.; Offermanns, S. PUMA-G and HM74 are receptors for nicotinic acid and mediate its anti-lipolytic effect. *Nat. Med.* **2003**, *9*, 352–355. [CrossRef] [PubMed]
88. Wise, A.; Foord, S.M.; Fraser, N.J.; Barnes, A.A.; Elshourbagy, N.; Eilert, M.; Ignar, D.M.; Murdock, P.R.; Steplewski, K.; Green, A.; et al. Molecular identification of high and low affinity receptors for nicotinic acid. *J. Biol. Chem.* **2003**, *278*, 9869–9874. [CrossRef] [PubMed]
89. Soga, T.; Kamohara, M.; Takasaki, J.; Matsumoto, S.; Saito, T.; Ohishi, T.; Hiyama, H.; Matsuo, A.; Matsushime, H.; Furuichi, K. Molecular identification of nicotinic acid receptor. *Biochem. Biophys. Res. Commun.* **2003**, *303*, 364–369. [CrossRef]
90. Gille, A.; Bodor, E.T.; Ahmed, K.; Offermanns, S. Nicotinic acid: Pharmacological effects and mechanisms of action. *Annu. Rev. Pharmacol. Toxicol.* **2008**, *48*, 79–106. [CrossRef] [PubMed]
91. Blad, C.C.; Ahmed, K.; IJzerman, A.P.; Offermanns, S. Biological and pharmacological roles of HCA receptors. *Adv. Pharmacol.* **2011**, *62*, 219–250. [PubMed]
92. Singh, N.; Gurav, A.; Sivaprakasam, S.; Brady, E.; Padia, R.; Shi, H.; Thangaraju, M.; Prasad, P.D.; Manicassamy, S.; Munn, D.H.; et al. Activation of Gpr109a, receptor for niacin and the commensal metabolite butyrate, suppresses colonic inflammation and carcinogenesis. *Immunity* **2014**, *40*, 128–139. [CrossRef] [PubMed]
93. Macia, L.; Tan, J.; Vieira, A.T.; Leach, K.; Stanley, D.; Luong, S.; Maruya, M.; Ian McKenzie, C.; Hijikata, A.; Wong, C.; et al. Metabolite-sensing receptors GPR43 and GPR109A facilitate dietary fibre-induced gut homeostasis through regulation of the inflammasome. *Nat. Commun.* **2015**, *6*, 6734. [CrossRef] [PubMed]
94. Elinav, E.; Strowig, T.; Kau, A.L.; Henao-Mejia, J.; Thaiss, C.A.; Booth, C.J.; Peaper, D.R.; Bertin, J.; Eisenbarth, S.C.; Gordon, J.I.; et al. NLRP6 inflammasome regulates colonic microbial ecology and risk for colitis. *Cell* **2011**, *145*, 745–757. [CrossRef] [PubMed]
95. Sawzdargo, M.; George, S.R.; Nguyen, T.; Xu, S.; Kolakowski, L.F.; O'Dowd, B.F. A cluster of four novel human G protein-coupled receptor genes occurring in close proximity to CD22 gene on chromosome 19q13.1. *Biochem. Biophys. Res. Commun.* **1997**, *239*, 543–547. [CrossRef] [PubMed]
96. Senga, T.; Iwamoto, S.; Yoshida, T.; Yokota, T.; Adachi, K.; Azuma, E.; Hamaguchi, M.; Iwamoto, T. LSSIG is a novel murine leukocyte-specific GPCR that is induced by the activation of STAT3. *Blood* **2003**, *101*, 1185–1187. [CrossRef] [PubMed]
97. Hatanaka, H.; Tsukui, M.; Takada, S.; Kurashina, K.; Choi, Y.L.; Soda, M.; Yamashita, Y.; Haruta, H.; Hamada, T.; Ueno, T.; et al. Identification of transforming activity of free fatty acid receptor 2 by retroviral expression screening. *Cancer Sci.* **2010**, *101*, 54–59. [CrossRef] [PubMed]
98. Vinolo, M.A.; Ferguson, G.J.; Kulkarni, S.; Damoulakis, G.; Anderson, K.; Bohlooly, Y.M.; Stephens, L.; Hawkins, P.T.; Curi, R. SCFAs induce mouse neutrophil chemotaxis through the GPR43 receptor. *PLoS ONE* **2011**, *6*, e21205. [CrossRef] [PubMed]

99. Sina, C.; Gavrilova, O.; Förster, M.; Till, A.; Derer, S.; Hildebrand, F.; Raabe, B.; Chalaris, A.; Scheller, J.; Rehmann, A.; et al. G protein-coupled receptor 43 is essential for neutrophil recruitment during intestinal inflammation. *J. Immunol.* **2009**, *183*, 7514–7522. [CrossRef] [PubMed]
100. Tang, Y.; Chen, Y.; Jiang, H.; Robbins, G.T.; Nie, D. G-protein-coupled receptor for short-chain fatty acids suppresses colon cancer. *Int. J. Cancer* **2011**, *128*, 847–856. [CrossRef] [PubMed]
101. Masui, R.; Sasaki, M.; Funaki, Y.; Ogasawara, N.; Mizuno, M.; Iida, A.; Izawa, S.; Kondo, Y.; Ito, Y.; Tamura, Y.; et al. G protein-coupled receptor 43 moderates gut inflammation through cytokine regulation from mononuclear cells. *Inflamm. Bowel Dis.* **2013**, *19*, 2848–2856. [CrossRef] [PubMed]
102. Sivaprakasam, S.; Gurav, A.; Paschall, A.V.; Coe, G.L.; Chaudhary, K.; Cai, Y.; Kolhe, R.; Martin, P.; Browning, D.; Huang, L.; et al. An essential role of Ffar2 (Gpr43) in dietary fibre-mediated promotion of healthy composition of gut microbiota and suppression of intestinal carcinogenesis. *Oncogenesis* **2016**, *5*, e238. [CrossRef] [PubMed]
103. Psichas, A.; Sleeth, M.L.; Murphy, K.G.; Brooks, L.; Bewick, G.A.; Hanyaloglu, A.C.; Ghatei, M.A.; Bloom, S.R.; Frost, G. The short chain fatty acid propionate stimulates GLP-1 and PYY secretion via free fatty acid receptor 2 in rodents. *Int. J. Obes.* **2015**, *39*, 424–429. [CrossRef] [PubMed]
104. Tolhurst, G.; Heffron, H.; Lam, Y.S.; Parker, H.E.; Habib, A.M.; Diakogiannaki, E.; Cameron, J.; Grosse, J.; Reimann, F.; Gribble, F.M. Short-chain fatty acids stimulate glucagon-like peptide-1 secretion via the G-protein-coupled receptor FFAR2. *Diabetes* **2012**, *61*, 364–371. [CrossRef] [PubMed]
105. Kaji, I.; Karaki, S.; Kuwahara, A. Short-chain fatty acid receptor and its contribution to glucagon-like peptide-1 release. *Digestion* **2014**, *89*, 31–36. [CrossRef] [PubMed]
106. Tazoe, H.; Otomo, Y.; Karaki, S.; Kato, I.; Fukami, Y.; Terasaki, M.; Kuwahara, A. Expression of short-chain fatty acid receptor GPR41 in the human colon. *Biomed. Res.* **2009**, *30*, 149–156. [CrossRef] [PubMed]
107. Kimura, I.; Inoue, D.; Maeda, T.; Hara, T.; Ichimura, A.; Miyauchi, S.; Kobayashi, M.; Hirasawa, A.; Tsujimoto, G. Short-chain fatty acids and ketones directly regulate sympathetic nervous system via G protein-coupled receptor 41 (GPR41). *Proc. Natl. Acad. Sci. USA* **2011**, *108*, 8030–8035. [CrossRef] [PubMed]
108. Stockinger, B.; Di Meglio, P.; Gialitakis, M.; Duarte, J.H. The aryl hydrocarbon receptor: Multitasking in the immune system. *Annu. Rev. Immunol.* **2014**, *32*, 403–432. [CrossRef] [PubMed]
109. Xie, G.; Raufman, J.P. Role of the aryl hydrocarbon receptor in colon neoplasia. *Cancers* **2015**, *7*, 1436–1446. [CrossRef] [PubMed]
110. Munn, D.H.; Mellor, A.L. IDO in the tumor microenvironment: Inflammation, counter-regulation, and tolerance. *Trends Immunol.* **2016**, *37*, 193–207. [CrossRef] [PubMed]

18

Effects of Higher Dietary Protein and Fiber Intakes at Breakfast on Postprandial Glucose, Insulin and 24-h Interstitial Glucose in Overweight Adults

Akua F. Amankwaah [1,2], R. Drew Sayer [3], Amy J. Wright [1], Ningning Chen [4], Megan A. McCrory [5] and Wayne W. Campbell [1,*]

1 Department of Nutrition Science, Purdue University, West Lafayette, IN 47907, USA; aamankwaah@calbaptist.edu (A.F.A.); amyjwright2@purdue.edu (A.J.W.)
2 Department of Public Health Sciences, College of Health Science, California Baptist University, Riverside, CA 92504, USA
3 Anschutz Health and Wellness Center, University of Colorado—Denver | Anschutz Medical Campus, Aurora, CO 80045, USA; drew.sayer@ucdenver.edu
4 Department of Statistics, Purdue University, West Lafayette, IN 47907, USA; chen929@purdue.edu
5 Department of Health Sciences, College of Health & Rehabilitation Sciences: Sargent College, Boston University, Boston, MA 02215, USA; mamccr@bu.edu
* Correspondence: campbellw@purdue.edu;

Abstract: Dietary protein and fiber independently influence insulin-mediated glucose control. However, potential additive effects are not well-known. Men and women (n = 20; age: 26 ± 5 years; body mass index: 26.1 ± 0.2 kg/m^2; mean ± standard deviation) consumed normal protein and fiber (NPNF; NP = 12.5 g, NF = 2 g), normal protein and high fiber (NPHF; NP = 12.5 g, HF = 8 g), high protein and normal fiber (HPNF; HP = 25 g, NF = 2 g), or high protein and fiber (HPHF; HP = 25 g, HF = 8 g) breakfast treatments during four 2-week interventions in a randomized crossover fashion. On the last day of each intervention, meal tolerance tests were completed to assess postprandial (every 60 min for 240 min) serum glucose and insulin concentrations. Continuous glucose monitoring was used to measure 24-h interstitial glucose during five days of the second week of each intervention. Repeated-measures ANOVA was applied for data analyses. The HPHF treatment did not affect postprandial glucose and insulin responses or 24-h glucose total area under the curve (AUC). Higher fiber intake reduced 240-min insulin AUC. Doubling the amount of protein from 12.5 g to 25 g/meal and quadrupling fiber from 2 to 8 g/meal at breakfast was not an effective strategy for modulating insulin-mediated glucose responses in these young, overweight adults.

Keywords: dietary protein; dietary fiber; breakfast; overweight; continuous glucose monitoring; meal tolerance test

---

1. Introduction

Type 2 diabetes (T2D) is a chronic metabolic disease that is impacted by insulin resistance, glucose intolerance, and dyslipidemia [1–3]. Dietary factors that influence blood glucose control may modify these metabolic abnormalities [3–6]. Total dietary energy intake and macronutrient composition are well-known to modulate glycemia [4,7]. Restricting energy intake and the resultant reductions in body weight improves these modifiable risk factors for T2D [8–10]. Nevertheless, maintaining energy restriction and weight loss over the long-term is challenging [11]. Manipulating dietary macronutrient composition without restricting energy has also been shown to be an effective dietary strategy for prevention of T2D [12,13].

The quantity and quality of carbohydrate and protein in a mixed meal modulate postprandial glucose and insulin concentrations, with the total amount and the type of carbohydrate consumed being the major contributors to postprandial glucose concentration [14–16]. An increased amount of digestible/metabolizable carbohydrate consumed is associated with higher postprandial glycemia [17–19], which increases the risk of developing T2D [20,21]. On the other hand, a higher amount of complex/indigestible carbohydrates, such as soluble, viscous, and gel-forming fibers [22–24] may attenuate postprandial glucose concentrations [25–29]. Among different forms of soluble fibers, psyllium fiber is known to consistently attenuate fasting and postprandial glucose and insulin [30,31] and distinctly exert a laxation effect when consumed with meals [32]. Dietary protein appears to stimulate insulin secretion in people with normal glucose tolerance and T2D [33–35] and this insulinotropic effect of protein is related to secretagogue amino acids, such as arginine and leucine [33]. Eggs are a complete protein source with a relatively high leucine content [36]. Evidence supporting a glucose lowering effect of eggs is inconclusive [37–39]. Experimental evidence supports metabolic effects of protein and fiber in blunting postprandial and long-term glucose responses independently [7,12,13,35,40]. However, the extent to which the effects of protein and fiber intakes on postprandial glucose when co-consumed may be additive are uncertain, particularly in overweight individuals, who may be at risk of developing T2D.

While traditional meal tolerance tests adequately assess the impact of meals/diets on postprandial glucose and insulin responses, this method does not support the assessment of daylong glucose control. Continuous glucose monitoring (CGM) is an emerging technique that is used to determine the 24-h pattern of interstitial glucose concentrations in community-dwelling individuals [41,42]. The CGM technique may be preferred to inpatient meal tolerance tests to track the impact of dietary intake on daylong glucose responses, particularly when the impact of self-selected dietary intake on glycemia is of interest. By using this approach, the suggested extended favorable effects of protein and fiber intakes on daylong glucose control can be assessed.

We conducted a randomized controlled crossover trial to assess the independent and combined effects of normal versus higher egg-based protein and fiber intakes at breakfast on postprandial glycemic and insulinemic responses as well as 24-h glucose patterns with CGM. The study focused on breakfast because the typical intakes of protein and fiber at this meal are lower than at lunch and dinner [43]. In addition, some previous studies suggest that higher protein [13,44,45] or fiber [46,47] intake at breakfast, particularly protein, may have favorable metabolic benefits by enhancing insulin-mediated glucose disposal due to increased insulin secretion. We hypothesized that co-consumption of higher quantities of egg-based protein and fiber at breakfast would lower postprandial glucose and 24-h glucose responses.

2. Materials and Methods

2.1. Participants

Overweight male and female adults were recruited from the Greater Lafayette, Indiana, USA, area through advertisement to participate in the study. The inclusion criteria for selection of participants were: age 21–45 years; body mass index (BMI) 25–29.9 kg/m^2; females with regular menstrual cycles; non-smoking; not taking medications or dietary/herbal supplements known to affect energy regulation or appetite; not pregnant or lactating within the past 1 year or planning a pregnancy; weight stable ($\pm$3 kg) for the past 3 months; not following a vigorous exercise regimen or weight loss program within the past 6 months; no acute illness; not diabetic (fasting blood glucose $\leq$126 mg/dL (7 mmol/L); not severely claustrophobic; willing to eat study foods; and not skipping breakfast >2 day/week. Eligible individuals were approved by the study physician to participate based on routine blood chemistry assessments. All participants gave written informed consent and the study had approval from the Purdue University Biomedical Institutional Review Board. Figure 1 shows participants' flow through the study. Baseline participant characteristics were not statistically different ($p > 0.05$)

between groups of participants who did versus did not complete the study. Two male participants were withdrawn from the study after randomization by the investigators due to an inability to fully comply with study procedures. These participants did not find the CGM comfortable to wear (one after three days of wearing the device and the other at the end of first intervention period). Four participants had scheduling conflicts. One of these individuals was not able to show up for the first test day appointment. The other three withdrew from the study after completing one or two testing periods. Data for these three participants were not included in the analysis. We obtained and included data from the 20 study completers in the postprandial glucose and insulin analysis. However, one of these 20 participants was unable to wear the CGM because it interfered with his farming occupation. This trial was registered on ClinicalTrials.gov (NCT02169245).

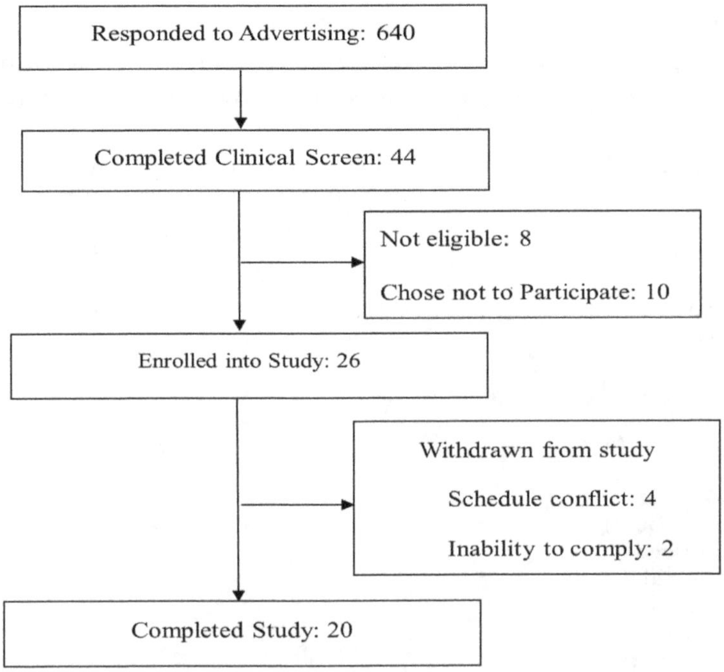

Figure 1. Consort diagram of the study.

2.2. Experimental Design

Participants completed this randomized crossover trial in approximately 15 weeks. Participants consumed four breakfast meals that varied in protein and fiber amounts daily for 2 weeks in random order. The breakfast types were normal protein and fiber (NPNF), normal protein and high fiber (NPHF), high protein and normal fiber (HPNF), and high protein and fiber (HPHF). During each 2-week intervention period, participants consumed the designated breakfast type every morning, but foods and beverages outside of breakfast were otherwise uncontrolled and self-chosen. Testing days were scheduled to occur on the last day of each 2-week intervention period. Twenty-four-hour interstitial glucose patterns were assessed by CGM during the second week of each 2-week intervention period. On the last day of each intervention period, a meal tolerance test was performed. Participants arrived at our clinical research facility after a 10-h overnight fast. Upon arrival, a fasting blood draw was obtained. Participants next consumed the same breakfast type (NPNF, NPHF, HPNF, and HPHF) that they had eaten for the preceding 2-week dietary intervention period. Participants were asked to consume the entire breakfast in no more than 15 min. Postprandial blood draws were obtained hourly for 4 h after the completion of breakfast. Fasting and postprandial serum samples were analyzed for glucose and insulin concentrations. Each 2-week period of dietary intervention was separated by $\geq$15 days (mean: 17 days, range: 15–36 days) during which time the participants were asked to consume their habitual diets. Study investigators (with the exception of the research dietitian, AJW) and participants were blinded to the protein and fiber content of the breakfast treatments during the study data collection period.

2.3. Breakfast Characteristics

All breakfast recipes (Tables S1–S16 were designed by a research dietitian (AJW) using ProNutra (Release 3.2, Viocare Technologies, Inc., Princeton, NJ, USA) and were prepared by metabolic research kitchen staff in conjunction with the NIH-supported bionutrition center at Purdue University. Breakfasts were provided to the participants to consume either on-site or at a self-chosen location. Four varieties (egg and potato casserole, quiche, breakfast sandwich, and breakfast burrito) of each breakfast type were provided within each 2-week intervention period to provide variety. Within each breakfast variety, pilot testing was completed to ensure comparable palatability and textural characteristics across NPNF, NPHF, HPNF, and HPHF breakfasts. While all breakfast varieties were designed to achieve the similar energy, macronutrient, and fiber amounts, the breakfast burrito was consumed on all testing days to provide additional consistency (Table 1).

Table 1. Energy and macronutrient distribution of provided breakfast treatments.

Dietary Variables	Breakfast Treatments			
	NPNF	HPNF	NPHF	HPHF
* Energy (kcal)	396	397	387	386
Available Carbohydrate (g)	51	50	51	48
Sugar (g)	18	22	11	14
Total Fiber (g)	2	2	8	8
Soluble Fiber (g)	0	1	6	7
Insoluble Fiber (g)	2	1	2	1
Total Protein (g)	12.5	25	12.5	25
Total Fat (g)	16	10	14	10
Saturated Fat (g)	4	3	4	3
Monounsaturated Fat (g)	6	3	6	3
Polyunsaturated Fat (g)	3	1	2	1
Trans Fat (g)	0	0	0	0
Cholesterol (mg)	114	325	114	325
Sodium (mg)	767	723	765	720

* Metabolizable energy. Data are based on information from ProNutra, Release 3.2, Viocare Technologies, Inc., Princeton, NJ, USA. NPNF: Normal Protein + Normal Fiber; HPNF: High Protein + Normal Fiber; NPHF: Normal Protein + High Fiber; HPHF: High Protein + High Fiber.

All four breakfast types (NPNF, NPHF, HPNF, and HPHF) provided ~400 kcals of metabolizable energy and contained ~50 g of available carbohydrate. High and normal protein were defined as 25 g and 12.5 g of protein, respectively. The increases in breakfast protein content for HPNF and HPHF were achieved by the addition of whole eggs and/or egg products such as egg white powder; and fat content was reduced to maintain similar total energy content among breakfast types. The high and normal fiber intakes were defined as 8 g, and 2 g, respectively. The additional fiber in NPHF and HPHF was achieved by adding powdered psyllium husk to the meals, which was shown to reduce postprandial glucose responses [30,31] and can easily be incorporated into meals for participant and investigator blinding. The energy, protein, and fiber content of the NPNF breakfasts were designed to resemble reported breakfast characteristics for adult males and females as described in the 2013–2014 What We Eat in America data tables [43]. The protein contents of HPNF and HPHF were doubled to 25 g (25% of energy at breakfast), which is consistent with published definitions of HP diets [48,49].

2.4. Dietary Intake

Self-selected food and beverage intakes during each intervention period were determined using the multiple-pass approach on three unscheduled days (one weekend day and two non-consecutive weekdays) and analyzed by the research dietitian using Nutrition Data System for Research

(NDSR) software, version 2013 (Nutrition Coordinating Center, Univ. MN, Minneapolis, MN, USA). Two-dimensional food portion visuals (Nutrition Coordinating Center, Univ. MN, Minneapolis, MN, USA) were used to assist subjects in estimating portion sizes.

2.5. Body Composition

Standing height without shoes was measured during baseline with a wall-mounted stadiometer. Whole body mass, fat mass, and lean mass were also determined at baseline using air displacement plethysmography (BOD POD, COSMED USA, Concord, CA, USA). Body mass index was calculated as body mass divided by height squared (kg/m^2).

2.6. 24-h Glucose (CGM)

A Medtronic iPro2 Professional CGM device (Northridge, CA, USA) was used to obtain 24-h continuous interstitial glucose concentration data from study participants during the last 7 days of each dietary intervention period. The glucose oxidase-based sensor inserted into the abdominal area at least 5 cm away from the umbilicus obtain an interstitial glucose measurement every 10 s and a recorder stored a smoothed and filtered average of these values every 5 min. Data obtained on the first and last day while participants wore the CGM device were excluded to obtain 24-h glucose data within periods where CGM sensor functional life was ideal. We considered 24-h glucose data valid when three or more self-monitoring glucose reading (finger sticks) were documented for calibration of CGM sensor glucose data [50]. CGM data were used to calculate 24-h interstitial glucose peak, mean, coefficient of variation (CV) and total area under the curve (AUC). The group mean and peak glucose were calculated from the individual participants' means of 2–5 days of useable CGM data. Similarly, group CV was calculated as mean of the ratio of the individual participants' standard deviation to mean. Also, in a subset of participants, the CGM data were used to document the postprandial glucose responses for 75 min after participants consumed the same trial-specific breakfast test treatment (breakfast burrito) as consumed during the corresponding meal tolerance test and also consumed their next meal or beverage by 75 min after consuming the test-specific breakfast treatment. Only participants who provided these data (obtained on different days) were used to graphically show the postprandial glucose responses in more detail (interstitial fluid samples every 5 min) to complement blood sampling (serum samples every hour) during the meal tolerance tests.

2.7. Biochemical Analyses and Calculation

Each blood sample was collected into vials containing serum separator and silica clot activator that were inverted several times and maintained at room temperature for 45 min to allow clotting and then centrifuged at 4 °C for 10 min at 4400 rpm. The resulting serum aliquots were stored at −80 °C until thawed for measurements of glucose by enzymatic colorimetry using an oxidase method on a COBAS Integra 400 analyzer (Roche Diagnostic Systems USA, Indianapolis, Indiana) and insulin by an electrochemiluminescence immunoassay method on the Elecsys 2010 analyzer (Roche Diagnostic USA, Indianapolis, Indiana). The trapezoidal method [51] was used to calculate total AUC for glucose and insulin at 0–120 min, 120–240 min, and 0–240 min time periods. The homeostatic model assessment (HOMA) insulin resistance (HOMA-IR), HOMA β-cell function (HOMA-%β) and whole-body (composite) insulin sensitivity index (ISI) were calculated as previously described [52,53].

2.8. Statistical Analysis

Independent *t*-test was used to assess baseline metabolic health indices between the individuals who completed vs. those who did not complete the study. Doubly repeated-measures ANOVA (PROC MIXED) was used to assess the effects of protein intake (normal vs. high), fiber intake (normal vs. high), and time (fasting-state (0) vs. 60 vs. 120 vs. 180 vs. 240 min), protein × time, fiber × time, and protein × fiber × time interactions on serum fasting and postprandial glucose and insulin. The 2 repeated factors in our model were time and intervention period. Repeated-measures

ANOVA (PROC MIXED) was used to assess the effects of breakfast meal treatments on 0–120, 120–240, and 0–240 min AUCs; 24-h interstitial glucose peak, mean, and CV, and predictive indices of glucose control measures HOMA-IR, HOMA-%β, and ISI. Data are presented as unadjusted mean ± standard deviation (SD) for participant characteristics and mean ± standard error of the mean (SEM) for all other results. We adjusted for fasting-dependent variable values (only when the outcome variable was expressed as AUC), sex, breakfast treatment order (chronological testing order: Period 1 vs. Period 2 vs. Period 3 vs. Period 4), and intervention carryover effect, as previously described [54]. Post hoc analyses were performed using Tukey–Kramer adjustment for multiple comparisons. Statistical significance was set using $\alpha = 0.05$, two-tailed. Statistical Analysis Systems software, version 9.3 (SAS Institute Inc., Cary, NC, USA) was used to perform all statistical analyses.

3. Results

3.1. Participant Characteristics

Participants were apparently healthy young overweight adults (seven females, 13 males). Baseline fasting glucose, lipid and lipoprotein concentrations were within the clinically normal reference ranges (Table 2).

Table 2. Baseline participant characteristics.

Variable	Mean ± SD
Age (years)	26 ± 5
Height (cm)	175 ± 10
Body Mass (kg)	83.4 ± 10.2
BMI (kg/m^2)	27.0 ± 1.3
% Body Fat	26.4 ± 9.5
Serum glucose (mmol/L)	5.2 ± 0.3
Total cholesterol (mmol/L)	4.3 ± 0.5
Low-density lipoprotein cholesterol (mmol/L)	2.6 ± 0.5
High-density lipoprotein cholesterol (mmol/L)	1.2 ± 0.2
Triglycerides (mmol/L)	1.1 ± 0.4

Values are means ± standard deviation (SD) for $n = 20$ participants. BMI: body mass index.

3.2. Breakfast Treatments Effect on Outcome Measures

3.2.1. The Effect of Breakfast Treatment on Fasting Glucose and Insulin Variables

Fasting serum glucose, insulin, and predictive indices of glucose control including HOMA-IR, ISI, and HOMA-β (%) measured on the last day of each two-week breakfast treatment were not different among treatments (Table 3).

Table 3. Fasting serum glucose, insulin, and indices of glucose control after two weeks of breakfast meals consumption.

Fasting Variables	Breakfast Treatments				
	NPNF	HPNF	NPHF	HPHF	p
Glucose (mmol/L)	5.3 ± 0.2	5.3 ± 0.2	5.2 ±0.1	5.2 ± 0.2	0.924
Insulin (pmol/L)	36 ± 6	36 ± 6	42 ± 6	42 ± 6	0.695
HOMA-IR	1.39 ± 0.1	1.51 ± 0.2	1.55 ± 0.2	1.54 ± 0.2	0.713
ISI	33 ± 5.2	32 ± 4.7	30 ± 5.6	31 ± 4.3	0.803
HOMA-β (%)	79 ± 10.2	79 ± 9.5	115 ± 36.9	88 ± 18.2	0.740

$n = 20$. Estimates are mean ± SEM. Homeostatic model assessment (HOMA) insulin resistance (HOMA-IR), HOMA β-cell function (HOMA-%β); whole-body (composite) insulin sensitivity index (ISI). The main effects of protein (high vs. low) and fiber (high vs. low) and their interaction on these fasting variables were assessed using a repeated-measures PROC mixed effects model, adjusting for sex, dietary treatment order, and carryover effect. NPNF: Normal Protein + Normal Fiber; HPNF: High Protein + Normal Fiber; NPHF: Normal Protein + High Fiber; HPHF: High Protein + High Fiber.

3.2.2. Time Course of Postprandial Glucose and Insulin Responses (AUC)

Results from meal tolerance testing showed that over time, postprandial glucose ($p = 0.005$) and insulin ($p < 0.0001$) responses occurred. Compared to fasting (time 0), insulin was higher at 60 and 120 min and glucose was lower at 60 min. The protein and/or fiber contents of the breakfast treatments did not affect 240-min glucose AUC. Protein intake did not affect 240-min insulin AUC, while higher fiber intake lowered 240-min insulin AUC ($p = 0.030$). Further analysis of the insulin AUCs indicated that higher fiber intake reduced insulin AUC at 120–240 min ($p = 0.002$), but not at 0–120 min ($p = 0.245$) (Figures 2 and 3). The apparent lack of a postprandial rise in glucose prompted an assessment of CGM-based interstitial glucose data from days that participants consumed the same treatment-specific breakfast burritos. Indeed, interstitial glucose increased after consumption of each breakfast meal treatment, peaking after about 30 min, and decreasing to baseline concentrations by 60–75 min (Figure 4). An effect was observed for fiber ($p = 0.017$) but not protein ($p = 0.631$) or their interaction ($p = 0.795$).

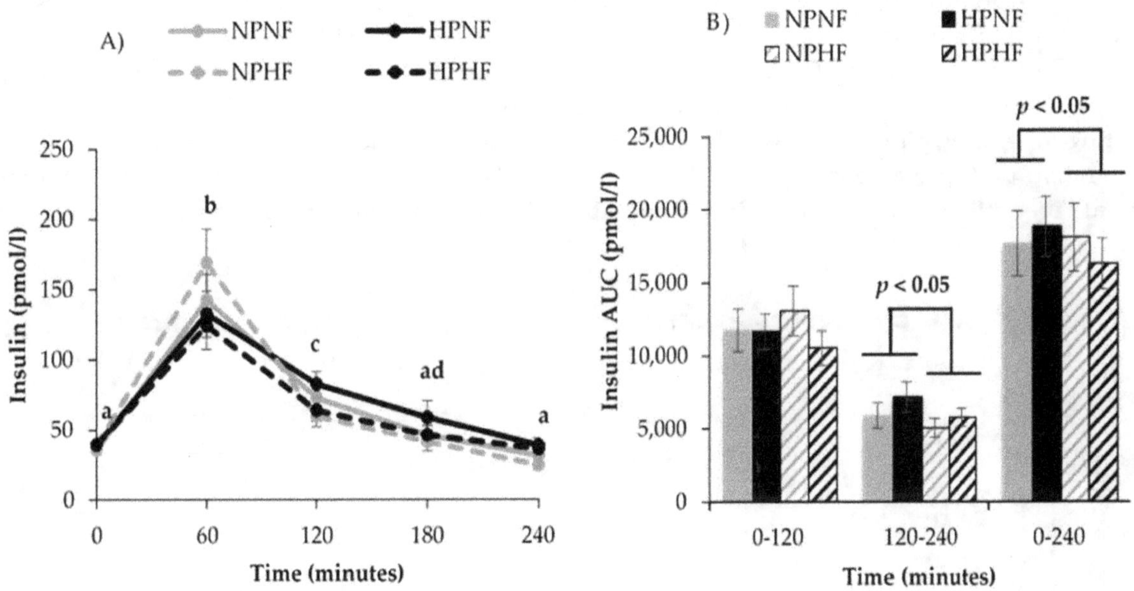

Figure 2. Postprandial time course (**A**) and total area under the curve (AUC) (**B**) for insulin response to breakfast treatments. Postprandial time points with different letters are statistically different (main effect of time, $p < 0.05$). $n = 20$, Estimates are unadjusted mean ± SEM. The main effects of protein (high vs. low) and fiber (high vs. low) and their interaction on postprandial insulin were assessed using a repeated-measures PROC mixed effects model, adjusting with fasting glucose (AUC only), for sex, dietary treatment order, and carryover effect. An effect was observed for fiber at 120–240 min ($p = 0.002$) and 0–240 min ($p = 0.030$) but not protein at 120–240 min ($p = 0.113$) or 0–240 min ($p = 0.569$) or their interaction ($p = 0.944$). NPNF: Normal Protein + Normal Fiber; HPNF: High Protein + Normal Fiber; NPHF: Normal Protein + High Fiber; HPHF: High Protein + High Fiber.

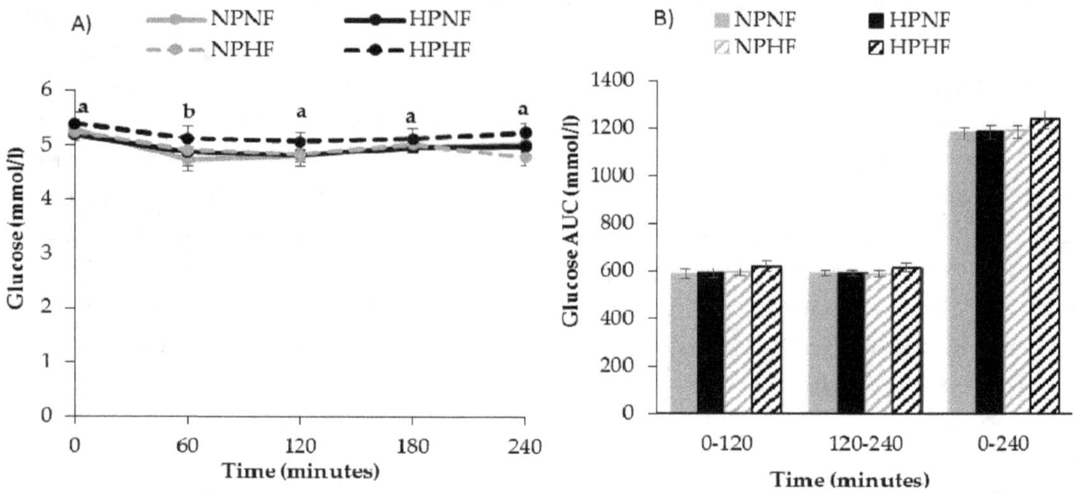

Figure 3. Postprandial time course (**A**) and total area under the curve (AUC) (**B**) for glucose response to breakfast treatments. $n = 20$, Estimates are unadjusted mean ± SEM. Values without a common letter are different, $p < 0.05$. The main effects of protein (high vs. low) and fiber (high vs. low) and their interaction on glucose were assessed using a repeated-measures PROC mixed effects model, adjusting for fasting glucose (AUC only), sex, dietary treatment order, and carryover effects. No effect or interaction effect was observed. NPNF: Normal Protein + Normal Fiber; HPNF: High Protein + Normal Fiber; NPHF: Normal Protein + High Fiber; HPHF: High Protein + High Fiber.

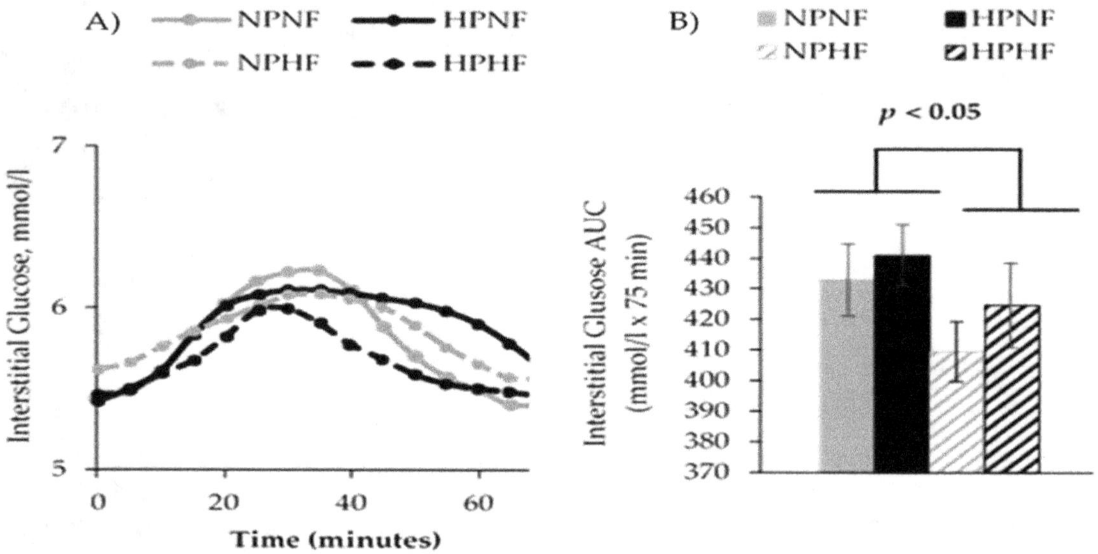

Figure 4. Postprandial time course (**A**) and total area under the curve (AUC) (**B**) for continuous glucose monitoring (CGM)-measured interstitial glucose after treatment-specific breakfast test meals (breakfast burrito) were consumed. Estimates are unadjusted mean ± SEM. The main effects of protein (high vs. low) and fiber (high vs. low) and their interaction on postprandial interstitial glucose were assessed using a repeated-measures PROC mixed effects model, adjusting with fasting glucose (AUC only), for sex, dietary treatment order, and carryover effect. An effect was observed for fiber ($p = 0.017$) but not protein ($p = 0.631$) or their interaction ($p = 0.795$). NPNF: Normal Protein + Normal Fiber; HPNF: High Protein + Normal Fiber; NPHF: Normal Protein + High Fiber; HPHF: High Protein + High Fiber. NPNF: $n = 11$, HPNF: $n = 15$, NPHF: $n = 14$, HPHF: $n = 14$.

3.3. 24-h Interstitial Glucose Variables

Among the four breakfast treatments, we did not observe differential responses in the interstitial glucose 24-h peak (p = 0.768), mean (p = 0.255), and CV (p = 0.534) and AUC (p = 0.179) (Table 4). Comparable 24-h interstitial glucose profiles were observed for all breakfast treatments (Supplementary Figure S1).

Table 4. Breakfast treatment effects on 24-h interstitial glucose variables.

Glucose Variables	Breakfast Treatments				
	NPNF	HPNF	NPHF	HPHF	p
Peak (mmol/L)	7.4 ± 0.2	7.1 ± 0.2	7.2 ± 0.1	7.2 ± 0.2	0.768
Mean (mmol/L)	5.5 ± 0.1	5.5 ± 0.1	5.5 ± 0.1	5.2 ± 0.1	0.255
Variability (CV)	0.99 ± 0.54	0.33 ± 0.23	0.30 ± 0.24	0.60 ± 0.38	0.534
AUC (mmol/L × 1440 min)	7982 ± 109	7977 ± 123	7755 ± 109	7860 ± 104	0.179

n = 19. Estimates are mean ± SEM. CV, coefficient of variation. AUC: total area under the curve. The main effects of protein (high vs. low) and fiber (high vs. low) and their interaction on 24-h interstitial glucose variables were assessed using a repeated-measures PROC mixed effects model, adjusting for sex, dietary treatment order, and carryover effect. No effect was observed for fiber and protein or their interaction. NPNF: Normal Protein + Normal Fiber; HPNF: High Protein + Normal Fiber; NPHF: Normal Protein + High Fiber; HPHF: High Protein + High Fiber.

3.4. Daily Energy and Macronutrients Intake

Among the four breakfast treatments, we did not observe differential responses in either the non-breakfast energy intake (self-chosen energy intake) (p = 0.421) or daily energy intakes (breakfast energy + self-chosen energy intakes after breakfast meals) (p = 0.394) (Supplementary Table S17 and S18), respectively. While we did not observe differences with the non-breakfast macronutrients intakes (Supplementary Table S17), we did observe differences in the daily total dietary fiber (p = 0.021), soluble fiber ($p < 0.0001$), and polyunsaturated fatty acids (p = 0.015) intakes but not the other macronutrients assessed (Supplementary Table S18).

4. Discussion

We conducted this study with the primary aim to assess the combined effect of higher intakes of protein and fiber consumed daily at breakfast over a 2-week period on postprandial glucose and insulin responses. We hypothesized that increasing protein and fiber amounts at breakfast would blunt postprandial serum glucose responses compared to increasing either protein or fiber alone. Contrary to our hypotheses, we observed that increasing protein and fiber amounts at breakfast did not influence postprandial glucose responses in overweight young adults. However, we observed an effect of fiber on insulin response (AUC). Increasing fiber lowered both the last two hours (120–240 min) and the composite 240-min insulin AUCs. Also, we did not observe protein and/or fiber breakfast meal effects on 24-h interstitial glucose or indices of glucose control.

Results from the meal tolerance tests suggested the lack of a postprandial glucose response that may be explained by the timing of blood sampling in the current study. Specifically, it is likely that postprandial glucose concentrations peaked and began returning to baseline levels before the first postprandial sample 60 min after breakfast. This is supported by interstitial glucose data obtained via CGM that showed peak glucose concentrations approximately 30 min after breakfast and declining to baseline concentration by 60–75 min. Generally, the expected postprandial glucose peak occurs one hour postprandial in overweight and obese adults [46]. This supported our choice of hourly blood sampling for the meal tolerance testing because our study participants were overweight adults. Other studies that included varying amounts of fiber [55] and protein [44,56] to meals also reported shorter postprandial glucose peaks occurring within 30–45 min but declining to either baseline or below baseline glucose concentration by 60 min. However, a modestly elevated postprandial insulin at 60 min was concurrently reported by those studies with meal tolerance testing. Our results are consistent with such studies. We observed that glucose concentration 60 min after breakfast was slightly, but statistically, lower than the fasting serum glucose concentration. Our results, together with others, suggest that future studies must always use frequent blood sampling (15-min interval within the first hour of feeding), particularly when both fiber and protein amounts are varied in test meals, to possibly avoid missing important data points within the first hour after feeding.

Studies assessing whether the consumption of higher amounts of protein and fiber simultaneously would better attenuate postprandial glucose response compared to when either protein or fiber is increased and consumed separately are lacking. To our knowledge, only one study assessed the effects of a moderate protein (from egg source) and high fiber (whole grains) breakfast treatment (protein = 20 g, fiber = 7 g, carbohydrates = 45 g) compared with a refined rice cereal breakfast (protein = 10 g, fiber = 1 g, carbohydrate = 55 g) [57]. Bonnema et al. [57] reported an attenuation of 3.5-h AUC glucose with the moderate protein and high fiber breakfast. Results of insulin AUC were not reported. Of note, the difference in carbohydrate content of those breakfasts may explain the glucose results as opposed to the combined effect of protein and fiber. In contrast, one previous study [58] systematically assessed the individual and combined effects of low vs. high glycemic index (GI) and protein breakfast treatments on postprandial insulin and glucose responses. Makris et al. [58] found that combining higher amounts of protein and low GI simultaneously did not have an effect on postprandial insulin and glucose responses. However, intake of higher amounts of the low GI breakfast meal attenuated postprandial insulin and glucose responses. We also did not observe an additive effect with intake of higher amounts of protein and fiber on postprandial insulin and glucose. Collectively, the expected favorable additive effect with increasing the amount of protein and either low GI carbohydrates or fiber from whole grains sources and fiber per se on postprandial insulin and glucose responses is inconclusive.

Our results partially supported the favorable metabolic effects established for soluble viscous fibers. The 6-g difference between the normal fiber (2 g) and high fiber (8 g) breakfast treatments was achieved by adding psyllium husk powder, which is known as a soluble fiber. We observed that increasing soluble fiber intake attenuated the postprandial insulin response. Other studies noted that increasing soluble fiber when a meal had greater amounts of high glycemic index foods/metabolizable carbohydrate content attenuated postprandial glucose [55,59] and insulin [55] responses. The lowering of insulin with increasing dietary fiber intake that was observed in our study is consistent with previous findings [27,55,60]. Reducing postprandial insulin with higher fiber intakes has beneficial metabolic effects in healthy overweight individuals who are at risk of developing hyperinsulinemia, an early abnormality preceding the development of type 2 diabetes. Insulin resistance with concurrent compensatory hyperinsulinemia is a major feature that underlies the development of metabolic morbidities, particularly, type 2 diabetes [61]. This compensatory elevation of insulin secretion is usually needed to achieve a normal postprandial glucose response in overweight and obese individuals [62] after a meal. Intervention strategies that alleviate the need for elevated insulin secretion for glucose clearance are beneficial. While dietary interventions that vary dietary macronutrient composition without inducing weight lost do not consistently improve insulin resistance, manipulating the dietary macronutrient content has been documented to impact the insulin resistance-induced hyperinsulinemia [46]. Therefore, increasing dietary fiber supported improvement in insulin sensitivity (lower insulin concentration to normalize blood glucose) as previously established [24,47].

In addition to assessing postprandial glucose and insulin responses by meal tolerance testing, our study design allowed us to evaluate potential "second meal effects" with CGM. Jenkins et al. [63] defined second meal effects as an effect of a first meal on the postprandial glucose response after eating the second meal. Consuming higher amounts of fiber and protein were previously shown to elicit "second meal effects" by reducing postprandial glucose responses following a second meal [64–67]. Other studies also reported an attenuation of daylong glucose (lunch and dinner meals) with intake of low GI foods [68]. Assessing such a prolonged effect of consuming a breakfast with controlled protein and fiber amounts on subsequent and uncontrolled meals was an important and novel aim of the current study. However, 24-h interstitial glucose variables, including AUC, were not influenced by the 4 breakfast treatments used in the current study, which suggests a lack of a "second meal effect". Our results may be due to the observed large variability between participants' self-selected intake after the breakfast meal (Tables S17 and S18). Our findings could also suggest that the inclusion of fiber in multiple meals across the day may be needed with the intake of a typical Western diet to improve daily glycemic control.

One limitation of the study was that the lack of provision of a standard meal the night before the acute measurement to metabolically stabilize our study participants may have confounded our study outcomes. Previous studies suggest a residual effect from dinner meals may impact the next morning glucose profile [68] particularly with high fiber intake. Another limitation was the fact that we could not match sugar, MUFA, PUFA, and total fat, across normal vs. the high breakfast treatment meals although these nutrients may influence our results. However, the magnitude of the differences in the amounts of the afore-mentioned nutrients between the normal vs. high protein and fiber breakfast treatments where not numerically substantial. Lastly, our study findings are only generalizable to overweight young adults. A strength of this study is that both researchers and study participants were blinded to the study dietary treatment. This potentially eliminates any biases with our dietary manipulation that may influence our study outcomes. Another strength is that the 2-week dietary acclimation period before our postprandial responses were assessed allowed us to determine the prolonged effects of consumption of protein and fiber breakfasts beyond a single meal.

5. Conclusions

In conclusion, consumption of a breakfast meal with both higher protein and fiber content did not differentially influence postprandial glucose response and 24-h glucose peak and AUC compared to the other three breakfast treatments. However, increasing fiber had an attenuation effect on the postprandial insulin response. Therefore, doubling the amount of protein from 12.5 g to 25 g/meal and quadrupling fiber from 2 to 8 g/meal simultaneously at breakfast may not be an effective therapeutic strategy to improve insulin and glucose responses acutely; however, higher fiber intake at breakfast may be effective for lowering the postprandial insulin response in healthy overweight, young adults.

Supplementary Materials:
Figure S1: 24-hour time course interstitial glucose from CGM to breakfast treatments and self-selected intakes after provided breakfast. n = 19, Estimates are unadjusted means. NPNF: Normal Protein + Normal Fiber; HPNF: High Protein + Normal Fiber; NPHF: Normal Protein + High Fiber; HPHF: High Protein + High Fiber, Table S1: NPNF breakfast burrito recipe, Table S2: HPNF breakfast burrito recipe, Table S3: NPHF breakfast burrito recipe, Table S4: HPHF breakfast burrito recipe, Table S5: NPNF breakfast sandwich recipe, Table S6: NPHP breakfast sandwich recipe, Table S7: NPHF breakfast sandwich recipe, Table S8: HPHF breakfast sandwich recipe, Table S9: NPNF breakfast casserole recipe, Table S10: HPNF breakfast casserole recipe, Table S11: NPHF breakfast casserole recipe, Table S12: HPHF breakfast casserole recipe, Table S13: NPNF breakfast quiche recipe, Table S14: HPNF breakfast quiche recipe, Table S15: NPHF breakfast quiche recipe, Table S16: HPHF breakfast quiche recipe: Table S17: Non-breakfast energy and macronutrient distribution, Table S18: Daily energy and macronutrient distribution.

Acknowledgments: Funding: American Egg Board/Egg Nutrition Center; NIH Indiana Clinical and Translational Sciences Institute, Clinical Research Center (Grant #UL1TR001108); USDA 2011-38420-20038. Financial supporters had no role in the design and conduct of the study or collection, analysis, and interpretation of the data. We are also grateful for Doug Maish EMS-P, CCRC for his assistance with clinical testing and Gerald W. Wehr (MD), IU School of Medicine-West Lafayette, our study physician.

Author Contributions: M.A.M., W.W.C., and R.D.S. designed the research project; A.F.A. and R.D.S. conducted the research; A.J.W. designed the intervention diets; N.C. conducted statistical analysis; A.F.A. and W.W.C. wrote the manuscript; A.F.A., W.W.W., M.A.M. have primary responsibility for the final content. All authors take responsibility for the final content of the manuscript.

References

1. Geiss, L.S.; Pan, L.; Cadwell, B.; Gregg, E.W.; Benjamin, S.M.; Engelgau, M.M. Changes in Incidence of Diabetes in U.S. Adults, 1997–2003. *Am. J. Prev. Med.* **2006**, *30*, 371–377. [CrossRef] [PubMed]
2. Cowie, C.C.; Rust, K.F.; Byrd-Holt, D.D.; Eberhardt, M.S.; Flegal, K.M.; Engelgau, M.M.; Saydah, S.H.; Williams, D.E.; Geiss, L.S.; Gregg, E.W. Prevalence of diabetes and impaired fasting glucose in adults in the U.S. population: National Health And Nutrition Examination Survey 1999–2002. *Diabetes Care* **2006**, *29*, 1263–1268. [CrossRef] [PubMed]
3. Eckel, R.H.; Kahn, R.; Robertson, R.M.; Rizza, R.A. Preventing Cardiovascular Disease and Diabetes: A Call to Action From the American Diabetes Association and the American Heart Association. *Circulation* **2006**, *113*, 2943–2946. [CrossRef] [PubMed]
4. Thomas, T.; Pfeiffer, A.F. Foods for the prevention of diabetes: How do they work? *Diabetes Metab. Res. Rev.* **2012**, *28*, 25–49. [CrossRef] [PubMed]
5. Salas-Salvado, J.; Martinez-Gonzalez, M.A.; Bullo, M.; Ros, E. The role of diet in the prevention of type 2 diabetes. *Nutr. Metab. Cardiovasc. Dis.* **2011**, *21*, B32–B48. [CrossRef] [PubMed]
6. Wyness, L. Understanding the role of diet in type 2 diabetes prevention. *Br. J. Community Nurs.* **2009**, *14*, 374–379. [CrossRef] [PubMed]
7. Wheeler, M.L.; Dunbar, S.A.; Jaacks, L.M.; Karmally, W.; Mayer-Davis, E.J.; Wylie-Rosett, J.; Yancy, W.S., Jr. Macronutrients, food groups, and eating patterns in the management of diabetes: A systematic review of the literature, 2010. *Diabetes Care* **2012**, *35*, 434–445. [CrossRef] [PubMed]
8. Most, J.; Tosti, V.; Redman, L.M.; Fontana, L. Calorie restriction in humans: An update. *Ageing Res. Rev.* **2016**. [CrossRef] [PubMed]
9. Omodei, D.; Fontana, L. Calorie restriction and prevention of age-associated chronic disease. *FEBS Lett.* **2011**, *585*, 1537–1542. [CrossRef] [PubMed]
10. Cox, K.L.; Burke, V.; Morton, A.R.; Beilin, L.J.; Puddey, I.B. Independent and additive effects of energy restriction and exercise on glucose and insulin concentrations in sedentary overweight men. *Am. J. Clin. Nutr.* **2004**, *80*, 308–316. [PubMed]
11. Heymsfield, S.B.; Harp, J.B.; Reitman, M.L.; Beetsch, J.W.; Schoeller, D.A.; Erondu, N.; Pietrobelli, A. Why do obese patients not lose more weight when treated with low-calorie diets? A mechanistic perspective. *Am. J. Clin. Nutr.* **2007**, *85*, 346–354. [PubMed]
12. Blom, W.A.; Lluch, A.; Stafleu, A.; Vinoy, S.; Holst, J.J.; Schaafsma, G. Effect of a high-protein breakfast on the postprandial ghrelin response. *Am. J. Clin. Nutr.* **2006**, *83*, 211–220. [PubMed]
13. Erdmann, J.; Topsch, R.; Lippl, F.; Gussmann, P.; Schusdziarra, V. Postprandial response of plasma ghrelin levels to various test meals in relation to food intake, plasma insulin, and glucose. *J. Clin. Endocr. Metab.* **2004**, *89*, 3048–3054. [CrossRef] [PubMed]
14. Sheard, N.F.; Clark, N.G.; Brand-Miller, J.C.; Franz, M.J.; Pi-Sunyer, F.X.; Mayer-Davis, E.; Kulkarni, K.; Geil, P. Dietary carbohydrate (amount and type) in the prevention and management of diabetes: A statement by the american diabetes association. *Diabetes Care* **2004**, *27*, 2266–2271. [CrossRef] [PubMed]
15. Franc, S.; Dardari, D.; Peschard, C.; Riveline, J.-P.; Biedzinski, M.; Boucherie, B.; Petit, C.; Requeda, E.; Mistretta, F.; Varroud-Vial, M.; Charpentier, G. Can Postprandial Blood Glucose Excursion Be Predicted in Type 2 Diabetes? *Diabetes Care* **2010**, *33*, 1913–1918. [CrossRef] [PubMed]
16. AlEssa, H.B.; Bhupathiraju, S.N.; Malik, V.S.; Wedick, N.M.; Campos, H.; Rosner, B.; Willett, W.C.; Hu, F.B. Carbohydrate quality and quantity and risk of type 2 diabetes in US women. *Am. J. Clin. Nutr.* **2015**, *102*, 1543–1553. [CrossRef] [PubMed]
17. Gross, L.S.; Li, L.; Ford, E.S.; Liu, S. Increased consumption of refined carbohydrates and the epidemic of type 2 diabetes in the United States: An ecologic assessment. *Am. J. Clin. Nutr.* **2004**, *79*, 774–779. [PubMed]
18. Hu, F.B. Are refined carbohydrates worse than saturated fat? *Am. J. Clin. Nutr.* **2010**, *91*, 1541–1542. [CrossRef] [PubMed]
19. Liu, S. Intake of Refined Carbohydrates and Whole Grain Foods in Relation to Risk of Type 2 Diabetes Mellitus and Coronary Heart Disease. *J. Am. Coll. Nutr.* **2002**, *21*, 298–306. [CrossRef] [PubMed]
20. Lichtenstein, A.H.; Appel, L.J.; Brands, M.; Carnethon, M.; Daniels, S.; Franch, H.A.; Franklin, B.; Kris-Etherton, P.; Harris, W.S.; Howard, B.; et al. Diet and Lifestyle Recommendations Revision 2006: A Scientific Statement From the American Heart Association Nutrition Committee. *Circulation* **2006**, *114*, 82–96. [CrossRef] [PubMed]

21. Beulens, J.W.J.; de Bruijne, L.M.; Stolk, R.P.; Peeters, P.H.M.; Bots, M.L.; Grobbee, D.E.; van der Schouw, Y.T. High Dietary Glycemic Load and Glycemic Index Increase Risk of Cardiovascular Disease Among Middle-Aged Women: A Population-Based Follow-Up Study. *J. Am. Coll. Cardiol.* **2007**, *50*, 14–21. [CrossRef] [PubMed]
22. McRorie, J.W. Evidence-Based Approach to Fiber Supplements and Clinically Meaningful Health Benefits, Part 1: What to Look for and How to Recommend an Effective Fiber Therapy. *Nutr. Today* **2015**, *50*, 82–89. [CrossRef] [PubMed]
23. Chutkan, R.; Fahey, G.; Wright, W.L.; McRorie, J. Viscous versus nonviscous soluble fiber supplements: Mechanisms and evidence for fiber-specific health benefits. *J. Am. Acad. Nurse Pract.* **2012**, *24*, 476–487. [CrossRef] [PubMed]
24. Jenkins, D.J.; Wolever, T.M.; Leeds, A.R.; Gassull, M.A.; Haisman, P.; Dilawari, J.; Goff, D.V.; Metz, G.L.; Alberti, K.G. Dietary fibres, fibre analogues, and glucose tolerance: Importance of viscosity. *Br. Med. J.* **1978**, *1*, 1392–1394. [CrossRef] [PubMed]
25. Jenkins, D.J.A.; Kendall, C.W.C.; Vuksan, V.; Vidgen, E.; Parker, T.; Faulkner, D.; Mehling, C.C.; Garsetti, M.; Testolin, G.; Cunnane, S.C.; et al. Soluble fiber intake at a dose approved by the US Food and Drug Administration for a claim of health benefits: Serum lipid risk factors for cardiovascular disease assessed in a randomized controlled crossover trial. *Am. J. Clin. Nutr.* **2002**, *75*, 834–839. [PubMed]
26. Dall'Alba, V.; Silva, F.M.; Antonio, J.P.; Steemburgo, T.; Royer, C.P.; Almeida, J.C.; Gross, J.L.; Azevedo, M.J. Improvement of the metabolic syndrome profile by soluble fibre–guar gum–in patients with type 2 diabetes: A randomised clinical trial. *Br. J. Nutr.* **2013**, *110*, 1601–1610. [CrossRef] [PubMed]
27. Cicero, A.G.; Derosa, G.; Bove, M.; Imola, F.; Borghi, C.; Gaddi, A. Psyllium improves dyslipidaemia, hyperglycaemia and hypertension, while guar gum reduces body weight more rapidly in patients affected by metabolic syndrome following an AHA Step 2 diet. *Mediterr. J. Nutr. Metab.* **2010**, *3*, 47–54. [CrossRef]
28. Gunness, P.; Gidley, M.J. Mechanisms underlying the cholesterol-lowering properties of soluble dietary fibre polysaccharides. *Food Funct.* **2010**, *1*, 149–155. [CrossRef] [PubMed]
29. Wolever, T.M.; Tosh, S.M.; Gibbs, A.L.; Brand-Miller, J.; Duncan, A.M.; Hart, V.; Lamarche, B.; Thomson, B.A.; Duss, R.; Wood, P.J. Physicochemical properties of oat beta-glucan influence its ability to reduce serum LDL cholesterol in humans: A randomized clinical trial. *Am. J. Clin. Nutr.* **2010**, *92*, 723–732. [CrossRef] [PubMed]
30. Gibb, R.D.; McRorie, J.W.; Russell, D.A.; Hasselblad, V.; D'Alessio, D.A. Psyllium fiber improves glycemic control proportional to loss of glycemic control: A meta-analysis of data in euglycemic subjects, patients at risk of type 2 diabetes mellitus, and patients being treated for type 2 diabetes mellitus. *Am. J. Clin. Nutr.* **2015**, *102*, 1604–1614. [CrossRef] [PubMed]
31. Pal, S.; Radavelli-Bagatini, S. Effects of psyllium on metabolic syndrome risk factors. *Obes. Rev.* **2012**, *13*, 1034–1047. [CrossRef] [PubMed]
32. McRorie, J.W. Evidence-Based Approach to Fiber Supplements and Clinically Meaningful Health Benefits, Part 2: What to Look for and How to Recommend an Effective Fiber Therapy. *Nutr. Today* **2015**, *50*, 90–97. [CrossRef] [PubMed]
33. Layman, D.K.; Baum, J.I. Dietary Protein Impact on Glycemic Control during Weight Loss. *J. Nutr.* **2004**, *134*, 968S–973S. [PubMed]
34. Salehi, A.; Gunnerud, U.; Muhammed, S.J.; Östman, E.; Holst, J.J.; Björck, I.; Rorsman, P. The insulinogenic effect of whey protein is partially mediated by a direct effect of amino acids and GIP on β-cells. *Nutr. Metab.* **2012**, *9*, 48. [CrossRef] [PubMed]
35. Nuttall, F.Q.; Gannon, M.C. Metabolic response of people with type 2 diabetes to a high protein diet. *Nutr. Metab. (Lond.)* **2004**, *1*, 6. [CrossRef] [PubMed]
36. Norton, L.E.; Wilson, G.J.; Layman, D.K.; Moulton, C.J.; Garlick, P.J. Leucine content of dietary proteins is a determinant of postprandial skeletal muscle protein synthesis in adult rats. *Nutr. Metab.* **2012**, *9*, 67. [CrossRef] [PubMed]
37. Djoussé, L.; Gaziano, J.M.; Buring, J.E.; Lee, I.M. Egg Consumption and Risk of Type 2 Diabetes in Men and Women. *Diabetes Care* **2009**, *32*, 295–300. [CrossRef] [PubMed]
38. Virtanen, J.K.; Mursu, J.; Tuomainen, T.-P.; Virtanen, H.E.K.; Voutilainen, S. Egg consumption and risk of incident type 2 diabetes in men: The Kuopio Ischaemic Heart Disease Risk Factor Study. *Am. J. Clin. Nutr.* **2015**, *101*, 1088–1096. [CrossRef] [PubMed]

39. Blesso, C.N.; Andersen, C.J.; Barona, J.; Volek, J.S.; Fernandez, M.L. Whole egg consumption improves lipoprotein profiles and insulin sensitivity to a greater extent than yolk-free egg substitute in individuals with metabolic syndrome. *Metabolism* **2013**, *62*, 400–410. [CrossRef] [PubMed]
40. Livesey, G.; Tagami, H. Interventions to lower the glycemic response to carbohydrate foods with a low-viscosity fiber (resistant maltodextrin): Meta-analysis of randomized controlled trials. *Am. J. Clin. Nutr.* **2009**, *89*, 114–125. [CrossRef] [PubMed]
41. Bell, K.J.; Smart, C.E.; Steil, G.M.; Brand-Miller, J.C.; King, B.; Wolpert, H.A. Impact of Fat, Protein, and Glycemic Index on Postprandial Glucose Control in Type 1 Diabetes: Implications for Intensive Diabetes Management in the Continuous Glucose Monitoring Era. *Diabetes Care* **2015**, *38*, 1008–1015. [CrossRef] [PubMed]
42. Baek, Y.H.; Jin, H.Y.; Lee, K.A.; Kang, S.M.; Kim, W.J.; Kim, M.G.; Park, J.H.; Chae, S.W.; Baek, H.S.; Park, T.S. The Correlation and Accuracy of Glucose Levels between Interstitial Fluid and Venous Plasma by Continuous Glucose Monitoring System. *Korean Diabetes J.* **2010**, *34*, 350–358. [CrossRef] [PubMed]
43. United States Department of Agriculture Agricultural Research Service. *What We Eat in America, NHANES Service*; United States Department of Agriculture Agricultural Research Service: Washington, DC, USA, 2011–2012. Available online: https://www.ars.usda.gov/northeast-area/beltsville-md/beltsville-human-nutrition-research-center/food-surveys-research-group/docs/wweia-data-tables/ (accessed on 31 March 2017).
44. Rains, T.M.; Leidy, H.J.; Sanoshy, K.D.; Lawless, A.L.; Maki, K.C. A randomized, controlled, crossover trial to assess the acute appetitive and metabolic effects of sausage and egg-based convenience breakfast meals in overweight premenopausal women. *J. Nutr.* **2015**, *14*, 17. [CrossRef] [PubMed]
45. Park, Y.-M.; Heden, T.D.; Liu, Y.; Nyhoff, L.M.; Thyfault, J.P.; Leidy, H.J.; Kanaley, J.A. A High-Protein Breakfast Induces Greater Insulin and Glucose-Dependent Insulinotropic Peptide Responses to a Subsequent Lunch Meal in Individuals with Type 2 Diabetes. *J. Nutr.* **2015**, *145*, 452–458. [CrossRef] [PubMed]
46. Jenkins, A.L.; Jenkins, D.J.A.; Wolever, T.M.S.; Rogovik, A.L.; Jovanovski, E.; Božikov, V.; Rahelić, D.; Vuksan, V. Comparable Postprandial Glucose Reductions with Viscous Fiber Blend Enriched Biscuits in Healthy Subjects and Patients with Diabetes Mellitus: Acute Randomized Controlled Clinical Trial. *Croat. Med. J.* **2008**, *49*, 772–782. [CrossRef] [PubMed]
47. Wolever, T.M.S.; Campbell, J.E.; Geleva, D.; Anderson, G.H. High-Fiber Cereal Reduces Postprandial Insulin Responses in Hyperinsulinemic but not Normoinsulinemic Subjects. *Diabetes Care* **2004**, *27*, 1281–1285. [CrossRef] [PubMed]
48. Halton, T.L.; Hu, F.B. The effects of high protein diets on thermogenesis, satiety and weight loss: A critical review. *J. Am. Coll. Nutr.* **2004**, *23*, 373–385. [CrossRef] [PubMed]
49. Kim, J.E.; O'Connor, L.E.; Sands, L.P.; Slebodnik, M.B.; Campbell, W.W. Effects of dietary protein intake on body composition changes after weight loss in older adults: A systematic review and meta-analysis. *Nutr. Rev.* **2016**, *74*, 210–224. [CrossRef] [PubMed]
50. Medtronic. *A Practical Guide to Continuous Glucose Monitoring*; Medtronic: North Ryde, Australia, 2011.
51. Potteiger, J.A.; Jacobsen, D.J.; Donnelly, J.E. A comparison of methods for analyzing glucose and insulin areas under the curve following nine months of exercise in overweight adults. *Int. J. Obes. Relat. Metab. Disord.* **2002**, *26*, 87–89. [CrossRef] [PubMed]
52. Matthews, D.R.; Hosker, J.P.; Rudenski, A.S.; Naylor, B.A.; Treacher, D.F.; Turner, R.C. Homeostasis model assessment: Insulin resistance and beta-cell function from fasting plasma glucose and insulin concentrations in man. *Diabetologia* **1985**, *28*, 412–419. [CrossRef] [PubMed]
53. Matsuda, M.; DeFronzo, R.A. Insulin sensitivity indices obtained from oral glucose tolerance testing: Comparison with the euglycemic insulin clamp. *Diabetes Care* **1999**, *22*, 1462–1470. [CrossRef] [PubMed]
54. Sayer, R.D.; Amankwaah, A.F.; Tamer, G.G.; Chen, N.; Wright, A.J.; Tregellas, J.R.; Cornier, M.-A.; Kareken, D.A.; Talavage, T.M.; McCrory, M.A.; et al. Effects of Dietary Protein and Fiber at Breakfast on Appetite, ad Libitum Energy Intake at Lunch, and Neural Responses to Visual Food Stimuli in Overweight Adults. *Nutrients* **2016**, *8*, 21. [CrossRef] [PubMed]
55. Potter, J.G.; Coffman, K.P.; Reid, R.L.; Krall, J.M.; Albrink, M.J. Effect of Test Meals of Varying Dietary Fiber Content on Plasma-Insulin and Glucose Response. *Am. J. Clin. Nutr.* **1981**, *34*, 328–334. [PubMed]

56. Acheson, K.J.; Blondel-Lubrano, A.; Oguey-Araymon, S.; Beaumont, M.; Emady-Azar, S.; Ammon-Zufferey, C.; Monnard, I.; Pinaud, S.; Nielsen-Moennoz, C.; Bovetto, L. Protein choices targeting thermogenesis and metabolism. *Am. J. Clin. Nutr.* **2011**, *93*, 525–534. [CrossRef] [PubMed]
57. Bonnema, A.L.; Altschwager, D.K.; Thomas, W.; Slavin, J.L. The effects of the combination of egg and fiber on appetite, glycemic response and food intake in normal weight adults—A randomized, controlled, crossover trial. *Int. J. Food Sci. Nutr.* **2016**, *67*, 723–731. [CrossRef] [PubMed]
58. Makris, A.P.; Borradaile, K.E.; Oliver, T.L.; Cassim, N.G.; Rosenbaum, D.L.; Boden, G.H.; Homko, C.J.; Foster, G.D. The Individual and Combined Effects of Glycemic Index and Protein on Glycemic Response, Hunger, and Energy Intake. *Obesity* **2011**, *19*, 2365–2373. [CrossRef] [PubMed]
59. Aller, R.; de Luis, D.A.; Izaola, O.; La Calle, F.; del Olmo, L.; Fernandez, L.; Arranz, T.; Hernandez, J.M.G. Effect of soluble fiber intake in lipid and glucose leves in healthy subjects: A randomized clinical trial. *Diabetes Res. Clin. Pract.* **2004**, *65*, 7–11. [CrossRef] [PubMed]
60. Karhunen, L.J.; Juvonen, K.R.; Flander, S.M.; Liukkonen, K.H.; Lahteenmaki, L.; Siloaho, M.; Laaksonen, D.E.; Herzig, K.H.; Uusitupa, M.I.; Poutanen, K.S. A Psyllium Fiber-Enriched Meal Strongly Attenuates Postprandial Gastrointestinal Peptide Release in Healthy Young Adults. *J. Nutr.* **2010**, *140*, 737–744. [CrossRef] [PubMed]
61. Reaven, G.M. The insulin resistance syndrome: Definition and dietary approaches to treatment. *Annu. Rev. Nutr.* **2005**, *25*, 391–406. [CrossRef] [PubMed]
62. Kn, F. *Metabolic Regulation*, 3rd ed.; Blackwell Publishing: Hoboken, NJ, USA, 2010.
63. Jenkins, D.J.A.; Wolever, T.M.S.; Nineham, R.; Sarson, D.L.; Bloom, S.R.; Ahern, J.; Alberti, K.G.M.M.; Hockaday, T.D.R. Improved glucose tolerance four hours after taking guar with glucose. *Diabetologia* **1980**, *19*, 21–24. [CrossRef] [PubMed]
64. O'Connor, L.E.; Campbell, W.W. A novel fiber composite ingredient incorporated into a beverage and bar blunts postprandial serum glucose and insulin responses: A randomized controlled trial. *Nutr. Res.* **2016**, *36*, 253–261. [CrossRef] [PubMed]
65. Chen, M.J.; Jovanovic, A.; Taylor, R. Utilizing the Second-Meal Effect in Type 2 Diabetes: Practical Use of a Soya-Yogurt Snack. *Diabetes Care* **2010**, *33*, 2552–2554. [CrossRef] [PubMed]
66. Clark, C.A.; Gardiner, J.; McBurney, M.I.; Anderson, S.; Weatherspoon, L.J.; Henry, D.N.; Hord, N.G. Effects of breakfast meal composition on second meal metabolic responses in adults with type 2 diabetes mellitus. *Eur. J. Clin. Nutr.* **2006**, *60*, 1122–1129. [CrossRef] [PubMed]
67. Jovanovic, A.; Gerrard, J.; Taylor, R. The Second-Meal Phenomenon in Type 2 Diabetes. *Diabetes Care* **2009**, *32*, 1199–1201. [CrossRef] [PubMed]
68. Nilsson, A.C.; Östman, E.M.; Granfeldt, Y.; Björck, I.M.E. Effect of cereal test breakfasts differing in glycemic index and content of indigestible carbohydrates on daylong glucose tolerance in healthy subjects. *Am. J. Clin. Nutr.* **2008**, *87*, 645–654. [PubMed]

Permissions

All chapters in this book were first published by MDPI; hereby published with permission under the Creative Commons Attribution License or equivalent. Every chapter published in this book has been scrutinized by our experts. Their significance has been extensively debated. The topics covered herein carry significant findings which will fuel the growth of the discipline. They may even be implemented as practical applications or may be referred to as a beginning point for another development.

The contributors of this book come from diverse backgrounds, making this book a truly international effort. This book will bring forth new frontiers with its revolutionizing research information and detailed analysis of the nascent developments around the world.

We would like to thank all the contributing authors for lending their expertise to make the book truly unique. They have played a crucial role in the development of this book. Without their invaluable contributions this book wouldn't have been possible. They have made vital efforts to compile up to date information on the varied aspects of this subject to make this book a valuable addition to the collection of many professionals and students.

This book was conceptualized with the vision of imparting up-to-date information and advanced data in this field. To ensure the same, a matchless editorial board was set up. Every individual on the board went through rigorous rounds of assessment to prove their worth. After which they invested a large part of their time researching and compiling the most relevant data for our readers.

The editorial board has been involved in producing this book since its inception. They have spent rigorous hours researching and exploring the diverse topics which have resulted in the successful publishing of this book. They have passed on their knowledge of decades through this book. To expedite this challenging task, the publisher supported the team at every step. A small team of assistant editors was also appointed to further simplify the editing procedure and attain best results for the readers.

Apart from the editorial board, the designing team has also invested a significant amount of their time in understanding the subject and creating the most relevant covers. They scrutinized every image to scout for the most suitable representation of the subject and create an appropriate cover for the book.

The publishing team has been an ardent support to the editorial, designing and production team. Their endless efforts to recruit the best for this project, has resulted in the accomplishment of this book. They are a veteran in the field of academics and their pool of knowledge is as vast as their experience in printing. Their expertise and guidance has proved useful at every step. Their uncompromising quality standards have made this book an exceptional effort. Their encouragement from time to time has been an inspiration for everyone.

The publisher and the editorial board hope that this book will prove to be a valuable piece of knowledge for researchers, students, practitioners and scholars across the globe.

List of Contributors

Mihir Parikh, Thane G. Maddaford, J. Alejandro Austria and Grant N. Pierce
Department of Physiology and Pathophysiology, College of Medicine, Faculty of Health Sciences, University of Manitoba, Winnipeg, MB R3E 0W3, Canada
Canadian Centre for Agri-Food Research in Health and Medicine (CCARM), Albrechtsen Research Centre, St Boniface Hospital, 351 Taché Avenue, Winnipeg, MB R2H 2A6, Canada
Institute of Cardiovascular Sciences, Albrechtsen Research Centre, St. Boniface Hospital, 351 Taché Avenue, Winnipeg, MB R2H 2A6, Canada

Michel Aliani
Canadian Centre for Agri-Food Research in Health and Medicine (CCARM), Albrechtsen Research Centre, St Boniface Hospital, 351 Taché Avenue, Winnipeg, MB R2H 2A6, Canada
Department of Human Nutritional Sciences, Faculty of Agricultural and Food Sciences, University of Manitoba, Winnipeg, MB R3T 2N2, Canada

Thomas Netticadan
Department of Physiology and Pathophysiology, College of Medicine, Faculty of Health Sciences, University of Manitoba, Winnipeg, MB R3E 0W3, Canada
Canadian Centre for Agri-Food Research in Health and Medicine (CCARM), Albrechtsen Research Centre, St Boniface Hospital, 351 Taché Avenue, Winnipeg, MB R2H 2A6, Canada
Morden Research and Development Centre, Agriculture and Agri-Food Canada, Morden, MB R6M 1Y5, Canada

Olatz Mompeo, Tim D. Spector, Marisa Matey Hernandez, Caroline Le Roy and Cristina Menni
Department of Twin Research & Genetic Epidemiology, King's College London, St Thomas' Hospital Campus, Westminster Bridge Road, London SE1 7EH, UK

Geo rey Istas, Melanie Le Sayec and Ana Rodriguez-Mateos
Department of Nutritional Sciences, King's College London, Franklin-Wilkins Building, Stamford St, London SE1 9NH, UK

Massimo Mangino
Department of Twin Research & Genetic Epidemiology, King's College London, St Thomas' Hospital Campus, Westminster Bridge Road, London SE1 7EH, UK
NIHR Biomedical Research Centre at Guy's and St Thomas' Foundation Trust, London SE1 9RT, UK

Amy Jennings
Norwich Medical School, University of East Anglia, Norwich NR4 7TJ, UK

Ana M. Valdes
Department of Twin Research & Genetic Epidemiology, King's College London, St Thomas' Hospital Campus, Westminster Bridge Road, London SE1 7EH, UK
Academic Rheumatology, University of Nottingham, Hucknall Road, Nottingham NG5 1PB, UK

Katharina Miller and Markus Schmid
Faculty of Life Sciences, Albstadt-Sigmaringen University, Anton-Günther-Str. 51, 72488 Sigmaringen, Germany

Walter Feucht
Unit of Fruit Science, TUM School of Life Sciences Weihenstephan, Technical University of Munich, Dürnast 2, 85354 Freising, Germany

Simon J. Reider, Nicole Przysiecki and Alexander R. Moschen
Christian Doppler Laboratory for Mucosal Immunology, Medical University Innsbruck, 6020 Innsbruck, Austria
Department of Internal Medicine I, Gastroenterology, Hepatology, Endocrinology & Metabolism, Medical University Innsbruck, 6020 Innsbruck, Austria

Judith Tragust
Christian Doppler Laboratory for Mucosal Immunology, Medical University Innsbruck, 6020 Innsbruck, Austria

Herbert Tilg
Department of Internal Medicine I, Gastroenterology, Hepatology, Endocrinology & Metabolism, Medical University Innsbruck, 6020 Innsbruck, Austria

Simon Moosmang, Sonja Sturm and Hermann Stuppner
Institute of Pharmacy/Pharmacognosy & Center for Molecular Biosciences Innsbruck, Leopold-Franzens Universität, 6020 Innsbruck, Austria

Lovro Trgovec-Greif, Lorenz Perschy and Thomas Rattei
Division of Computational Systems Biology, Department of Microbiology, University of Vienna, 1010 Vienna, Austria

Simon Tragust
General Zoology Institute of Biology, University Halle, 06108 Halle, Germany

Lulu Jing, Jiaojiao Gu, Meihong Xu, Zhaofeng Zhang and Yong Li
Department of Nutrition and Food Hygiene, School of Public Health, Peking University, Beijing 100191, China

Xue Li
Department of Nutrition and Food Hygiene, School of Public Health, Peking University, Beijing 100191, China
Centre for Population Health Sciences, University of Edinburgh, Edinburgh EH8 9AG, UK

Xiaxia Cai
Department of Nutrition and Food Hygiene, School of Public Health, Peking University, Beijing 100191, China
Department of Nutrition and Food Hygiene, School of Public Health, Capital Medical University, Beijing 100191, China

Xiaotao Ma
Department of Nutrition and Food Hygiene, School of Public Health, Peking University, Beijing 100191, China
Department of Clinical Nutrition, China-Japan Friendship Hospital, Peking University, Beijing 100191, China

Lei Bao
Department of Nutrition and Food Hygiene, School of Public Health, Peking University, Beijing 100191, China
Department of Clinical Nutrition, International Hospital, Peking University, Beijing 100191, China

Jun Li
The 153 Hospital of People's Liberation Army, Zhengzhou 450001, China

Rui Xu, Zhi Ding, Ping Zhao, Lingchao Tang, Xiaoli Tang and Shuomeng Xiao
Department of Gastrointestinal Surgery, Sichuan Cancer Hospital, Chengdu 610041, China

Sebely Pal and Suleen Ho
School of Public Health, Curtin University, Perth 6845, Australia

Roland J. Gahler
Factors Group Research, Burnaby, BC V3N 4S9, Canada

Simon Wood
Food, Nutrition and Health Program, University of British Columbia, Vancouver, BC V6T 1Z4, Canada

Chao Ding, Xiaolong Ge, Xueying Zhang, Hongliang Tian, Lili Gu, Jianfeng Gong, Weiming Zhu and Ning Li
Department of General Surgery, Jinling Hospital, Medical School of Nanjing University, Nanjing 210002, China

Hongkan Wang
First Affiliated Hospital, School of Medicine, Zhejiang University, Hangzhou 310003, China

Isabel Halnes, Katherine J. Baines, Bronwyn S. Berthon, Peter G. Gibson and Lisa G. Wood
Centre for Healthy Lungs, Hunter Medical Research Institute, University of Newcastle, Callaghan, NSW 2308, Australia

Lesley K. MacDonald-Wicks
School of Health Sciences, University of Newcastle, Callaghan, NSW 2305, Australia

Sarina Pacifici
Department of Animal Sciences, Cornell University, Ithaca, NY 14853, USA

Jaehong Song
Department of Biological Sciences, Cornell University, Ithaca, NY 14853, USA

Cathy Zhang
Division of Nutritional Sciences, Cornell University, Ithaca, NY 14853, USA

Qiaoye Wang
Department of Food Science and Technology, Cornell University, Ithaca, NY 14853, USA

Raymond P. Glahn, Nikolai Kolba and Elad Tako
USDA-ARS, Robert W. Holley Center for Agriculture and Health, Cornell University, Ithaca, NY 14853, USA

Huawei Zeng, David P. Taussig and Lu Ann K. Johnson
United States Department of Agriculture, Agricultural Research Service, Grand Forks Human Nutrition Research Center, Grand Forks, ND 58203, USA

Wen-Hsing Cheng
Department of Food Science, Nutrition and Health Promotion, Mississippi State University, Starkville, MS 39762, USA

Reza Hakkak
Departments of Dietetics and Nutrition, University of Arkansas for Medical Sciences, Little Rock, AR 72205, USA
Arkansas Children Research Institute, Little Rock, AR 72202, USA

Eric Francelino Andrade, Paula Novato Gondim and Márcio Gilberto Zangeronimo
Department of Veterinary Medicine, Federal University of Lavras, Lavras 37200-000, Brazil

Andressa Ribeiro Veiga Lima, Fernando Henrique Ferrari Alves and Luciano José Pereira
Department of Health Sciences, Federal University of Lavras, Lavras 37200-000, Brazil

Ingrid Edwiges Nunes
Department of Animal Sciences, Federal University of Lavras, Lavras 37200-000, Brazil

Débora Ribeiro Orlando
Department of Agricultural Sciences, Federal University of Jequitinhonha and Mucuri Valleys, Rua Vereador João Narciso, 1380—Bairro Cachoeira, Unaí 3861-000, Brazil

Lise Deroover, Anja Luypaerts and Greet Vandermeulen
Translational Research in Gastrointestinal Disorders, KU Leuven, Leuven 3000, Belgium

Christophe M. Courtin and Joran Verspreet
Centre for Food and Microbial Technology, KU Leuven, Leuven 3000, Belgium
Leuven Food Science and Nutrition Research Centre, KU Leuven, Leuven 3000, Belgium

Kristin Verbeke
Translational Research in Gastrointestinal Disorders, KU Leuven, Leuven 3000, Belgium
Leuven Food Science and Nutrition Research Centre, KU Leuven, Leuven 3000, Belgium

Bruno Annibale and Edith Lahner
Medical-Surgical Department of Clinical Sciences and Translational Medicine, University Sapienza, Via di Grottarossa 1035, 00189 Rome, Italy

Marilia Carabotti
Medical-Surgical Department of Clinical Sciences and Translational Medicine, University Sapienza, Via di Grottarossa 1035, 00189 Rome, Italy
Department of Internal Medicine and Medical Specialties, University Sapienza, Viale del Policlinico 155, 00161 Rome, Italy

Carola Severi
Department of Internal Medicine and Medical Specialties, University Sapienza, Viale del Policlinico 155, 00161 Rome, Italy

Liliana G. González-Rodríguez and José Miguel Perea Sánchez
Department of Nutrition and Dietetics, Faculty of Health Sciences, University Alfonso X El Sabio, Madrid 28691, Spain
VALORNUT Research Group, Department of Nutrition, Faculty of Pharmacy, Complutense University, Madrid 28040, Spain

Javier Aranceta-Bartrina
Department of Preventive Medicine and Public Health, University of Navarra, Pamplona, Navarra 31008, Spain
Biomedical Research Networking Center for Physiopathology of Obesity and Nutrition (CIBEROBN), Carlos III Health Institute, Madrid 28029, Spain

Ángel Gil
Biomedical Research Networking Center for Physiopathology of Obesity and Nutrition (CIBEROBN), Carlos III Health Institute, Madrid 28029, Spain
Department of Biochemistry and Molecular Biology II and Institute of Nutrition and Food Sciences, University of Granada, Granada 18100, Spain

Marcela González-Gross
Biomedical Research Networking Center for Physiopathology of Obesity and Nutrition (CIBEROBN), Carlos III Health Institute, Madrid 28029, Spain
ImFINE Research Group, Department of Health and Human Performance, Technical University of Madrid, Madrid 28040, Spain

Lluis Serra-Majem
Biomedical Research Networking Center for Physiopathology of Obesity and Nutrition (CIBEROBN), Carlos III Health Institute, Madrid 28029, Spain
Research Institute of Biomedical and Health Sciences, University of Las Palmas de Gran Canaria, Faculty of Health Sciences, c/Doctor Pasteur s/n Trasera del Hospital, Las Palmas de Gran Canaria, 35016 Las Palmas, Spain

Gregorio Varela-Moreiras
Department of Pharmaceutical and Health Sciences, Faculty of Pharmacy, CEU San Pablo University, Madrid 28668, Spain
Spanish Nutrition Foundation (FEN), Madrid 28010, Spain

Rosa M. Ortega
VALORNUT Research Group, Department of Nutrition, Faculty of Pharmacy, Complutense University, Madrid 28040, Spain
Department of Nutrition, Faculty of Pharmacy, Madrid Complutense University, Madrid 28040, Spain

Caleigh M. Sawicki and Nicola M. McKeown
Nutritional Epidemiology, Jean Mayer USDA Human Nutrition Research Center on Aging at Tufts University, Boston, MA 02111, USA
Friedman School of Nutrition Science and Policy, Tufts University, Boston, MA 02111, USA

Kara A. Livingston
Nutritional Epidemiology, Jean Mayer USDA Human Nutrition Research Center on Aging at Tufts University, Boston, MA 02111, USA

Martin Obin
Nutrition & Genomics Laboratory, Jean Mayer USDA Human Nutrition Research Center on Aging at Tufts University, Boston, MA 02111, USA

Susan B. Roberts
Energy Metabolism Laboratory, Jean Mayer USDA Human Nutrition Research Center on Aging at Tufts University, Boston, MA 02111, USA

Mei Chung
Nutrition/Infection Unit, Department of Public Health and Community Medicine, Tufts University School of Medicine, Boston, MA 02111, USA

Sathish Sivaprakasam, Yangzom D. Bhutia, Sabarish Ramachandran and Vadivel Ganapathy
Department of Cell Biology and Biochemistry, Texas Tech University Health Sciences Center, Lubbock, TX 79430, USA

Akua F. Amankwaah
Department of Nutrition Science, Purdue University, West Lafayette, IN 47907, USA
Department of Public Health Sciences, College of Health Science, California Baptist University, Riverside, CA 92504, USA

Amy J. Wright and Wayne W. Campbell
Department of Nutrition Science, Purdue University, West Lafayette, IN 47907, USA

R. Drew Sayer
Anschutz Health and Wellness Center, University of Colorado—Denver | Anschutz Medical Campus, Aurora, CO 80045, USA

Ningning Chen
Department of Statistics, Purdue University, West Lafayette, IN 47907, USA

Megan A. McCrory
Department of Health Sciences, College of Health & Rehabilitation Sciences: Sargent College, Boston University, Boston, MA 02215, USA

Index

www.ingramcontent.com/pod-product-compliance
Lightning Source LLC
LaVergne TN
LVHW080929210926
848485LV00004B/762